I0038033

ENDOCRINE BOARD REVIEW

Serge A. Jabbour, MD, Program Chair
Professor and Division Director
Division of Endocrinology
Sidney Kimmel Medical College
Thomas Jefferson University

Richard J. Auchus, MD, PhD
Professor of Internal Medicine
Division of Metabolism,
Endocrinology & Diabetes
University of Michigan Medical School

Carolyn B. Becker, MD
Associate Professor of Medicine
and Master Clinician
Division of Endocrinology,
Diabetes and Hypertension
Brigham and Women's Hospital

Andrea D. Coviello, MD
Associate Professor of Medicine
Division of Endocrinology,
Metabolism, and Nutrition
Duke University School of Medicine

Frances J. Hayes, MD
Clinical Director
Endocrine Division
Massachusetts General Hospital

Laurence Katznelson, MD
Professor and Division Director
Division of Endocrinology
Stanford University

Michelle F. Magee, MD
Associate Professor of Medicine
Georgetown University
School of Medicine

Kathryn A. Martin, MD
Professor of Medicine
Division of Endocrinology, Metabolism,
and Molecular Medicine
Massachusetts General Hospital

Elizabeth N. Pearce, MD, MSc
Associate Professor
Endocrinology, Diabetes
& Nutrition Section
Boston University School of Medicine

Abbie L. Young, MS, CGC, ELS(D)
Medical Editor

Endocrine Society
2055 L Street NW, Suite 600, Washington, DC 20036
1-888-ENDOCRINE • www.endocrine.org

ENDOCRINE
SOCIETY

ENDOCRINE
SOCIETY
Hormone Science to Health

The Endocrine Society is the world's largest, oldest, and most
active organization working to advance the clinical practice of
endocrinology and hormone research. Founded in 1916, the Society
now has more than 18,000 global members across a range of
disciplines. The Society has earned an international reputation for
excellence in the quality of its peer-reviewed journals, educational
resources, meetings, and programs that improve public health
through the practice and science of endocrinology.

Visit us at:
education.endocrine.org
endocrine.org

Other Publications:
https://www.endocrine.org/
publications

On the Cover: © Shutterstock. Close-up of students writing and
reading examination answer sheets in classroom of school with stress.
(By arrowsmith2).

OVERVIEW

Endocrine Board Review (EBR) 10th Edition (2018) is a board examination preparation book designed for endocrine fellows who have completed or are nearing completion of their fellowship and are preparing to sit for the board certification exam, and for practicing endocrinologists in search of a comprehensive self-assessment of endocrinology, either to prepare for recertification or to update their practice. EBR consists of approximately 240 case-based, American Board of Internal Medicine (ABIM) style, multiple-choice questions. Each section follows the ABIM Endocrinology, Diabetes, and Metabolism Certification Examination blueprint, covering the breadth and depth of the certification and recertification examinations. Each case is discussed in detail with detailed answer explanations and references provided.

The EBR 10th Edition (2018) reference book is intended primarily for consultation and self-assessment of knowledge relating to endocrinology. As a reference book, educational credits are not available upon completion of the multiple-choice questions included. For information on educational products that include educational credit, please visit endocrine.org/store.

LEARNING OBJECTIVES

Upon completion of this educational activity, learners will be able to demonstrate enhanced medical knowledge and clinical skills across all major areas of endocrinology; apply knowledge and skills in diagnosing, managing, and treating a wide spectrum of endocrine disorders; and successfully complete the board examination for certification or recertification in the subspecialty of endocrinology, diabetes, and metabolism.

TARGET AUDIENCE

This activity should be of substantial interest to endocrinologists, internists, and endocrine fellows preparing for the board examination or recertification or to endocrinologists and other health care practitioners seeking a review in endocrinology.

STATEMENT OF INDEPENDENCE

The Endocrine Society has a policy of ensuring that the content and quality of this educational activity are balanced, independent, objective, and scientifically rigorous. The scientific content of this activity was developed under the supervision of the Endocrine Society's Endocrine Board Review Chair on the Clinical Endocrinology Update Steering Committee. The commercial supporters of this activity have no influence over the planning of this activity.

DISCLOSURE POLICY

The faculty, committee members, and staff who are in position to control the content of this activity are required to disclose to the Endocrine Society and to learners any relevant financial relationship(s) of the individual or spouse/partner that have occurred within the last 12 months with any commercial interest(s) whose products or services are related to the content. Financial relationships are defined by remuneration in any amount from the commercial interest(s) in the form of grants; research support; consulting fees; salary; ownership interest (eg, stocks, stock options, or ownership interest excluding diversified mutual funds); honoraria or other payments for participation in speakers' bureaus, advisory boards, or boards of directors; or other financial benefits. The intent of this disclosure is not to prevent planners with relevant financial relationships from planning or delivery of content, but rather to provide learners with information that allows them to make their own judgments of whether these financial relationships may have influenced the educational activity with regard to exposition or conclusion.

The Endocrine Society has reviewed all disclosures and resolved or managed all identified conflicts of interest, as applicable.

The faculty reported the following relevant financial relationship(s) during the content development process for this activity:

> **Richard J. Auchus, MD, PhD:** Novartis Pharmaceuticals: *Contracted Research Support & Consultant*; Strongbridge Biopharma: *Contracted Research Support & Consultant*; Millendo Therapeutics: *Consultant*; Quest Diagnostics: *Consultant*; Corcept Therapeutics: *Consultant*; Janssen Pharmaceuticals: *Consultant*; Spruce Biosciences: *Contracted Research Support and Consultant*; Neurocrine Biosciences: *Contracted Research Support*; Diurnal, LTD: *Contracted Research Support and Consultant*; Viamet Pharmaceuticals: *Consultant*
>
> **Andrea D. Coviello, MD:** Novo Nordisk Inc.: *Consultant and Speaker*
>
> **Serge A. Jabbour, MD:** *AstraZeneca, Eli Lilly & Janssen: Consultant/Advisory boards*
>
> **Michelle F. Magee, MD:** Lilly and Sanofi: *Funding for conduct of research studies to the MedStar Health Research Institute*; Sanofi: *Speaker/Honoraria*

The following faculty reported no relevant financial relationships: Carolyn B. Becker, MD; Frances J. Hayes, MD; Laurence Katznelson, MD; Kathryn A. Martin, MD; Elizabeth Pearce, MD

The medical editor for this activity reported no relevant financial relationships: Abbie L. Young, MS, CGC, ELS(D)

Endocrine Society staff associated with the development of content for this activity reported no relevant financial relationships.

DISCLAIMERS

The information presented in this activity represents the opinion of the faculty and is not necessarily the official position of the Endocrine Society.

USE OF PROFESSIONAL JUDGMENT:

The educational content in this activity relates to basic principles of diagnosis and therapy and does not substitute for individual patient assessment based on the health care provider's examination of the patient and consideration of laboratory data and other factors unique to the patient. Standards in medicine change as new data become available.

DRUGS AND DOSAGES:

When prescribing medications, the physician is advised to check the product information sheet accompanying each drug to verify conditions of use and to identify any changes in drug dosage schedule or contraindications.

POLICY ON UNLABELED/OFF-LABEL USE

The Endocrine Society has determined that disclosure of unlabeled/off-label or investigational use of commercial product(s) is informative for audiences and therefore requires this information to be disclosed to the learners at the beginning of the presentation. Uses of specific therapeutic agents, devices, and other products discussed in this educational activity may not be the same as those indicated in product labeling approved by the Food and Drug Administration (FDA). The Endocrine Society requires that any discussions of such "off-label" use be based on scientific research that conforms to generally accepted standards of experimental design, data collection, and data analysis. Before recommending or prescribing any therapeutic agent or device, learners should review the complete prescribing information, including indications, contraindications, warnings, precautions, and adverse events.

ACKNOWLEDGMENT OF COMMERCIAL SUPPORT

The activity is not supported by educational grant(s) or other funds from any commercial supporter.

Publication Date: August 2018

Contents

QUESTIONS   ANSWERS

DIABETES MELLITUS, SECTION 1 BOARD REVIEW 7 88
Serge A. Jabbour, MD

ADRENAL BOARD REVIEW 17 107
Richard J. Auchus, MD, PhD

CALCIUM AND BONE BOARD REVIEW 28 125
Carolyn B. Becker, MD

OBESITY/LIPIDS BOARD REVIEW 40 146
Andrea D. Coviello, MD

PITUITARY BOARD REVIEW 47 166
Laurence Katznelson, MD

DIABETES MELLITUS, SECTION 2 BOARD REVIEW 55 178
Michelle F. Magee, MD

FEMALE REPRODUCTION BOARD REVIEW 64 195
Kathryn A. Martin, MD

MALE REPRODUCTION BOARD REVIEW 70 206
Frances J. Hayes, MD

THYROID BOARD REVIEW 77 219
Elizabeth N. Pearce, MD, MSc

APPENDIX A: LABORATORY REFERENCE RANGES 236

**APPENDIX B: COMMON ABBREVIATIONS
USED IN ENDOCRINE BOARD REVIEW** 240

ENDOCRINE BOARD REVIEW

Diabetes Mellitus, Section 1 Board Review

Serge A. Jabbour, MD • Thomas Jefferson University

1 A 47-year-old man asks you whether he should be screened for diabetes mellitus. He has no symptoms, and he does not have hypertension, dyslipidemia, or history of cardiovascular disease. His only medications are a daily multivitamin, omega-3 fatty acids, and calcium. His family history is negative for diabetes. He does not smoke cigarettes or drink alcohol. He exercises on a regular basis.

On physical examination, his blood pressure is 120/70 mm Hg and BMI is 24.0 kg/m². The rest of his examination findings are unremarkable.

When should you screen this patient for diabetes?
  A. Now
  B. At age 50 years
  C. Only if he develops cardiovascular risk factors
  D. Only if BMI becomes greater than 25 kg/m²

2 A 54-year-old man is referred to you for management of diabetes mellitus. He has had diabetes for 4 years and is treated with metformin, 1000 mg twice daily, and glimepiride, 2 mg twice daily. He also has hypertension treated with ramipril, 10 mg daily, and dyslipidemia treated with atorvastatin, 20 mg daily. Moderate nonproliferative diabetic retinopathy was diagnosed at his last eye examination 8 months ago. He has a history of multinodular goiter and benign findings on FNA biopsy 2 years ago. He has no concerns except that he has been unable to lose weight despite trying various diets.

On physical examination, his blood pressure is 130/80 mm Hg and BMI is 32 kg/m². He has a goiter with a left dominant nodule of approximately 2 cm.

Laboratory test results:
  Hemoglobin A_{1c} = 8.7% (4.0%-5.6%)
    (72 mmol/mol [20-38 mmol/mol])
  Creatinine = 0.7 mg/dL (0.7-1.3 mg/dL)
    (61.9 μmol/L [61.9-114.9 μmol/L])
  Complete blood cell count, normal
  Electrolytes, normal
  Liver function tests, normal
  TSH, normal

You decide to add once-weekly semaglutide. Which of the following should be done at his follow-up visit, assuming he remains asymptomatic?
  A. Amylase and lipase measurement
  B. Calcitonin measurement
  C. Monofilament testing
  D. Creatinine measurement
  E. Eye examination

3 A 64-year-old man with an 8-year history of type 2 diabetes mellitus is self-referred to discuss newer therapies with good cardiovascular outcome data. He also has hypertension and dyslipidemia. He experienced a myocardial infarction 3 years ago. His current medications include metformin, glipizide, lisinopril, metoprolol, rosuvastatin, and aspirin.

On physical examination, his blood pressure is 122/75 mm Hg and BMI is 33 kg/m². His examination findings are otherwise unremarkable.

Laboratory test results:
  Hemoglobin A_{1c} = 8.3% (4.0%-5.6%)
    (67 mmol/mol [20-38 mmol/mol])
  Creatinine = 0.9 mg/dL (0.7-1.3 mg/dL)
    (SI: 79.6 μmol/L [61.9-114.9 μmol/L])
  Complete blood cell count, normal
  Electrolytes, normal
  Liver function tests, normal
  TSH, normal

You recommend adding an agent that, besides improving his hemoglobin A_{1c}, has been shown in cardiovascular outcome trials to significantly lower the 3-point major adverse cardiovascular events.

Which of the following agents would you add?
   A. Lixisenatide
   B. Once-weekly exenatide
   C. Sitagliptin
   D. Liraglutide
   E. Alogliptin

4 A 63-year-old woman with a 10-year history of type 2 diabetes mellitus presents for follow-up. She has no specific concerns. Her medical history is notable for hypertension, dyslipidemia, nonproliferative diabetic retinopathy, toe amputation, and congestive heart failure. She is currently being treated for bladder cancer with intravesical Bacillus Calmette-Guerin therapy.

Her current medications are metformin, 500 mg twice daily; insulin detemir, 20 units at bedtime; ramipril, 10 mg daily; metoprolol, 50 mg daily; spironolactone, 25 mg daily; furosemide, 40 mg daily; atorvastatin, 40 mg daily; and aspirin.

On physical examination, her blood pressure is 138/85 mm Hg and BMI is 36 kg/m^2. She has acanthosis nigricans on her neck, a 2/6 systolic ejection murmur, weak dorsalis pedis pulses bilaterally, and absence of the left great toe. Her lungs are clear to auscultation.

Laboratory test results:
   Hemoglobin A_{1c} = 8.2% (4.0%-5.6%)
      (66 mmol/mol [20-38 mmol/mol])
   Estimated glomerular filtration rate = 53 mL/min
      per 1.73 m^2 (>60 mL/min per 1.73 m^2)
   Complete blood cell count, normal
   Electrolytes, normal
   Liver function tests, normal
   TSH, normal

Which of the following agents would you add next?
   A. Dapagliflozin
   B. Canagliflozin
   C. Saxagliptin
   D. Ertugliflozin
   E. Lixisenatide

5 A 44-year-old woman is referred to you for consultation to start insulin pump therapy. Gestational diabetes mellitus requiring insulin was diagnosed at age 23 years. Her glucose tolerance normalized after delivery, and diabetes was not diagnosed until 7 years later at age 30 years. Her diabetes was initially managed with metformin and glyburide without success, so her treatment was switched to insulin. Her current regimen consists of insulin glargine, 22 units at bedtime, and insulin glulisine with meals, 1 unit for every 10 g of carbohydrates. Additional medications include flecainide, ramipril, atorvastatin, and coenzyme Q10.

Her medical history is notable for bilateral sensorineural hearing loss, macular pattern dystrophy with retinal pigmentation, Wolf-Parkinson-White syndrome, proteinuria, muscle weakness, and intolerance to exercise improved after coenzyme Q10 supplementation. Her family history is notable for a sister who has insulin-dependent diabetes, profound hearing deficit, proteinuria, and renal impairment. Her brother is healthy. She has one child, a 21-year-old daughter, who is healthy.

On physical examination, her blood pressure is 118/65 mm Hg, and BMI is 22 kg/m^2. She has decreased sensation on monofilament testing of her feet.

Laboratory test results:
   Hemoglobin A_{1c} = 7.8% (4.0%-5.6%)
      (62 mmol/mol [20-38 mmol/mol])
   Estimated glomerular filtration rate = 55 mL/min
      per 1.73 m^2 (>60 mL/min per 1.73 m^2)
   Urine albumin-to-creatinine ratio = 265 mg/g creat
      (<30 mg/g creat)

Which of the following tests is most likely be positive?
   A. Zinc transporter 8 (ZnT8) antibodies
   B. *GCK* (glucokinase) gene mutation
   C. Glutamic acid decarboxylase 65 antibodies
   D. A3243G mutation in mitochondrial DNA
   E. *HNF1A* (hepatocyte nuclear factor 1α) gene mutation

6 A 19-year-old woman with type 1 diabetes mellitus, well controlled on basal/mealtime insulins, presents for follow-up. She delivered a healthy baby 2 weeks ago. She asks you about environmental factors that could increase her child's risk of having type 1 diabetes.

Which of the following should her child should avoid?
   A. Vitamin D supplementation
   B. Intake of omega-3 fatty acids
   C. Intake of cow milk
   D. Low nitrates in drinking water
   E. Exposure to rhinovirus

7 A 45-year-old man sees you for management of uncontrolled type 2 diabetes mellitus. He has had diabetes for 3 years, initially controlled on metformin, but recently his hemoglobin A_{1c} level increased to 8.0% (4.0%-5.6%) (64 mmol/mol [20-38 mmol/mol]).

He tells you that he is interested in adding an SGLT-2 inhibitor to lower his hemoglobin A_{1c}, reduce his weight, and improve his blood pressure. He asks you to clarify the mechanism of action of SGLT-2 inhibitors at the kidney level.

You explain to him that SGLT-2 inhibitors:
   A. Block and up-regulate SGLT-2 in the S3 segment of the proximal renal tubule
   B. Lower the renal threshold for glucose excretion from 220 mg/dL to 180 mg/dL
   C. Down-regulate SGLT-2 in the S1 segment of the distal renal tubule
   D. Lower the renal threshold for glucose excretion from 220 mg/dL to less than 100 mg/dL

8 A 54-year-old woman is referred to you for discrepancy in her laboratory results. She has had type 2 diabetes mellitus for 8 years, which was initially treated with metformin. Glimepiride was then added 6 months ago when her hemoglobin A_{1c} level was 9.2% (4.0%-5.6%) (77 mmol/mol [20-38 mmol/mol]). Currently, her fasting blood glucose fingerstick measurements are on average 150 to 220 mg/dL (8.3-12.2 mmol/L) and her postprandial measurements are 200 to 280 mg/dL (11.1-15.4 mmol/L) postprandially. She also has a medical history of hypertension, dyslipidemia, and iron-deficiency anemia.

Her medications include metformin, 1000 mg twice daily; glimepiride, 2 mg twice daily; simvastatin, 40 mg daily; enalapril, 20 mg daily; iron; and cinnamon.

On physical examination, her blood pressure is 140/85 mm Hg and BMI is 34 kg/m². Examination findings are otherwise unremarkable.

Recent laboratory test results:
   Hemoglobin A_{1c} = 8.0% (4.0%-5.6%)
      (64 mmol/mol [20-38 mmol/mol])
   Serum 1,5-anhydroglucitol = 5 µg/mL (optimal
      range for patients with diabetes >10 µg/mL)
   Estimated glomerular filtration rate = 71 mL/min
      per 1.73 m² (>60 mL/min per 1.73 m²)
   Serum creatinine = 1.1 mg/dL (0.6-1.1 mg/dL)
      (SI: 97.2 µmol/L [53.0-97.2 µmol/L])
   Hemoglobin = 10.5 g/dL (12.1-15.1 g/dL)
      (SI: 105 g/L [121-151 g/L])
   Urine albumin-to-creatinine ratio = 125 mg/g creat
      (<30 mg/g creat)

You add canagliflozin, 100 mg daily, and see her back in 3 months.

Her blood glucose fingerstick measurements are on average 80 to 130 mg/dL (4.4-7.2 mmol/L) fasting in the morning and 120-170 mg/dL (6.7-9.4 mmol/L) postprandially.

Laboratory test results:
   Hemoglobin A_{1c} = 6.8% (51 mmol/mol)
   Serum 1,5-anhydroglucitol = 4 µg/mL

Her primary care physician cannot explain why her 1,5-anhydroglucitol level remains less than 10 µg/mL despite her hemoglobin A_{1c} being less than 7.0% and her blood glucose fingerstick measurements being at goal.

The laboratory discrepancy is most likely being caused by interference from which of the following?
   A. Anemia
   B. Iron
   C. Undiagnosed sickle cell trait
   D. Cinnamon
   E. Canagliflozin

9 A 26-year-old man with a 5-year history of type 1 diabetes mellitus is referred to you because he is interested in insulin pump therapy. He travels often for work, and he has an erratic eating schedule. However, he has good glycemic control, and he does not want to be on multiple daily injections anymore. His current insulin regimen consists of insulin glargine, 22 units at bedtime, and insulin lispro, 6 units with each meal (total daily insulin dose: 40 units).

Self-monitoring of blood glucose shows values ranging between 80 and 130 mg/dL (4.4-7.2 mmol/L). He rarely has hypoglycemic events.

On physical examination, his BMI is 23.5 kg/m^2. Examination findings are unremarkable.

A recent hemoglobin A_{1c} measurement is 6.9% (4.0%-5.6%) (52 mmol/mol [20-38 mmol/mol]).

After he undergoes intensive education (basal/bolus concept, carbohydrate counting, etc), you recommend switching his current injection regimen to insulin pump therapy (with lispro) with which of the following parameters?

Answer	Basal Rate (X units/h)	Carbohydrate Ratio (1 unit/X g)	Sensitivity Factor (1 unit/X mg/dL)
A.	0.9	20	60
B.	0.6	15	55
C.	1.2	15	45
D.	1.4	10	30
E.	1.0	10	60

10 A 45-year-old woman has a skin lesion on her left lower extremity (*see image*). A similar but smaller lesion is also present on her right lower extremity.

Biopsy shows an inflammatory granulomatous dermatitis with collagen degeneration and fat deposition.

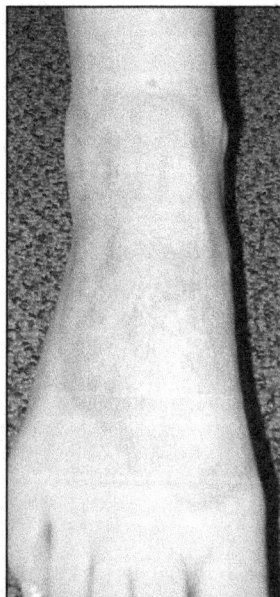

Which of the following diagnoses does this patient most likely have?
A. Type 1 diabetes mellitus
B. Graves disease
C. Glucagonoma
D. Pseudohypoparathyroidism
E. Familial hypercholesterolemia

11 An 18-year-old woman is seen for erratic blood glucose values. Type 1 diabetes mellitus was diagnosed 2 years ago, and a regimen of basal and mealtime insulins was initiated. Her glycemic control has always been adequate, with hemoglobin A_{1c} values around 7.0% (4.0%-5.6%) (53 mmol/mol [20-38 mmol/mol]). However, a few weeks ago, she started to notice unpredictable blood glucose values with recurrent hypoglycemic episodes (blood glucose values between 45 and 60 mg/dL [2.5-3.3 mmol/L]) that occur mainly after meals, accompanied by symptoms. Despite eating more snacks to prevent hypoglycemia, she has lost 4 lb (1.8 kg) in the past 2 weeks. She has no gastrointestinal complaints or dizziness. Her menses are regular.

Her current medications are insulins glargine and lispro. Her blood pressure is 110/70 mm Hg, and BMI is 22 kg/m^2.

Physical examination findings are unremarkable.

Laboratory test results:
Hemoglobin A_{1c} = 6.7% (4.0%-5.6%) (50 mmol/mol [20-38 mmol/mol])
Serum cortisol (8 AM) = 20 µg/dL (5-25 µg/dL) (551.8 nmol/L [137.9-689.7 nmol/L])
Complete blood cell count, normal
Electrolytes, normal
Creatinine, normal
Liver function tests, normal

Further workup is done.

An elevation in which of the following would most likely explain her hypoglycemia?
A. ACTH
B. Free T_4
C. Tissue transglutaminase IgA antibodies
D. 21-Hydroxylase antibodies
E. Glutamic acid decarboxylase 65 antibodies

12 A 56-year-old man with a 28-year history of type 1 diabetes mellitus has been using an insulin pump for 11 years with a rapid-acting insulin analogue. He has recently been experiencing recurrent high fasting blood glucose values. His diabetes is complicated by proliferative retinopathy, microalbuminuria with a stable creatinine concentration of 1.1 mg/dL (97.2 μmol/L), and peripheral sensory neuropathy. You examine his logbook, which documents self-monitored blood glucose levels 4 to 5 times daily before meals. He has a bedtime snack most days. You note there are a few glucose values at random times in the 40s and 50s, and fasting levels most mornings are in the high 100s to low 200s. On questioning the patient, you learn that he has no symptoms associated with the low blood glucose values. He is seeking guidance about achieving better glycemic control.

Which of the following is the best recommendation?
 A. Increase the basal insulin rate 2 hours before the time fasting hyperglycemia is occurring
 B. Eliminate the bedtime snack
 C. Change the method of insulin delivery to multiple daily injections
 D. Begin monitoring glucose levels with a continuous glucose sensor

13 A 32-year-old woman with a 21-year history of type 1 diabetes mellitus is feeling stressed and frustrated because she is having unpredictable hypoglycemia occurring at various times of the day, often within an hour or two after eating. She reports adherence to her insulin regimen and has had nutrition education multiple times, most recently 2 months ago. She performs carbohydrate counting and appropriate insulin adjustment. She has a history of diabetic peripheral neuropathy and diabetic retinopathy.

Review of systems reveals blurred vision, intermittent gastric fullness, and fluctuating weight. Her blood pressure is 121/79 mm Hg.

A basic metabolic panel is unremarkable. Her glucose meter reveals glucose checks 6 to 7 times daily and highly variable glucose levels ranging from the 40s to over 300 mg/dL (>16.7 mmol/L) at various times during the day, with no appreciable pattern.

Which of the following is most likely to uncover the etiology of her hypoglycemia and glycemic variability?
 A. Psychiatric evaluation
 B. ACTH stimulation test
 C. Gastric emptying study
 D. Review of carbohydrate counting skills

14 A 31-year-old woman with a 2-year history of type 1 diabetes mellitus is asking for advice on how to reduce her risk for future heart disease. Her 53-year-old father, who also has type 1 diabetes, just had a myocardial infarction. The patient is on multiple daily insulin injection therapy, but she does not count carbohydrates or make insulin adjustments before meals. She has experienced several episodes of mild hypoglycemia in the past 6 months, and 1 severe episode that occurred overnight. She did not bring her glucose meter or a log to this visit. Her blood pressure is 120/69 mm Hg, and pulse rate is 78 beats/min.

Laboratory test results (sample drawn while fasting):
 Hemoglobin A_{1c} = 8.7% (4.0%-5.6%)
  (72 mmol/mol [20-38 mmol/mol])
 LDL cholesterol = 98 mg/dL (<100 mg/dL
  [optimal]) (SI: 2.54 mmol/L [<2.59 mmol/L])
 HDL cholesterol = 64 mg/dL (>60 mg/dL
  [optimal]) (SI: 1.66 mmol/L [>1.55 mmol/L])
 Serum creatinine, normal
 Spot urine albumin, normal

On the basis of data from clinical trials, which intervention would be most useful for reducing her cardiovascular disease risk?
 A. Improve glucose control to achieve a hemoglobin A_{1c} level <7.0% (<53 mmol/mol)
 B. Start treatment with a statin
 C. Start treatment with an ACE inhibitor
 D. Decrease her long-acting insulin dose by 20% to avoid hypoglycemia

15 A 47-year-old man with a 19-year history of type 1 diabetes mellitus has no diabetes complications and no specific concerns. He is treated with insulins glargine and aspart and a baby aspirin daily. His blood pressure is 129/68 mm Hg, and BMI is 25.5 kg/m^2.

Laboratory test results:

Hemoglobin A_{1c} = 7.2% (4.0%-5.6%) (55 mmol/mol [20-38 mmol/mol])

Total cholesterol = 173 mg/dL (<200 mg/dL [optimal]) (SI: 4.48 mmol/L [<5.18 mmol/L])

LDL cholesterol = 92 mg/dL (<100 mg/dL [optimal]) (SI: 2.38 mmol/L [<2.59 mmol/L])

HDL cholesterol = 45 mg/dL (>60 mg/dL [optimal]) (SI: 1.17 mmol/L [>1.55 mmol/L])

Triglycerides = 178 mg/dL (<150 mg/dL [optimal]) (SI: 2.01 mmol/L [<1.70 mmol/L])

Serum creatinine = 0.86 mg/dL (0.7-1.3 mg/dL) (SI: 76.0 μmol/L [61.9-114.9 μmol/L])

Urinary albumin-to-creatinine ratio = 19 mg/g creat (<30 mg/g creat)

How should you advise this patient regarding the best course of action to reduce his risk for cardiovascular disease?

A. Intensify his treatment regimen to attain a target hemoglobin A_{1c} level <7.0% (<53 mmol/mol)

B. Start treatment with a statin

C. Start treatment with an ACE inhibitor

D. Refer to a nutritionist for dietary instruction for weight loss

16 In the 17-year follow-up of the Epidemiology of Diabetes Interventions and Complications (EDIC) study (an extension of the Diabetes Control and Complications Trials [DCCT]), which of the following significant trends were observed?

Answer	Myocardial Infarction	Stroke	Cardiovascular Death
A.	↓	↓	No change
B.	↓	↑	↓
C.	↓	↓	↓
D.	↓	↓	↑

17 A 28-year-old woman with a 20-year history of type 1 diabetes mellitus has been on insulin pump therapy for 6 years. She describes recurrent episodes of mild hypoglycemia in the midafternoon that are characterized by sweating and anxiety. You examine her logbook and see documented hypoglycemic values between 50 and 64 mg/dL (2.8 and 3.6 mmol/L) approximately 4 times per week around 3 to 4 PM. The patient uses insulin aspart in her pump.

There has been no change in physical activity.

Current pump settings:

Basal rates:

Midnight to 6 AM = 1.0 units/h

6 AM to midnight = 1.2 units/h

Correction (sensitivity) factor = 1 unit:40 mg/dL glucose

Insulin-to-carbohydrate ratio = 1 unit:10 g

The patient weighs 156 lb (70.9 kg) (BMI = 26 kg/m²).

Which of the following is the best advice now to alleviate her hypoglycemic episodes?

A. Increase her carbohydrate intake at lunch

B. Eat a carbohydrate snack at 2 or 3 PM

C. Change the prelunch carbohydrate ratio to 1:8

D. Perform basal rate testing from breakfast until dinner

18 A 24-year-old woman with type 1 diabetes mellitus diagnosed 4 months ago presents with recent onset of recurrent hypoglycemia. She is on basal-bolus insulin therapy, approximately 0.35 units/kg per day, with long- and short-acting insulin analogues. Her weight is 121 lb (55 kg). Her current hemoglobin A_{1c} level is 6.3% (45 mmol/mol), down from 12.4% (112 mmol/mol) at diagnosis. She performs self-monitoring of blood glucose 4 to 6 times daily, before meals and at bedtime, but also frequently after meals because she often has symptoms of hypoglycemia 1.5 to 2 hours after meals confirmed by low blood glucose values (between 50 and 60 mg/dL [2.8-3.3 mmol/L]). She also has fasting hypoglycemia (into the 50s and 60s) once or twice a week.

How should you advise this patient regarding the best course of action now?

A. Reduce basal insulin doses by 10% to 20%

B. Reduce all insulin doses by 10% to 20%

C. Reduce premeal insulin by 10% to 20%

D. Increase carbohydrate intake to at least 50 g with each meal

19 A 34-year-old man with type 1 diabetes mellitus is in the clinic waiting room when the receptionist notes he seems confused when his name is called, speaks with slurred words, and is unable to follow commands. He is found to have a fingerstick blood glucose value of 39 mg/dL (2.2 mmol/L). After recovery with oral glucose, he reports that despite careful monitoring, including use of his continuous glucose sensor, he has had 5 or 6 episodes of hypoglycemia with blood glucose levels between 40 and 50 mg/dL (2.2-2.8 mmol/L) in the past 2 weeks, without any warning symptoms that he can recall. Over his 16-year history of diabetes, he has always aimed for tight glycemic control because he fears developing long-term complications. His current hemoglobin A_{1c} level is 5.9% (41 mmol/mol), and his treatment regimen consists of multiple daily insulin injections.

Which of the following is the most important next step in this patient's care?
   A. Temporarily relax his tight glucose targets
   B. Instruct him to always carry a glucagon emergency kit
   C. Begin using an insulin pump for insulin administration
   D. Attend a diabetes education class focused on hypoglycemia avoidance

20 A 33-year-old woman presents for management of recently diagnosed type 2 diabetes mellitus. Three months ago, a hemoglobin A_{1c} value of 8.9% (74 mmol/mol) was documented. Because she had longstanding obesity (BMI = 34 kg/m²), she enrolled in a hospital-based, dietitian-led, group weight-loss program, and she has since lost 5 lb (2.3 kg). She has also been engaged in lifestyle modification efforts while on metformin monotherapy, 1500 mg daily, for the past 3 months.

Laboratory test results from today's visit:
   Hemoglobin A_{1c} = 7.8% (4.%-5.6%) (62 mmol/mol [20-38 mmol/mol])
   Fasting blood glucose = 146 mg/dL (70-99 mg/dL) (SI: 8.1 mmol/L [3.9-5.5 mmol/L])

Which of the following is the best next step to improve her glycemic control?
   A. Stop metformin; begin insulin glargine, 10 units at bedtime
   B. Add sitagliptin, 100 mg daily, to current metformin therapy
   C. Increase metformin dosage to 2000 mg daily
   D. Stop metformin; begin sitaglipin, 100 mg daily

21 A 62-year-old man with a 10-year history of type 2 diabetes mellitus presents for a follow-up visit. He has a personal history of cardiovascular disease, with a myocardial infarction that occurred at age 58 years. He also has a family history of heart disease. His current medications are lisinopril, 20 mg daily; metformin, 1000 mg daily; insulin lispro, 4 units before each meal; and insulin glargine, 20 units in the morning. He quit smoking 5 years ago after a 20 pack-year history. On physical examination, his seated blood pressure is 140/90 mm Hg and BMI is 30 kg/m².

Recent laboratory test results:
   Hemoglobin A_{1c} = 6.8% (4.0%-5.6%) (51 mmol/mol [20-38 mmol/mol])
   Fasting plasma glucose = 94 mg/dL (70-99 mg/dL) (SI: 5.2 mmol/L [3.9-5.5 mmol/L])
   Total cholesterol = 189 mg/dL (<200 mg/dL [optimal]) (SI: 4.90 mmol/L [<5.18 mmol/L])
   Triglycerides = 120 mg/dL (<150 mg/dL [optimal]) (SI: 1.36 mmol/L [<1.70 mmol/L])
   LDL cholesterol = 135 mg/dL (<100 mg/dL [optimal]) (SI: 3.50 mmol/L [<2.59 mmol/L])
   HDL cholesterol = 40 mg/dL (>60 mg/dL [optimal]) (SI: 1.04 mmol/L [>1.55 mmol/L])

Which of the following is the best treatment to address his lipid profile?
   A. Pravastatin, 40 mg daily
   B. Rosuvastatin, 20 mg daily
   C. Lovastatin, 40 mg daily
   D. Simvastatin, 20 mg daily

22 Diabetes mellitus was recently diagnosed in a 43-year-old woman when she was noted on routine clinical evaluation to have a fasting plasma glucose level of 154 mg/dL (8.5 mmol/L).

Other abnormal laboratory values:
AST = 119 U/L (20-48 U/L) (SI: 2.0 μkat/L [0.33-0.80 μkat/L])
ALT = 134 U/L (10-40 U/L) (SI: 2.3 μkat/L [0.17-0.67 μkat/L])
Hemoglobin A_{1c} = 6.9% (4.0%-5.6%) (52 mmol/mol [20-38 mmol/mol])

She has no family history of diabetes, but several relatives have had liver disease of uncertain cause. Review of systems is notable for oligomenorrhea for 2 years and amenorrhea for 3 months. On physical examination, she has a mildly enlarged, nontender liver, no ascites or other signs of chronic liver disease, and no edema. Liver ultrasonography shows a mildly enlarged liver without masses, no evidence of steatosis, and no biliary disease. Hepatitis (A, B, C) serologies are negative or suggestive of previous infection.

Which of the following tests is most likely to reveal the etiology of her diabetes?
A. Hepatocyte nuclear factor 1 alpha (*HNF1A*) genetic testing
B. Zinc transporter 8 (ZnT8) antibody measurement
C. Transferrin saturation
D. Serum ceruloplasmin measurement
E. Mitochondrial antibody titers

23 An 81-year-old man with a history of chronic obstructive pulmonary disease, ulcerative colitis, and benign prostatic hypertrophy develops new-onset diabetes mellitus and presents with fatigue, a 22-lb (10-kg) weight loss, diarrhea, anorexia, and increasing nocturia. His fasting blood glucose level is 256 mg/dL (14.2 mmol/L). One year ago, a random blood glucose measurement was 113 mg/dL (6.3 mmol/L).

Physical examination reveals a cachectic elderly man with a violaceous skin rash across his feet (*see image*) that has been unsuccessfully treated with topical clotrimazole. Laboratory analysis is notable for anemia and low levels of zinc and essential fatty acids.

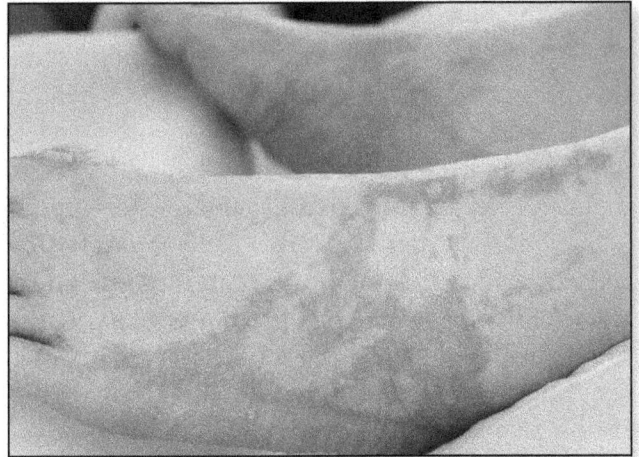

Measurement of which of the following is most likely to reveal the etiology of his diabetes?
A. Glucagon
B. CA 19-9
C. Somatostatin
D. 24-Hour urinary free cortisol

24 A 42-year-old black woman has sickle-cell disease and type 2 diabetes mellitus. Her hemoglobin A_{1c} level is consistently 4.8% (29 mmol/mol) with point-of-care testing despite suboptimal control of blood glucose levels on metformin, 1000 mg twice daily, and insulin detemir, 40 units at bedtime (fasting values on home glucose monitoring are 160 to 190 mg/dL [8.9-10.5 mmol/L]).

Which of the following tests would you use to assess the adequacy of her glycemic control?
A. A laboratory-based hemoglobin A_{1c} assay
B. 2-Hour postprandial glucose measurement
C. Urinary glucose testing
D. Fructosamine measurement
E. Continuous glucose monitoring

25 A 36-year-old woman is referred to you for glucosuria, which was documented by her primary care physician whom she saw for the first time after moving to the area. She has no concerns. She has no known history of diabetes mellitus or renal disease. Her only medications are an oral contraceptive and a proton-pump inhibitor. Her blood pressure is 112/63 mm Hg, and BMI is 23 kg/m².

Laboratory test results (fasting):
    Glucose = 88 mg/dL (70-99 mg/dL)
        (SI: 4.9 mmol/L [3.9-5.5 mmol/L])
    Hemoglobin A_{1c} = 5.1% (4.0%-5.6%)
        (32 mmol/mol [20-38 mmol/mol])
    Creatinine = 0.7 mg/dL (0.6-1.1 mg/dL)
        (SI: 61.9 µmol/L [53.0-97.2 µmol/L])
    Sodium = 141 mEq/L (136-142 mEq/L)
        (SI: 141 mmol/L [136-142 mmol/L])
    Potassium = 3.7 mEq/L (3.5-5.0 mEq/L)
        (SI: 3.7 mmol/L [3.5-5.0 mmol/L])
    Bicarbonate = 24 mEq/L (21-28 mEq/L)
        (SI: 24 mmol/L [21-28 mmol/L])
    Phosphate = 4.0 mg/dL (2.3-4.7 mg/dL)
        (SI: 1.3 mmol/L [0.7-1.5 mmol/L])
    Urinalysis results:
        pH = 5.5
        Protein and ketones, negative
        0 red blood cells/0 white blood cells
        Glucose, 3+

Which of the following is the most likely diagnosis?
    A. IgA nephropathy
    B. Renal Fanconi syndrome
    C. Familial renal glucosuria
    D. Galactosemia

26 A 57-year-old woman is referred by her primary care physician because of uncontrolled diabetes. The patient has a long history of severe asthma requiring multiple hospital admissions in the past and several episodes of respiratory failure. She has been treated with 40 to 60 mg of prednisone for the past 3 years. On this regimen, she has been able to avoid hospital stays, but she has developed diabetes that requires insulin therapy. After an initial favorable response to insulin, her hemoglobin A_{1c} level has climbed to greater than 11.0% (>97 mmol/mol) over the past year. Her insulin requirements have escalated, and she is now taking 100 units of insulin glargine in the morning, 75 to 80 units of insulin aspart before meals, and occasional coverage of snacks with 20 to 30 units. She is adherent to her injection regimen and misses only 2 to 3 doses per month. Recently, she has noticed fatigue and decreased appetite, with nocturia 2 to 3 times per night.

On physical examination, her BMI is 30 kg/m². She has acanthosis on the back of her neck and under her arms. There is no hepatomegaly or evidence of diabetic neuropathy.

Which of the following therapeutic interventions will lower this patient's blood glucose most effectively?
    A. Add insulin glargine in the evening
    B. Add liraglutide
    C. Add pioglitazone
    D. Change to U500 insulin
    E. Change the insulin delivery to an insulin pump

27 A 46-year-old man presents for advice on treatment of type 2 diabetes mellitus. He has been treated with metformin for 4 years, since an elevated blood glucose concentration was detected on a preoperative evaluation. His glucose control has varied, and a sulfonylurea was added last year when his hemoglobin A_{1c} level increased to greater than 8.0% (>64 mmol/mol). However, he gained 11 lb (5 kg) with this treatment and stopped the drug after 6 months. He is otherwise healthy and his only medications are metformin and lisinopril.

On physical examination, his blood pressure is 138/84 mm Hg and BMI is 33 kg/m². A repeated hemoglobin A_{1c} measurement is 8.4% (4.0%-5.6%) (68 mmol/mol [20-38 mmol/mol]).

Which of the following treatments is the best option for this patient?
    A. Repaglinide
    B. Dulaglutide
    C. Sitagliptin
    D. Pioglitazone
    E. Insulin glargine

28 A colleague in primary care calls you with a question about the diagnosis of diabetes mellitus. He had screened an overweight (BMI = 28 kg/m²) 44-year-old man who has a grandmother and sister with diabetes. Neither of his parents has diabetes. The patient's hemoglobin A_{1c} level is 5.9% (41 mmol/mol). Because this value is considered abnormal, your colleague had ordered a 75-g oral glucose tolerance test.

The following results were obtained:
    Fasting glucose = 116 mg/dL (6.4 mmol/L)
    1-hour glucose = 224 mg/dL (12.4 mmol/L)
    2-hour glucose = 188 mg/dL (10.4 mmol/L)

On the basis of these results, which of the following should you recommend?

A. Another oral glucose tolerance test with measurements of serum insulin to assess insulin resistance

B. Initiation of metformin to treat early type 2 diabetes

C. Weight loss and exercise to prevent type 2 diabetes

D. Another measurement of fasting glucose to exclude type 2 diabetes

E. Genetic screening for mutations involved in maturity-onset diabetes of the young

29 A 47-year-old black man is admitted to the intensive care unit with hyperglycemia. He presented to the emergency department with polyuria, polydipsia, and abdominal pain. He has no history of diabetes and has been treated only for hypertension and gout in the past. His mother, maternal aunt, and maternal grandmother all developed type 2 diabetes in their 60s, but none of his siblings or children are affected. He has a history of binge drinking but has not consumed alcohol recently. He has lost 15 to 20 lb (6.8 to 9.1 kg) over the last 2 months.

On physical examination, he is in no acute distress. His BMI is 31.2 kg/m^2. His pulse rate is 92 beats/min, and respiratory rate is 18 breaths/min. Findings on funduscopic and abdominal examinations are normal. There are no signs of neuropathy.

Laboratory test results (sample drawn at hospital admission):

Glucose = 617 mg/dL (70-99 mg/dL) (SI: 34.2 mmol/L [3.9-5.5 mmol/L])

Sodium = 139 mEq/L (136-142 mEq/L) (SI: 139 mmol/L [136-142 mmol/L])

Potassium = 3.3 mEq/L (3.5-5.0 mEq/L) (SI: 3.3 mmol/L [3.5-5.0 mmol/L])

Chloride = 97 mEq/L (96-106 mEq/L) (SI: 97 mmol/L [96-106 mmol/L])

Bicarbonate = 20 mEq/L (21-28 mEq/L) (SI: 20 mmol/L [21-28 mmol/L])

Serum acetone = 2+

AST = 77 U/L (20-48 U/L) (SI: 1.3 µkat/L [0.33-0.80 µkat/L])

ALT = 67 U/L (10-40 U/L) (SI: 1.1 µkat/L [0.17-0.67 µkat/L])

Serum urea nitrogen = 53 mg/dL (8-23 mg/dL) (SI: 18.9 mmol/L [2.9-8.2 mmol/L])

Creatinine = 1.7 mg/dL (0.7-1.3 mg/dL) (SI: 150.3 µmol/L [61.9-114.9 µmol/L])

Triglycerides = 750 mg/dL (<150 mg/dL [optimal]) (SI: 8.48 mmol/L [<1.70 mmol/L])

Venous pH = 7.28 (7.35-7.45)

Hemoglobin A$_{1c}$ = 10.7% (4.0%-5.6%) (93 mmol/mol [20-38 mmol/mol])

Lipase = 70 U/L (10-73 U/L) (SI: 1.17 µkat/L [0.17-1.22 µkat/L])

Amylase = 55 U/L (26-102 U/L) (SI: 0.92 µkat/L [0.43-1.70 µkat/L])

Which of the following is the most likely diagnosis?

A. Latent autoimmune diabetes in adults

B. Ketosis-prone diabetes

C. Maturity-onset diabetes of the young type 1

D. Alcoholic ketoacidosis

E. Pancreatitis

30 A 24-year-old woman is referred for evaluation after developing hyperglycemia during a hospitalization for pneumonia. She has cystic fibrosis and was admitted to the hospital last month for an exacerbation of chronic pulmonary disease thought to be due to bacterial infection. During the early period of her hospital stay for antibiotic treatment, several blood glucose values were documented to be greater than 200 mg/dL (>11.1 mmol/L), but fasting blood glucose levels had decreased to below 100 mg/dL (<5.6 mmol/L) the 2 days before discharge. She had been generally well in the year before hospitalization, but she did note an 8.8-lb (4-kg) weight loss over that time.

On physical examination, her BMI is 22 kg/m^2. She has a resonant chest with decreased breath sounds and decreased muscle mass and subcutaneous fat.

Which of the following is the most appropriate diagnostic strategy now?

A. Oral glucose tolerance test

B. Continuous glucose monitoring

C. Hemoglobin A$_{1c}$ measurement

D. A mixed-meal tolerance test

E. Measurement of fasting blood glucose on 2 occasions

Adrenal Board Review

Richard J. Auchus, MD, PhD ● University of Michigan

1 A 37-year-old woman is referred for evaluation of an incidental adrenal mass that was identified on CT performed as part of the workup for an episode of painless hematuria 4 weeks ago. In taking a history, you elicit a 14-lb (6.5-kg) weight gain over the past year associated with the onset of irregular menses, hirsutism, and poor sleep. She takes no medications.

On physical examination, her blood pressure is 140/88 mm Hg. She has mild to moderate facial fullness and plethora and supraclavicular fat accumulation.

CT demonstrates a 1.4-cm left adrenal mass (*see image; right and left adrenal glands are identified by arrows*).

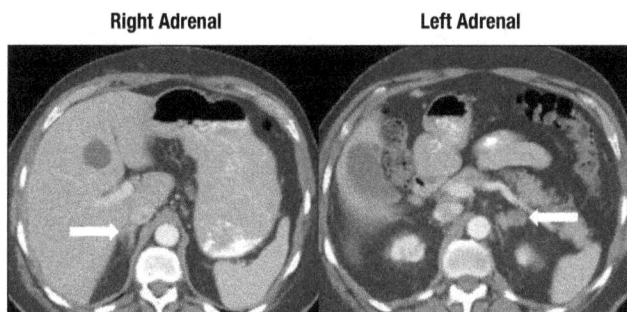

Right Adrenal   Left Adrenal

Laboratory test results:
    Sodium = 138 mEq/L (136-142 mEq/L)
      (SI: 138 mmol/L [136-142 mmol/L])
    Potassium = 3.7 mEq/L (3.5-5.0 mEq/L)
      (SI: 3.7 mmol/L [3.5-5.0 mmol/L])
    Late-night salivary cortisol (2 measurements) =
      0.43 µg/dL (11.8 nmol/L) and 0.62 µg/dL
      (17.0 nmol/L) (<0.13 µg/dL) (SI: <3.6 nmol/L)
    Serum cortisol after overnight 1-mg
      dexamethasone = 8.2 µg/dL (SI: 226.2 nmol/L)
    Serum aldosterone = 4 ng/dL (4-21 ng/dL)
      (SI: 111.0 pmol/L [111.0-582.5 pmol/L])
    Pregnancy test, negative

Which of the following studies should you order next?
    A. Plasma renin activity
    B. Adrenal MRI
    C. Dexamethasone corticotropin-releasing hormone test
    D. Biopsy of the adrenal tumor
    E. Plasma ACTH measurement

2 You are asked to evaluate a 17-year-old boy for adrenal insufficiency. For the last year, he has noticed weight loss, anorexia, salt craving, and orthostasis. He also describes weakness in his lower extremities, gait instability, slurred speech, and confusion. He has no fever, cough, or dyspnea.

On physical examination, he has orthostatic hypotension, hyperpigmentation (particularly in the palmar creases) without vitiligo, brisk deep tendon reflexes, clonus in the left ankle, and the bilateral Babinski sign.

Laboratory test results (sample drawn at 8 AM):
    Plasma ACTH = 220 pg/mL (10-60 pg/mL)
      (SI: 48.4 pmol/L [2.2-13.2 pmol/L])
    Serum cortisol = 1.3 µg/dL (5-25 µg/dL)
      (SI: 35.9 nmol/L [137.9-389.7 nmol/L])
    Free T_4 = 1.2 ng/dL (0.8-1.8 ng/dL)
      (SI: 15.4 pmol/L [10.30-23.17 pmol/L])
    TSH = 0.9 mIU/L (0.5-5.0 mIU/L)

Which of the following should you recommend to identify the most likely cause of adrenal insufficiency in this patient?
    A. Measure very-long-chain fatty acids
    B. Measure 21-hydroxylase antibodies
    C. Perform adrenal CT
    D. Measure serum aldosterone
    E. Perform an ACTH stimulation test

3 A primary care physician refers to you a 32-year-old man because of an elevated plasma ACTH concentration. He has a 10-year history of primary adrenal insufficiency due to autoimmune adrenalitis. He also has primary hypothyroidism due to Hashimoto thyroiditis. The patient feels well and has no concerns. His medications include hydrocortisone, 12.5 mg every morning and 5 mg every afternoon; fludrocortisone, 50 mcg daily; and levothyroxine, 125 mcg daily.

On physical examination, he is a healthy-appearing man with a blood pressure of 122/76 mm Hg, a regular pulse rate of 70 beats/min, and a BMI of 24 kg/m². His skin is well pigmented in sun-exposed areas. Examination findings are otherwise normal.

Laboratory test results:
    Electrolytes, normal
    Plasma renin activity = 2.1 ng/mL per h
      (0.6-4.3 ng/mL per h)
    Serum TSH = 2.8 mIU/L (0.5-5.0 mIU/L)
    Plasma ACTH = 312 pg/mL (10-60 pg/mL)
      (SI: 68.6 pmol/L [2.2-13.2 pmol/L])

In addition to reviewing sick-day corticosteroid management, which of the following should you recommend?
  A. Discontinue hydrocortisone and substitute prednisone, 5 mg in the morning and 2.5 mg in the afternoon
  B. Add dexamethasone, 0.75 mg orally at bedtime
  C. Increase the hydrocortisone dosage to 20 mg in the morning and 10 mg in the afternoon
  D. Increase the fludrocortisone dosage to 100 mcg daily
  E. Make no changes in his corticosteroid dosages

4 A 36-year-old woman presents with resistant hypertension, hypokalemia, and recurrent pregnancy losses. Her medications include amlodipine, labetalol, and potassium chloride. A hypertension specialist ordered a laboratory evaluation.

Laboratory test results:
    Sodium = 138 mEq/L (136-142 mEq/L)
      (SI: 138 mmol/L [136-142 mmol/L])
    Potassium = 3.0 mEq/L (3.5-5.0 mEq/L)
      (SI: 3.0 mmol/L [3.5-5.0 mmol/L])

    Serum aldosterone = 14 ng/dL (4-21 ng/dL)
      (SI: 388.4 pmol/L [111.0-582.5 pmol/L])
    Plasma renin activity = <0.6 ng/mL per h
      (0.6-4.3 ng/mL per h)

CT of the abdomen without contrast demonstrates a 3.4-cm right adrenal mass of –5 Hounsfield units and an atrophic left adrenal gland (*see image, arrows*).

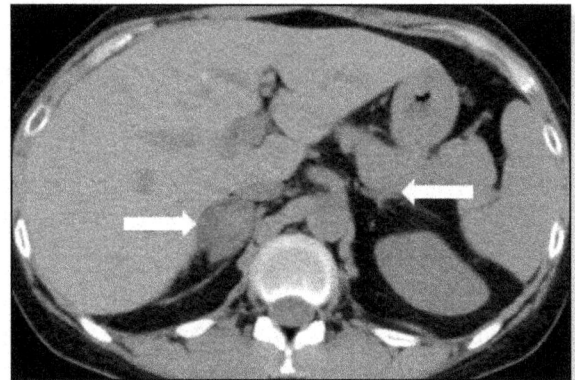

The patient is referred for adrenal venous sampling, which is performed under cosyntropin stimulation. The results are as follows:

Measurement	Right Adrenal Vein	Left Adrenal Vein	Inferior Vena Cava
Aldosterone	6845 ng/dL (189,880 pmol/L)	2806 ng/dL (77,838 pmol/L)	55 ng/dL (1525 pmol/L)
Cortisol	1382 µg/dL (38,127 nmol/L)	129 µg/dL (3559 nmol/L)	56 µg/dL (1545 nmol/L)
Aldosterone-to-Cortisol Ratio	5.0	21.8	0.98

Which of the following is the best next step in this patient's management?
  A. Manage her hypertension with spironolactone, 50 mg daily
  B. Perform a 1-mg overnight dexamethasone suppression test
  C. Perform a saline infusion test
  D. Perform left adrenalectomy
  E. Perform adrenal MRI

5 A 54-year-old man is referred for evaluation of fatigue and possible Cushing syndrome. His problems started after a back injury at work 1 year ago. He developed sudden lower back pain while lifting a heavy load and was sent home. He was evaluated and prescribed 6 weeks of physical therapy with some relief, and then he was given monthly back injections in a pain clinic for 6 months (these treatments ended 4 months ago). The injections markedly eased his pain, but he developed rapid weight gain, hunger, easy bruising, and facial fullness.

His initial evaluation with his primary care physician documented the following laboratory values:

Urinary free cortisol = <3 µg/24 h (4-50 µg/24 h)
(SI: <8.3 nmol/d [11-138 nmol/d])
Overnight 1-mg dexamethasone suppression test, cortisol = <0.2 µg/dL (SI: <5.5 nmol/L)

The patient is referred to you for further evaluation. He reports that his condition has not changed over the last 6 months. On physical examination, he has facial plethora and fullness, prominent supraclavicular fat pads, and dermal atrophy with diffuse bruising. His blood pressure is 125/80 mm Hg. His visual fields are full, and he has no pedal edema.

Which of the following diagnostic tests will reveal the etiology of his Cushing syndrome?
   A. Late-night salivary cortisol measurement
   B. Pituitary MRI with contrast
   C. Urine synthetic glucocorticoid testing
   D. CT scan of chest, abdomen, and pelvis
   E. ^{111}In-pentetreotide ("octreotide") scan

6 A 44-year-old woman presents with a 5-month history of rapidly progressive balding, voice deepening, and hirsutism. She has also had amenorrhea for 2 months and now has a new diagnosis of hypertension.

Her primary care physician obtained the following laboratory tests:

Sodium = 144 mEq/L (136-142 mEq/L)
(SI: 144 mmol/L [136-142 mmol/L])
Potassium = 3.2 mEq/L (3.5-5.0 mEq/L)
(SI: 3.2 mmol/L [3.5-5.0 mmol/L])
Serum aldosterone = <4 ng/dL (4-21 ng/dL)
(SI: <111.0 pmol/L [111.0-582.5 pmol/L])

Plasma renin activity = <0.6 ng/mL per h
(0.6-4.3 ng/mL per h)
Plasma ACTH = 15 pg/mL (10-60 pg/mL)
(3.3 pmol/L [2.2-13.2 pmol/L])
Serum cortisol = 14 µg/dL (5-25 µg/dL)
(386.2 nmol/L [137.9-389.7 nmol/L])
Serum DHEA-S = 1630 µg/dL (18-244 µg/dL)
(SI: 7.56 µmol/L [0.49-6.61 µmol/L])
Serum total testosterone = 279 ng/dL (8-60 ng/dL)
(9.7 nmol/L [0.3-2.1 nmol/L])
SHBG = 1.3 µg/mL (2.2-14.6 µg/mL)
(SI: 12 nmol/L [20-130 nmol/L])

Which of the following is the most likely diagnosis?
   A. Macronodular adrenocortical hyperplasia
   B. Nonclassic 11β-hydroxylase deficiency
   C. Adrenocortical carcinoma
   D. Licorice ingestion
   E. Anabolic steroid abuse

7 A 57-year-old man is referred for a second opinion about primary aldosteronism. He developed resistant hypertension in his early 50s and was found to be hypokalemic 6 months ago on routine blood testing.

Screening laboratory test results:
Sodium = 147 mEq/L (136-142 mEq/L)
(SI: 147 mmol/L [136-142 mmol/L])
Potassium = 3.2 mEq/L (3.5-5.0 mEq/L)
(SI: 3.2 mmol/L [3.5-5.0 mmol/L])
Serum aldosterone = 22 ng/dL (4-21 ng/dL)
(SI: 610.3 pmol/L [111.0-582.5 pmol/L])
Plasma renin activity = <0.6 ng/mL per h
(0.6-4.3 ng/mL per h)

On the third day of a high-salt diet, the 24-hour urine collection documents a sodium excretion of 280 mEq/24 h (280 mmol/d) and an aldosterone excretion of 20 µg/24 h (55.4 nmol/d). CT with fine cuts of the adrenals shows normal glands. He undergoes adrenal venous sampling with continuous infusion of cosyntropin at 50 mcg per h. The results are shown (*see table next page*).

Measurement	Right Adrenal Vein	Left Adrenal Vein	Inferior Vena Cava
Aldosterone	44 ng/dL (1220.6 pmol/L)	6400 ng/dL (177,536 pmol/L)	44 ng/dL (1220.6 pmol/L)
Cortisol	22 µg/dL (606.9 nmol/L)	2000 µg/dL (55,176 nmol/L)	20 µg/dL (551.8 nmol/L)
Aldosterone-to-Cortisol Ratio	2.0	3.2	2.2

He is told that the source is the left adrenal gland on the basis of the high left adrenal vein aldosterone concentration and the aldosterone-to-cortisol ratio.

How do you interpret the results of the adrenal venous sampling study?
  A. Unable to localize
  B. Left adrenal gland is the source (left adenoma)
  C. Both adrenal glands are sources (bilateral, idiopathic hyperaldosteronism)
  D. Insufficient information to interpret whether the study was successful

8 A 23-year-old woman with congenital adrenal hyperplasia (due to 21-hydroxylase deficiency) diagnosed at birth sees you as part of her care transition from her pediatric endocrinologist. Her current treatment consists of hydrocortisone, 10 mg 3 times daily with meals, and fludrocortisone acetate, 0.2 mg every evening. She has regular menses, is not sexually active, and is not attempting to become pregnant.

On physical examination, she has no acne or unwanted facial hair, purple striae, or skin thinning. Her BMI is 25.2 kg/m². Her blood pressure is 115/76 mm Hg. She feels well and has no complaints.

She took her hydrocortisone today at 6 AM and 12 PM, and her blood is drawn at 5:30 PM.

Laboratory test results (5:30 PM blood draw):
  Sodium = 138 mEq/L (136-142 mEq/L)
    (SI: 138 mmol/L [136-142 mmol/L])
  Potassium = 4.2 mEq/L (3.5-5.0 mEq/L)
    (SI: 4.2 mmol/L [3.5-5.0 mmol/L])
  Serum DHEA-S = <15 µg/dL (44-332 µg/dL)
    (SI: <0.4 µmol/L [1.19-9.00 µmol/L])
  Serum testosterone = 40 ng/dL (8-60 ng/dL)
    (SI: 1.4 nmol/L [0.3-2.1 nmol/L])

Plasma renin activity = 2.4 ng/mL per h
  (0.6-4.3 ng/mL per h)
Serum androstenedione = 90 ng/dL (80-240 ng/dL)
  (SI: 3.0 nmol/L [2.79-8.38 nmol/L])
Serum 17-hydroxyprogesterone = 4500 ng/dL
  (<80 ng/dL) (SI: 136.4 nmol/L [2.42 nmol/L])

Which of the following changes to her management would you recommend?
  A. No changes
  B. Increase the second dose of hydrocortisone to 15 mg
  C. Switch hydrocortisone to dexamethasone, 1 mg at bedtime
  D. Divide hydrocortisone as 7.5 mg 4 times daily
  E. Stop fludrocortisone acetate

9 A 45-year-old man presents for follow-up after removal of a paraganglioma along his left lower spine. Before surgery 6 months ago, his plasma plasma normetanephrine was elevated at 4500 pg/mL (24.6 pmol/L) and plasma metanephrine was normal at 6 pg/mL (0.03 pmol/L). He received α-adrenergic blockade and underwent uneventful surgery. Genetic testing revealed a common mutation in the *SDHB* gene, and he was counseled about the need to maintain long-term surveillance for metachronous and metastatic tumors. At his first postoperative visit 3 months ago, his plasma normetanephrine was slightly abnormal at 200 pg/mL (1.1 pmol/L), and today his plasma normetanephrine concentration is 380 pg/mL (2.1 pmol/L). You are concerned about his rising normetanephrine and recommend imaging.

Which of the following imaging modalities would be the most sensitive for detecting recurrent or residual disease in this patient?
  A. Chest/abdomen/pelvis MRI
  B. ^{123}I-metaiodobenzguanine scan
  C. Chest/abdomen/pelvis CT
  D. ^{68}Ga-DOTATATE PET/CT scan
  E. ^{99}Tc-sestabmibi scan

10 An 18-year-old man is referred from pediatric endocrinology for management of congenital adrenal hyperplasia due to 11β-hydroxylase deficiency. He was managed with hydrocortisone 3 times daily throughout childhood. During the past 2 years, his blood pressure was consistently high, and his regimen was changed to liquid prednisolone twice daily. This treatment normalized his blood pressure, but he gained a significant amount of weight and slept poorly. Six months ago, his dosage was reduced to 3.5 mg in the morning and 1 mg at bedtime and he has felt well. This is the minimum dosage he can tolerate without weight gain and poor sleep; however, his blood pressure is consistently elevated, on average 145/90 mm Hg.

Findings on physical examination are normal, including normal-sized testes without adrenal rest tumors.

Laboratory test results on his current regimen:
  Sodium = 143 mEq/L (136-142 mEq/L)
    (SI: 143 mmol/L [136-142 mmol/L])
  Potassium = 3.3 mEq/L (3.5-5.0 mEq/L)
    (SI: 3.3 mmol/L [3.5-5.0 mmol/L])
  Serum testosterone = 600 ng/dL (300-900 ng/dL)
    (SI: 20.8 nmol/L [10.4-31.2 nmol/L])
  Serum androstenedione = 300 ng/dL
    (65-210 ng/dL) (SI: 10.5 nmol/L
    [2.27-7.33 nmol/L])
  Serum LH = 3.1 mIU/mL (1.0-9.0 mIU/mL)
    (SI: 3.1 IU/L [1.0-9.0 IU/L])
  Plasma renin activity = <0.6 ng/mL per h
    (0.6-4.3 ng/mL per h)
  Serum aldosterone = <3 ng/dL (4-21 ng/dL)
    (SI: <83.2 pmol/L [111.0-582.5 pmol/L])
  Serum 11-deoxycortisol = 2600 ng/dL
    (10-79 ng/dL)

Which of the following changes to his management would you recommend?
  A. Add eplerenone, 50 mg twice daily
  B. Switch prednisolone to dexamethasone, 0.75 mg at bedtime
  C. Increase the prednisolone dosage to 4 mg in the morning and 1.5 mg at bedtime
  D. Add potassium chloride, 60 mEq daily
  E. Add spironolactone, 50 mg twice daily

11 A 39-year-old woman is evaluated for recurrent Cushing disease. She underwent transsphenoidal surgery 2 years ago with resolution of her hypercortisolemia and symptoms; however, she did not experience a phase of adrenal insufficiency. Over the last 6 months, easy bruising, weight gain, and depressed mood have returned.

Laboratory test results:
  Late-night salivary cortisol = 0.41 µg/dL
    (<0.13 µg/dL) (SI: 11.3 nmol/L [<3.6 nmol/L])
  Urinary free cortisol = 129 µg/24 h (4-50 µg/24 h)
    (SI: 356 nmol/d [11-138 nmol/d])
  Serum cortisol (8 AM) after overnight 1-mg
    dexamethasone suppression test = 17.4 µg/dL
    (SI: 480.0 nmol/L)
  DHEA-S = 400 µg/dL (31-228 µg/dL)
    (SI: 10.8 µmol/L [0.84-6.78 µmol/L])
  Basal plasma ACTH = 51 pg/mL (10-60 pg/mL)
    (SI: 11.2 pmol/L [2.2-13.2 pmol/L])
  Fasting glucose = 120 mg/dL (70-99 mg/dL)
    (SI: 6.7 mmol/L [3.9-5.5 mmol/L])
  Serum potassium = 3.7 mEq/L (3.5-5.0 mEq/L)
    (SI: 3.7 mmol/L [3.5-5.0 mmol/L])
  Serum ALT = 18 U/L (10-40 U/L) (SI: 0.30 µkat/L
    [0.17-0.67 µkat/L])

After a discussion with the patient, you decide to start therapy with pasireotide, 600 mcg twice daily.

Which of the following should be monitored most frequently in this patient after starting this therapy?
  A. Serum potassium
  B. Serum glucose
  C. Vaginal bleeding
  D. Serum ALT
  E. Blood pressure

12 A 58-year-old man is referred for evaluation of an incidentally discovered adrenal mass. He had not seen a physician in 10 years, and he sought medical attention for postprandial abdominal pain. Abdominal CT without contrast was obtained (*see image*). The official interpretation is "1.2-cm left adrenal mass, MRI can further characterize." The abdominal pain has since resolved with a 6-week course of omeprazole. His medical history is unremarkable.

On physical examination, he has no cushingoid stigmata. Blood pressure measurements obtained in the clinic since he first presented have ranged as follows: systolic 144-162 mm Hg and diastolic 92-98 mm Hg (even after resolution of his abdominal pain).

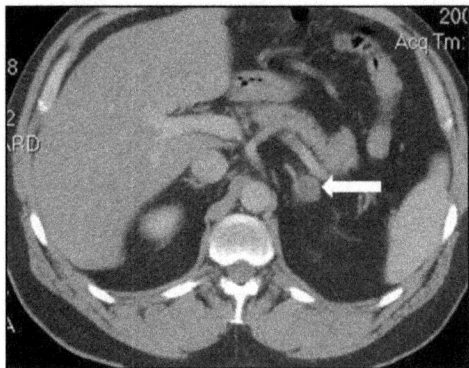

Laboratory test results:
Potassium = 3.8 mEq/L (3.5-5.0 mEq/L)
  (SI: 3.8 mmol/L [3.5-5.0 mmol/L])
Plasma normetanephrine = 150 pg/mL
  (<165 pg/mL) (SI: 0.82 pmol/L [<0.90 nmol/L])
Plasma metanephrine = 40 pg/mL (<99 pg/mL)
  (SI: 0.20 pmol/L [<0.50 nmol/L])
Serum cortisol (8 AM) after overnight 1-mg
  dexamethasone suppression test = 0.4 µg/dL
  (SI: 11.0 nmol/L)
Fasting glucose = 80 mg/dL (70-99 mg/dL)
  (SI: 4.4 mmol/L [3.9-5.5 mmol/L])

Which of the following is the best next step in this patient's management?
  A. Measure 24-hour urine for metanephrines
  B. Perform adrenal MRI
  C. Measure serum DHEA-S and plasma ACTH
  D. Repeat adrenal CT in 1 year
  E. Measure serum aldosterone and plasma renin activity

13 You are asked to evaluate for Cushing syndrome in a 49-year-old man in the intensive care unit. Small cell lung cancer was previously diagnosed, and he began chemotherapy 3 months ago. Over the last 4 weeks following his last cycle of chemotherapy, he has experienced rapid onset of hyperglycemia, hypertension, muscle weakness, and psychosis. He was taken to the emergency department by ambulance, where he was confused and hypoxic.

Laboratory test results:
Plasma ACTH = 420 pg/mL (10-60 pg/mL)
  (SI: 92.4 pmol/L [2.2-13.2 pmol/L])
Serum cortisol = 180 µg/dL (5-25 µg/dL)
  (SI: 4966 nmol/L [137.9-389.7 nmol/L])
Serum potassium = 2.4 mEq/L (3.5-5.0 mEq/L)
  (2.4 mmol/L [3.5-5.0 mmol/L])
ALT = 150 U/L (10-40 U/L) (SI: 2.5 µkat/L
  [0.17-0.67 µkat/L])

He was intubated and ventilated before transfer to the intensive care unit. You suspect ectopic ACTH syndrome, but the patient is too ill for further evaluation.

Which of the following medications do you recommend immediately to treat his hypercortisolemia?
  A. Mitotane
  B. Pasireotide
  C. Etomidate
  D. Ketoconazole
  E. Mifepristone

14 A 43-year-old woman is seeing you for follow-up of Cushing disease. She initially presented with hypertension, hypokalemia, muscle weakness, hirsutism, oligomenorrhea, and weight gain over the last 2 years.

Preoperative laboratory test results:
Late-night salivary cortisol = 0.82 µg/dL
  (<0.13 µg/dL) (SI: 22.6 nmol/L [<3.6 nmol/L])
Urinary free cortisol = 850 µg/24 h (4-50 µg/24 h)
  (SI: 2346 nmol/d [11-138 nmol/d])
Basal plasma ACTH = 102 pg/mL (10-60 pg/mL)
  (SI: 22.4 pmol/L [2.2-13.2 pmol/L])

Inferior petrosal sinus sampling and MRI confirmed a pituitary tumor, and she underwent transsphenoidal surgery 6 weeks ago. Postoperatively, serial morning cortisol values were less than 0.5 µg/dL (<13.8 nmol/L), and she was discharged on the third postoperative day and instructed to take hydrocortisone, 25 mg on arising and 10 mg in the early afternoon (without her antihypertensive medications).

Her blood pressure has normalized, and she has lost 8 lb (3.6 kg). She describes diffuse muscle aches, fatigue, and anorexia. She states, "I am sleeping all day and feel worse than when I had Cushing's."

On physical examination, her blood pressure is 120/80 mm Hg and pulse rate is 70 beats/min without orthostatic changes. Her cushingoid features are beginning to resolve.

Laboratory test results in clinic:
Serum sodium = 136 mEq/L (136-142 mEq/L)
(SI: 136 mmol/L [136-142 mmol/L])
Serum potassium = 4.4 mEq/L (3.5-5.0 mEq/L)
(SI: 4.4 mmol/L [3.5-5.0 mmol/L])
Fasting glucose = 80 mg/dL (70-99 mg/dL)
(SI: 4.4 mmol/L [3.9-5.5 mmol/L])
Serum cortisol (8 AM) before first dose of hydrocortisone = <0.5 µg/dL (5-25 µg/dL)
(SI: <13.8 nmol/L [137.9-389.7 nmol/L])
DHEA-S = <15 µg/dL (18-244 µg/dL)
(SI: <0.41 µmol/L [0.49-6.61 µmol/L])
Basal plasma ACTH = <4 pg/mL (10-60 pg/mL)
(SI: <0.9 pmol/L [2.2-13.2 pmol/L])

Which of the following should you do next to address her symptoms?
A. Repeat pituitary MRI
B. Add fludrocortisone, 0.1 mg daily
C. Measure late-night salivary cortisol
D. Increase the hydrocortisone dosage to 40 mg on arising and 20 mg in the early afternoon
E. Add DHEA, 25 mg daily

15 A 40-year-old woman with recurrent Cushing disease is commencing mifepristone therapy, 300 mg daily. Her comorbidities from Cushing disease include hypertension and diabetes mellitus for which she takes amlodipine, 5 mg daily, and metformin, 1500 mg daily. Her blood pressure is 135/85 mm Hg. Her menses have been irregular.

Laboratory test results:
Fasting glucose = 185 mg/dL (70-99 mg/dL)
(SI: 10.3 mmol/L [3.9-5.5 mmol/L])
Potassium = 3.7 mEq/L (3.5-5.0 mEq/L)
(SI: 3.7 mmol/L [3.5-5.0 mmol/L])

Serum cortisol = 18 µg/dL (5-25 µg/dL)
(SI: 496.6 nmol/L [137.9-389.7 nmol/L])
Hemoglobin A$_{1c}$ = 8.5% (4.0%-5.6%)
(69 mmol/mol [20-38 mmol/mol])
Plasma ACTH = 65 pg/mL (10-60 pg/mL)
(SI: 14.3 pmol/L [2.2-13.2 pmol/L])
Urinary free cortisol = 360 µg/24 h (4-50 µg/24 h)
(SI: 993.6 nmol/d [11-138 nmol/d])

Which of the following parameters should you use to titrate the mifepristone dosage in this patient?
A. Urinary free cortisol excretion
B. Return of regular monthly menses
C. Plasma ACTH level
D. Blood pressure
E. Serum glucose level

16 You are called for consultation on a 72-year-old man who is in the medical intensive care unit for hypovolemic shock from sepsis. Before hospital admission, his only medications were metformin, 1000 mg daily; lisinopril, 20 mg daily; and atorvastatin, 5 mg daily. He remains intubated and treated with pressors and saline boluses for 3 days. His systolic blood pressure is 85 mm Hg, and pulse rate is 118 beats/min. The team has performed an ACTH-stimulation test and asks for your interpretation.

Laboratory test results:
Basal serum cortisol = 15 µg/dL (5-25 µg/dL)
(SI: 413.8 nmol/L [137.9-389.7 nmol/L])
Stimulated serum cortisol = 16 µg/dL
(SI: 441.4 nmol/L)
Serum glucose = 134 mg/dL (70-99 mg/dL)
(SI: 7.4 mmol/L [3.9-5.5 mmol/L])
Serum albumin = 2.3 g/dL (3.5-5.0 g/dL)
(SI: 23 g/L [35-50 g/L])

Which of the following do you recommend as the best next step in this patient's evaluation and management?
A. Insulin tolerance test
B. Serum DHEA-S measurement
C. Plasma ACTH measurement
D. Low-dose ACTH-stimulation test
E. No further testing

17 You are evaluating a 23-year-old woman with a well-documented diagnosis of nonclassic 21-hydroxylase deficiency based on a cosyntropin-stimulated 17-hydroxyprogesterone concentration of 2800 ng/dL (84.8 nmol/L) with a simultaneous cortisol concentration of 23 μg/dL (634.5 nmol/L). She was married 12 months ago and she and her spouse want to have children soon. She has not become pregnant, however, despite regular monthly timed intercourse. She has had 4 menses during the past year at 8- to 15-week intervals.

Which of the following treatments do you recommend?
  A. Anastrozole, 1 mg daily
  B. Dexamethasone, 1 mg at bedtime, and fludrocortisone, 0.1 mg daily
  C. Clomiphene, 50 mg daily
  D. Hydrocortisone, 10 mg twice daily
  E. Metformin, 500 mg twice daily

18 A gynecologist colleague asks you to evaluate a 21-year-old woman for primary amenorrhea. The patient has recently moved from Brazil, and she was not previously evaluated before moving to the United States. The gynecologist could not palpate a uterine cervix during pelvic examination, and a karyotype analysis was 46,XY.

On physical examination, her height is 71 in (180 cm) and she has long arms and legs. Her blood pressure is 148/96 mm Hg. Cardiac examination reveals a 2/6 holosystolic, nonradiating murmur, and an S_4. She has no axillary or pubic hair, and breasts are Tanner stage 1.

Laboratory test results:
  Sodium = 144 mEq/L (136-142 mEq/L)
    (SI: 144 mmol/L [136-142 mmol/L])
  Potassium = 3.4 mEq/L (3.5-5.0 mEq/L)
    (SI: 3.4 mmol/L [3.5-5.0 mmol/L])
  Serum testosterone = <5 ng/dL (8-60 ng/dL)
    (SI: <0.2 nmol/L [0.3-2.1 nmol/L])
  Serum LH = 55 mIU/mL (1.0-18.0 mIU/mL)
    (SI: 55 IU/L [1.0-18.0 IU/L])
  Plasma ACTH = 105 pg/mL (10-60 pg/mL)
    (SI: 23.1 pmol/L [2.2-13.2 pmol/L])
  Serum aldosterone = <2 ng/dL (4-21 ng/dL)
    (SI: <55.5 pmol/L [111.0-582.5 pmol/L])

Plasma renin activity = <0.6 ng/mL per h
    (0.6-4.3 ng/mL per h)
  Serum cortisol = <1 μg/dL (5-25 μg/dL)
    (SI: <27.6 nmol/L [137.9-389.7 nmol/L])

Which of the following additional laboratory tests will reveal the diagnosis?
  A. Serum corticosterone and 11-deoxycorticosterone measurement
  B. Serum androstenedione and dihydrotestosterone measurement
  C. Sequencing of the androgen receptor gene
  D. Serum 17-hydroxypregnenolone and dehydroepiandrosterone measurement
  E. Serum estrone and estradiol measurement

19 Autoimmune adrenal insufficiency was diagnosed in a 34-year-old woman 6 months ago. In the year leading up to her diagnosis, she experienced progressive anorexia, 20-lb (9.1-kg) weight loss, weakness, and fatigue. She has been treated with hydrocortisone, 15 mg upon waking in the morning and 5 mg in the early afternoon, as well as fludrocortisone acetate, 0.1 mg at bedtime. On this regimen, she felt markedly better and regained 15 lb (6.8 kg). Despite these improvements, she still has persistent fatigue throughout the day, which does not change when she takes her hydrocortisone doses. She has regular monthly menses.

On physical examination, her blood pressure is 105/65 mm Hg and pulse rate is 82 beats/min. She has no purple striae, facial rounding, dermal atrophy, vitiligo, or bruises.

Laboratory test results:
  Sodium = 138 mEq/L (136-142 mEq/L)
    (SI: 138 mmol/L [136-142 mmol/L])
  Potassium = 4.8 mEq/L (3.5-5.0 mEq/L)
    (SI: 4.8 mmol/L [3.5-5.0 mmol/L])
  Plasma ACTH = 400 pg/mL (10-60 pg/mL)
    (SI: 88 pmol/L [2.2-13.2 pmol/L])
  Plasma renin activity = 13.4 ng/mL per h
    (0.6-4.3 ng/mL per h)
  Serum TSH = 2.2 mIU/L (0.5-5.0 mIU/L)

Which of the following changes do you recommend in her management?
- A. Distribute hydrocortisone, 10 mg upon waking, 5 mg at lunch, and 5 mg at the evening meal
- B. Switch hydrocortisone to prednisone, 10 mg upon waking
- C. Increase the fludrocortisone acetate dosage to 0.2 mg at bedtime
- D. Increase the hydrocortisone dosage to 25 mg upon waking and 10 mg in the early afternoon
- E. Reassure her that no changes are necessary

20 A 6-cm left adrenal pheochromocytoma is diagnosed in a 55-year-old man. His urine metanephrine and normetanephrine levels are 8 to 12 times the upper normal limit. His blood pressure is 165/105 mm Hg, and pulse rate is 85 beats/min. You start phenoxybenzamine, 10 mg at bedtime, and advance to 10 mg twice daily the next day. He calls you 4 days later with concerns of palpitations. His blood pressure is now 140/90 mm Hg, and pulse rate is 85 beats/min sitting. When standing, his blood pressure is 110/70 mm Hg, and pulse rate is 115 beats/min.

Which of the following is the most important next step in his management?
- A. Add metoprolol, 50 mg twice daily
- B. Increase the phenoxybenzamine dosage to 20 mg twice daily
- C. Substitute nicardipine for phenoxybenzamine
- D. Increase water intake
- E. Increase sodium intake

21 A 24-year-old man is referred by a urologist for evaluation before surgery for testicular masses. The patient gives a history of taking hydrocortisone and fludrocortisone throughout childhood, but he stopped all medications at age 21 years.

On physical examination, he is a normal-appearing young man with a blood pressure of 106/72 mm Hg and pulse rate of 84 beats/min. Both testes have firm, irregular masses that are 4 to 6 cm in maximal dimension. His 8-AM cortisol concentration is 4 μg/dL (110.4 nmol/L) by immunoassay and 1 μg/dL (27.6 nmol/L) by mass spectrometry. Semen analysis documents azoospermia.

Which of the following patterns do you predict for his other laboratory test results?

Answer	Testosterone	Androstenedione	LH
A.	↑	↑	↑
B.	↓	↓	↓
C.	Normal	↑	↓
D.	↓	↓	↑
E.	Normal	Normal	Normal

22 An 18-year-old young man presents with 18 months of weight gain, poor sleep, depression, muscle weakness, and easy bruising. He abruptly stopped growing when his symptoms began, and his pubertal progression slowed.

On physical examination, he has wide purple striae on his abdomen and flanks, central obesity, facial plethora, and moon facies.

Screening laboratory test results:
- Sodium = 142 mEq/L (136-142 mEq/L)
  (SI: 142 mmol/L [136-142 mmol/L])
- Potassium = 3.3 mEq/L (3.5-5.0 mEq/L)
  (SI: 3.3 mmol/L [3.5-5.0 mmol/L])
- Serum DHEA-S = 30 μg/dL (35-535 μg/dL)
  (SI: 0.8 μmol/L [0.9-14.5 μmol/L])
- Plasma ACTH = <5 pg/mL (10-60 pg/mL)
  (SI: <1.1 pmol/L [2.2-13.2 pmol/L])
  (same result on repeated measurement)
- Urinary free cortisol = 870 μg/24 h (4-50 μg/24 h)
  (SI: 2401 nmol/d [11-138 nmol/d])
- Serum aldosterone = <3 ng/dL (4-21 ng/dL)
  (SI: <83.2 pmol/L [111.0-582.5 pmol/L])
- Plasma renin activity = <0.6 ng/mL per h
  (0.6-4.3 ng/mL per h)
- Serum testosterone = 240 ng/dL (300-900 ng/dL)
  (SI: 8.3 nmol/L [10.4-31.2 nmol/L])
- Serum cortisol = 28 μg/dL (5-25 μg/dL)
  (SI: 772.5 nmol/L [137.9-389.7 nmol/L])

The serum cortisol concentration is 35 μg/dL (772.5 nmol/L) after 1 mg of dexamethasone the night before.

CT shows normal-sized but irregular adrenals (*see image, arrows*).

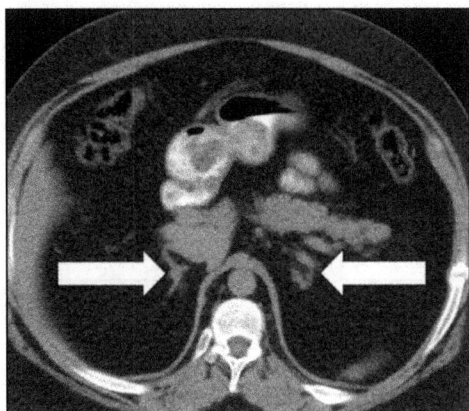

Which of the following forms of Cushing syndrome does this patient have?
A. Solitary adrenal adenoma
B. Pituitary tumor (Cushing disease)
C. Micronodular adrenocortical hyperplasia
D. Ectopic ACTH syndrome
E. Synthetic glucocorticoid therapy

23 A 48-year-old woman was diagnosed with medullary thyroid cancer 2 years ago. Following thyroidectomy and lymph node dissection, her calcitonin remained elevated at 1500 pg/mL (438 pmol/L). She has been managed with levothyroxine replacement and monitoring. She has felt well and has not experienced diarrhea or symptoms due to tumor mass effects. CT imaging has shown multiple metastases to the lung, liver, and bone (all smaller than 1.5 cm) with slight interval growth every 6 months. The calcitonin doubling time is approximately 18 months. In the 3 months since her last CT, she abruptly developed hypertension and hypokalemia, diabetes mellitus, poor sleep, muscle weakness, and depression.

On physical examination, her blood pressure is 160/94 mm Hg. She has a flat affect with slow response to commands, 2+ bilateral pedal edema, and muscle weakness.

Laboratory test results:
Serum potassium = 2.8 mEq/L (3.5-5.0 mEq/L)
    (SI: 2.8 mmol/L [3.5-5.0 mmol/L])
Serum cortisol = 130 µg/dL (5-25 µg/dL)
    (SI: 3586 nmol/L [137.9-389.7 nmol/L])

Plasma ACTH = 390 pg/mL (10-60 pg/mL)
    (SI: 85.8 pmol/L [2.2-13.2 pmol/L])
Serum calcitonin = 3200 pg/mL (<8 pg/mL)
    (SI: 934.4 pmol/L [<2.34 pmol/L])
Hemoglobin A_{1c} = 10.0% (4.0%-5.6%)
    (86 mmol/mol [20-38 mmol/mol])

On repeated CT, the metastases are not measurably changed from the scan 3 months ago. The adrenal glands are thickened but show no tumors.

Which of the following is the most appropriate next step in this patient's management?
A. Biopsy a liver metastasis
B. Perform bilateral adrenalectomy
C. Begin depot octreotide, 30 mg monthly
D. Refer to oncology for cytotoxic chemotherapy
E. Begin vandetanib, 300 mg daily

24 A 52-year-old man is referred for evaluation of resistant hypertension. Chlorthalidone was discontinued 1 month ago due to hypokalemia. He is currently treated with nifedipine, candesartan, nebivolol, and clonidine. On this regimen, he was screened for primary aldosteronism 1 week ago.

Laboratory test results:
Sodium = 144 mEq/L (136-142 mEq/L)
    (SI: 144 mmol/L [136-142 mmol/L])
Potassium = 2.9 mEq/L (3.5-5.0 mEq/L)
    (SI: 3.5 mmol/L [3.5-5.0 mmol/L])
Serum aldosterone = 8 ng/dL (4-21 ng/dL)
    (SI: 222 pmol/L [111.0-582.5 pmol/L])
Plasma renin activity = <0.6 ng/mL per h
    (0.6-4.3 ng/mL per h)

Which of the following is your conclusion about what needs to be done now on the basis of these screening tests?
A. No further testing; primary aldosteronism has been excluded
B. Rescreen after correcting hypokalemia
C. Rescreen after stopping candesartan
D. Rescreen after substituting doxazosin for nifedipine
E. No further testing; primary aldosteronism has been established

25 A 72-year-old man is referred to you for evaluation of primary aldosteronism. He has had resistant hypertension with difficult-to-control potassium for at least 15 years. You complete the evaluation, and you diagnose a 0.9-cm left aldosterone-producing adenoma with concordant lateralization on adrenal venous sampling.

You refer the patient for laparoscopic adrenalectomy. His preoperative blood pressure is 150/90 mm Hg.

Preoperative laboratory test results:
    Serum potassium = 3.9 mEq/L (3.5-5.0 mEq/L)
        (SI: 3.9 mmol/L [3.5-5.0 mmol/L])
    Baseline serum creatinine = 1.7 mg/dL
        (0.7-1.3 mg/dL) (SI: 150.3 μmol/L
        [61.9-114.9 μmol/L])
    Urine albumin = 220 mg/24 h (<30 mg/24 h)

For which of the following complications is he at risk postoperatively?
    A. Renal failure
    B. Refractory hypotension
    C. Prolonged hyperkalemia
    D. Persistent hyperaldosteronism
    E. Adrenal insufficiency

Calcium and Bone Board Review

Carolyn B. Becker, MD ● Brigham & Women's Hospital

1 A 25-year-old woman presents to her obstetrician during the second trimester of pregnancy with nausea and vomiting after eating at a restaurant. Her laboratory results return with an elevated calcium level of 11.0 mg/dL (2.8 mmol/L).

Laboratory test results one week later (after a full recovery):
Serum calcium = 10.9 mg/dL (8.2-10.2 mg/dL) (SI: 2.8 mmol/L [2.1-2.6 mmol/L])
PTH = 55 pg/mL (10-65 pg/mL) (SI: 55 ng/L [10-65 ng/L])
Serum 25-hydroxyvitamin D = 33 ng/mL (30-80 ng/mL [optimal]) (SI: 82.4 nmol/L [74.9-199.7 nmol/L])

From a morning fasting collection of blood and urine, the ratio of her calcium clearance to creatinine clearance is 0.016.

Her parents are deceased and she has no siblings or children. No previous laboratory results are available. Neck ultrasonography is negative for any parathyroid abnormalities. She has no other health issues.

Which of the following is the best next step?
A. Genetic testing for a calcium-sensing receptor (*CASR*) gene mutation
B. Referral for parathyroid surgery but delay surgery until the third trimester of pregnancy
C. Referral to a surgeon for immediate 4-gland parathyroid exploration
D. MRI of the neck and mediastinum
E. Genetic testing for an *MEN1* gene mutation

2 You are evaluating a 40-year-old man who presents with low-trauma bilateral midshaft femur fractures treated surgically with rods by the orthopedist. His medical history is positive for 3 previous metatarsal fractures and poor dentition. His mother was diagnosed with osteoporosis in her 60s. Physical examination reveals loss of 2 teeth and scars from recent femur surgery but findings are otherwise normal.

DXA reveals Z-scores of –4.0 at the total hip and –3.8 at the femoral neck.

Laboratory test results show:
Complete blood cell count, normal
Creatinine = 0.8 mg/dL (0.7-1.3 mg/dL) (SI: 70.7 μmol/L [61.9-114.9 μmol/L])
Albumin = 4.0 g/L (3.5-5.0 g/dL) (SI: 40 g/L [35-50 g/L])
Alkaline phosphatase = 20 U/L (50-120 U/L) (SI: 0.33 μkat/L [0.84-2.00 μkat/L])
Bone-specific alkaline phosphatase = 3.9 μg/L (≤20 μg/L)
Calcium = 9.8 mg/dL (8.2-10.2 mg/dL) (SI: 2.5 mmol/L [2.1-2.6 mmol/L])
PTH = 35 pg/mL (10-65 pg/mL) (SI: 35 ng/L [10-65 ng/L])
25-Hydroxyvitamin D = 28 ng/mL (30-80 ng/mL [optimal]) (SI: nmol/L [74.9-199.7 nmol/L])

Which of the following is the best next step in this patient's care?
A. Screen for *COL1A1/COL1A2* gene mutations
B. Begin alendronate
C. Measure fasting C-telopeptide
D. Refer for tetracycline-labeled iliac crest bone biopsy
E. Measure serum pyridoxal 5´-phosphate

3 A 60-year-old man with renal failure due to polycystic kidney disease has been receiving hemodialysis for 20 years. He underwent 3.5-gland parathyroidectomy 10 years ago because of tertiary hyperparathyroidism. Five years ago, type 2 diabetes was diagnosed, and he took glipizide briefly before switching to insulin. He comes to you because of multiple vertebral fractures, a pelvic fracture, and a hip fracture over the past 7 years.

DXA reveals a femoral neck T-score of −3.8. Physical examination is negative for retinopathy or neuropathy. His medications include once-daily insulin glargine and calcitriol, 0.5 mcg twice daily.

Laboratory test results:
Hemoglobin A_{1c} = 7.2% (4.0%-5.6%)
(SI: 55 mmol/mol [20-38 mmol/mol])
Serum calcium = 8.1 mg/dL (8.2-10.2 mg/dL)
(SI: 2.0 mmol/L [2.1-2.6 mmol/L])
Albumin = 3.5 g/L (3.5-5.0 g/dL) (SI: 35 g/L [35-50 g/dL])
Phosphate = 5.2 mg/dL (2.3-4.7 mg/dL)
(SI: 1.7 mmol/L [0.7-1.5 mmol/L])
Creatinine = 8.4 mg/dL (0.7-1.3 mg/dL)
(SI: 742.6 μmol/L [61.9-114.9 μmol/L])
25-Hydroxyvitamin D = 24 ng/mL (30-80 ng/mL [optimal]) (SI: 59.9 nmol/L [74.9-199.7 nmol/L])
PTH = 90 pg/mL (10-65 pg/mL) (SI: 90 ng/L [10-65 ng/L])
Total alkaline phosphatase = 12 U/L (50-120 U/L)
(SI: 0.20 μkat/L [0.84-2.00 μkat/L])

An iliac crest biopsy is done after double-tetracycline labeling and results are pending.

Which of the following is the most likely cause of this patient's fragility fractures?
A. Osteitis fibrosa cystica
B. Osteomalacia
C. Adynamic bone disease
D. Mixed renal osteodystrophy
E. Diabetes-related osteoporosis

4 A 51-year-old man with newly diagnosed HIV infection is admitted to the hospital with acute nausea, vomiting, and altered mental status. According to his friends, he has been ill for 3 months with fever, weight loss, night sweats, malaise, and cough. He is an undocumented immigrant from Central America who avoided seeking traditional medical care due to concerns about deportation.

On physical examination, he is a lethargic, cachectic man with tachycardia and diffuse lymphadenopathy.

Laboratory test results:
Calcium = 17.1 mg/dL (8.2-10.2 mg/dL)
(SI: 4.3 mmol/L [2.1-2.6 mmol/L])
Albumin = 3.3 g/dL (3.5-5.0 g/dL) (SI: 33 g/L [35-50 g/dL])
Intact PTH = <10 pg/mL (10-65 pg/mL)
(SI: <10 ng/L [10-65 ng/L])
PTHrP, undetectable
25-Hydroxyvitamin D = 525 ng/mL (30-80 ng/mL [optimal]) (SI: 1310.4 nmol/L [74.9-199.7 nmol/L])
1,25-Dihydroxyvitamin D = >180 pg/mL (16-65 pg/mL) (SI: >468 pmol/L [41.6-169.0 pmol/L])

Chest x-ray reveals multiple opacities. Bronchoscopy is positive for *Mycobacterium bovis*.

Which of the following is the most likely etiology of this patient's hypercalcemia?
A. *Mycobacterium bovis* infection
B. HIV-associated increase in vitamin D–binding protein
C. Occult lymphoma
D. Vitamin D intoxication
E. HIV-associated immune reconstitution syndrome

5 A 60-year-old woman presents with polyuria, nocturia, constipation, and fatigue.

Laboratory test results:
Serum total calcium = 12.9 mg/dL (8.2-10.2 mg/dL)
(SI: 3.2 mmol/L [2.1-2.6 mmol/L])
Albumin = 4.0 g/dL (3.5-5.0 g/dL) (SI: 40 g/L [35-50 g/dL])

Phosphate = 2.5 mg/dL (2.3-4.7 mg/dL)
(SI: 0.8 [0.7-1.5 mmol/L])
Intact PTH = 78 pg/mL (10-65 pg/mL)
(SI: 78 ng/L [10-65 ng/L])
25-Hydroxyvitamin D = 22 ng/mL (30-80 ng/mL
[optimal]) (SI: 54.9 nmol/L [74.9-199.7 nmol/L])

Neck ultrasonography reveals a 1.5-cm parathyroid mass below the right lower thyroid lobe. She undergoes minimally invasive parathyroidectomy and successful resection of the parathyroid mass. She is discharged home later that day when her serum calcium and PTH are documented to be 10.8 mg/dL (2.7 mmol/L) and 8 pg/mL (8 ng/L), respectively. Pathology is consistent with a "typical parathyroid adenoma."

One week later, she returns for blood work, still feeling fatigued. Her serum calcium concentration is 11.1 mg/dL (2.8 mmol/L) and PTH is 10 pg/mL (10 ng/L). She is given reassurance. At a follow-up appointment 3 months after parathyroidectomy, she reports polyuria, nocturia, constipation, worsening fatigue, and weight loss.

Laboratory test results:
Calcium = 16.5 mg/dL (8.2-10.2 mg/dL)
(SI: 4.1 mmol/L [2.1-2.6 mmol/L])
Ionized calcium = 1.77 mg/dL (4.60-5.08 mg/dL)
(SI: 0.4 mmol/L [1.2-1.3 mmol/L])
Creatinine = 2.2 mg/dL (0.6-1.1 mg/dL)
(SI: 194.5 µmol/L [53.0-97.2 µmol/L])
Phosphate = 3.0 mg/dL (2.3-4.7 mg/dL)
(SI: 10.0 mmol/L [0.7-1.5 mmol/L])
25-Hydroxyvitamin D = 23 ng/dL (30-80 ng/mL
[optimal]) (SI: 57.4 nmol/L [74.9-199.7 nmol/L])
1,25-Dihydroxyvitamin D = 12 pg/mL
(16-65 pg/mL) (SI: 31.2 pmol/L
[41.6-169.0 pmol/L])
Intact PTH = <10 pg/mL (10-65 pg/mL)
(SI: <10 ng/L [10-65 ng/L])
Alkaline phosphatase = 78 U/L (50-120 U/L)
(SI: 1.30 µkat/L [0.84-2.00 µkat/L])
Serum protein electrophoresis/urine protein
electrophoresis, normal

Which of the following is the best next test to perform?
A. PTHrP measurement
B. 4D CT of the neck and mediastinum
C. PTH antibody measurement
D. 24-Hour urinary calcium excretion
E. Total body bone scan

6 A 20-year-old homeless woman is taken to the emergency department for evaluation. She is unable to give a clear history due to mild intellectual disability but she does describe numbness and tingling of her hands.

On physical examination, she is short and obese. Hand film is shown (*see image*).

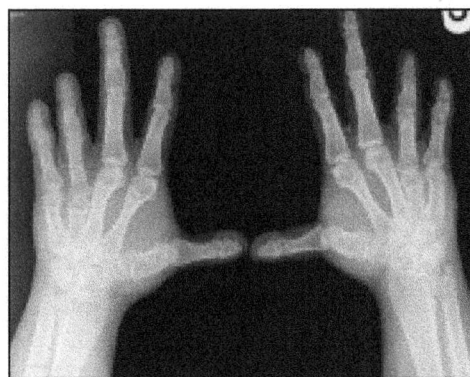

Laboratory test results:
Calcium = 6.0 mg/dL (8.2-10.2 mg/dL)
(SI: 1.5 mmol/L [2.1-2.6 mmol/L])
Albumin = 3.0 g/dL (3.5-5.0 g/dL) (SI: 30 g/L
[35-50 g/dL])
Phosphate = 5.9 mg/dL (2.3-4.7 mg/dL)
(SI: 1.9 mmol/L [0.7-1.5 mmol/L])
PTH = 420 pg/dL (10-65 pg/mL) (SI: 420 ng/L
[10-65 ng/L])
25-Hydroxyvitamin D =16 ng/mL (30-80 ng/mL
[optimal]) (SI: 39.9 nmol/L [74.9-199.7 nmol/L])
TSH = 5.9 mIU/L (0.5-5.0 mIU/L)
Free T$_4$ = 0.9 ng/dL (0.8-1.8 ng/dL)
(SI: 11.36 pmol/L [10.30-23.17 pmol/L])

Which of the following is the most likely diagnosis?
A. DiGeorge syndrome (22q11.2 deletion
syndrome)
B. Activating mutation in the gene encoding the
calcium-sensing receptor (*CASR*)
C. Autoimmune polyglandular syndrome type 1
D. Pseudohypoparathyroidism type 1A
E. Pseudopseudohypoparathyroidism

7 A 75-year-old woman comes for a follow-up visit after falling and breaking her wrist. Screening DXA at age 65 years showed osteoporosis, and she was prescribed weekly alendronate. After taking 2 doses, however, she had adverse effects and stopped the medication. She declined further treatment. In addition to osteoporosis, her medical history is notable for mild depression for which she has taken fluoxetine daily for several years.

On physical examination, she is a thin, frail, elderly woman wearing a cast on her right wrist. She has poor tandem gait and is unable to balance well on 1 foot.

DXA shows T-scores of –3.0 at the lumbar spine and –3.2 at the femoral neck. She is still very opposed to taking antiosteoporosis medication due to fears about cracking femurs and rotting jaws.

Laboratory test results:
Serum sodium = 131 mEq/L (136-142 mEq/L)
(SI: 131 mEq/L [136-142 mmol/L])
Serum potassium = 3.8 mEq/L (3.5-5.0 mEq/L)
(SI: 3.8 mEq/L [3.5-5.0 mmol/L])
Calcium = 9.5 mg/dL (8.2-10.2 mg/dL)
(SI: 2.4 mmol/L [2.1-2.6 mmol/L])
Intact PTH = 70 pg/mL (10-65 pg/mL)
(SI: 70 ng/L [10-65 ng/L])
25-Hydroxyvitamin D = 18 ng/mL (30-80 ng/mL [optimal]) (SI: 44.9 nmol/L [74.9-199.7 nmol/L])
Urine osmolality = 550 mOsm/kg
(150-1150 mOsm/kg) (SI: 550 mmol/kg [150-1150 mmol/kg]

In addition to optimizing calcium and vitamin D, which of the following would be a reasonable next step to improve her bone health?

A. Send her to a personal trainer for an intensive weightlifting program
B. Recommend that her antidepressant be changed to a different class
C. Treat her with daily salt tablets
D. Place her on a 1000 cc per day fluid restriction
E. Prescribe a very high-calorie diet to promote weight gain

8 A 78-year-old woman with severe chronic obstructive pulmonary disease and congestive heart failure is admitted to the hospital for acute renal failure, pneumonia, and new-onset atrial fibrillation.

On physical examination, she is febrile and lethargic but oriented to person, place, and time. She is in mild respiratory distress with rales and decreased breath sounds at the lung bases.

Laboratory test results:
Serum calcium = 12.8 mg/dL (8.2-10.2 mg/dL)
(SI: 3.2 mmol/L [2.1-2.6 mmol/L])
Serum creatinine = 1.8 mg/dL (0.6-1.1 mg/dL)
(SI: 159.1 µmol/L [53.0-97.2 µmol/L])
Estimated glomerular filtration rate = 27 mL/min per 1.73 m^2 (>60 mL/min per 1.73 m^2)
PTH = 176 pg/mL (10-65 pg/mL) (SI: 176 ng/L [10-65 ng/L])

Which of the following is the most appropriate management for her hypercalcemia?

A. Urgent exploratory parathyroid surgery
B. Zoledronic acid, 5 mg intravenously
C. Cinacalcet, 30 mg orally twice daily
D. Normal saline, 0.9% intravenously at 500 cc/h
E. Nasal calcitonin, 200 IU once daily

9 An 18-year-old man comes to you for follow-up of hypoparathyroidism. He initially presented at age 3 years with a seizure and severe hypocalcemia. Since then, he has been maintained on calcium and calcitriol. He has also been treated for intermittent oral candidiasis and fungal infections of his fingernails and toenails since childhood. Otherwise, he feels well.

On physical examination, he has some tinea of the nails and negative Chvostek and Trousseau signs.

An 8-AM cortisol measurement is 14 µg/dL (386.2 nmol/L).

In addition to measuring calcium, phosphate, renal function, and vitamin D, which of the following additional tests should you order now?

- A. Serum ceruloplasmin
- B. 21-Hydroxylase antibodies
- C. Glutamic acid decarboxylase (GAD$_{65}$) antibodies
- D. PTH antibodies
- E. TPO antibodies

10 A 74-year-old woman with severe osteoporosis (lumbar spine T-score of –3.2, compression fractures of T8 and T9 after minimal trauma) is being referred for anabolic therapy with teriparatide. She takes adequate calcium and vitamin D and is otherwise in good health. An extensive laboratory workup for secondary causes of osteoporosis comes back negative. You tell her that you plan to treat her for 18 to 24 months with teriparatide. Before she agrees, she would like to know more about the possible adverse effects from the drug.

Which of the following is most likely to occur in this patient during her course of treatment with teriparatide?

- A. Acute gout
- B. Osteosarcoma
- C. Nephrolithiasis
- D. Nephrocalcinosis
- E. Hypercalcemia

11 A 22-year-old male refugee from a wartorn country presents with severe, diffuse bone pain, joint deformities, and dental abscesses. His family history is unavailable because he was separated from his parents as an infant and grew up in a refugee camp.

On physical examination, he has short stature, severe genu varum (bow-leggedness), and very poor dentition.

Laboratory test results:
Calcium = 8.0 mg/dL (8.2-10.2 mg/dL)
 (SI: 2.0 mmol/L [2.1-2.6 mmol/L])
Albumin = 3.0 g/dL (3.5-5.0 g/dL) (SI: 30 g/L [35-50 g/L])
Phosphate = 1.3 mg/dL (2.3-4.7 mg/dL)
 (SI: 0.4 mmol/L [0.7-1.5 mmol/L])

25-Hydroxyvitamin D = 24 ng/mL (30-80 ng/mL [optimal]) (SI: 59.9 nmol/L [62.4-199.7 nmol/L])
1,25-Dihydroxyvitamin D = 30 pg/mL
 (16-65 pg/mL) (SI: 78 pmol/L [41.6-169.0 pmol/L])
Intact PTH = 85 pg/mL (10-65 pg/mL) (SI: 85 ng/L [10-65 ng/L])
Alkaline phosphatase = 234 U/L (50-120 U/L)
 (SI: 3.9 μkat/L [0.84-2.00 μkat/L])
Renal tubular reabsorption of phosphate, low

In addition to referring for dental care, which of the following treatments would you recommend for this patient?

- A. Calcitriol plus oral phosphate
- B. Calcitriol only
- C. Oral phosphate only
- D. Cinacalcet
- E. No additional treatment is necessary

12 A 60-year-old postmenopausal woman is referred for osteopenia. She has recently started prednisone, 15 mg daily, for chronic inflammatory arthritis and has derived tremendous benefit from this treatment. Attempts to lower the dosage have resulted in return of her pain syndrome. The plan is for her to continue on prednisone for up to 6 months. She is otherwise in excellent health, consumes adequate calcium and vitamin D, and exercises regularly. She has no personal or family history of fractures.

DXA documents that the patient's lowest T-score is –2.1 at the femoral neck. The FRAX calculator reveals a 10-year absolute risk for major osteoporotic fracture of 16% and a risk for hip fracture of 2.6%.

Laboratory evaluation is normal, including vitamin D.

On the basis of these results, which of the following is the best next step?

- A. Monitor her closely with a repeat DXA in 6 months
- B. Check fasting serum C-telopeptide now
- C. Adjust the FRAX scores upward by 15% at the spine and 20% at the hip
- D. Begin denosumab, 60 mg subcutaneously every 6 months
- E. Begin teriparatide, 20 mcg subcutaneously daily

13 You are evaluating an 82-year-old woman with osteoporosis who lives alone and is brought to her appointment by her daughter who lives over an hour away. The patient has been on oral alendronate, 70 mg weekly, for 5 years. She has missed her last 2 visits due to inability to get to the clinic. She has had no fractures, but feels she has lost some height.

Her current DXA shows T-scores of –1.5 at the lumbar spine, –2.8 at the femoral neck, and –2.6 at the total hip. Vertebral fracture assessment reveals moderate compression fractures at T10, L2, and L4. Her bone mineral density increased dramatically at the spine during the first 2 years on alendronate and then stabilized at the current level.

On physical examination, she appears frail. She is very cooperative but slightly confused. Back examination reveals moderate kyphosis without tenderness; her gait is slow, and she is unable to balance on 1 foot or rise from a chair without using her arms. She has had 3 falls since her visit nearly 2 years ago.

Laboratory test results:
Serum calcium, normal
Serum phosphate, normal
Serum creatinine, normal
Intact PTH, normal
Serum protein electrophoresis/urine protein electrophoresis, normal
25-Hydroxyvitamin D, normal
Fasting serum C-telopeptide = 658 pg/mL (104-1008 pg/mL)

She asks whether she can go on a "drug holiday."

In addition to referring her to physical therapy for gait and balance training, which of the following should you recommend for this patient's osteoporosis management?
A. Discontinue alendronate and reassess in 1 to 2 years
B. Continue alendronate for another 5 years
C. Switch to teriparatide
D. Switch to denosumab
E. Switch to zoledronic acid

14 You are called to see a 36-year-old woman with hypercalcemia. She comes to the emergency department following 24 hours of nausea, vomiting, and abdominal pain. Her medical history is notable for heavy alcohol use and severe gastroesophageal reflux disease. She takes no prescription medications but does take several over-the-counter therapies "for her stomach."

On physical examination, she is afebrile and lethargic with very dry mucous membranes and epigastric tenderness. Breast examination is negative for masses.

Chest x-ray and abdominal CT are normal.

Initial laboratory test results:
Calcium = 14.8 mg/dL (8.2-10.2 mg/dL) (SI: 3.7 mmol/L [2.1-2.6 mmol/L])
Phosphate = 3.5 mg/dL (2.3-4.74 mg/dL) (SI: 1.1 mmol/L [0.7-1.5 mmol/L])
Potassium = 3.0 mEq/L (3.5-5.0 mEq/L) (SI: 3.0 mmol/L [3.5-5.0 mmol/L])
Bicarbonate = 39 mEq/L (21-28 mEq/L) (SI: 39 mmol/L [21-28 mmol/L])
Serum urea nitrogen = 50 mg/dL (8-23 mg/dL) (SI: 17.9 mmol/L [2.9-8.2 mmol/L])
Creatinine = 3.5 mg/dL (0.7-1.3 mg/dL) (SI: 309.4 μmol/L [61.9-114.9 μmol/L])
Intact PTH = <10 pg/mL (10-65 pg/mL) (SI: <10 ng/L [10-65 ng/L])
Other labs, pending

In addition to making the patient nothing-by-mouth status, which of the following would be the most effective treatment for her hypercalcemia?
A. Intravenous zoledronic acid, 4 mg now and monthly as needed
B. Intravenous isotonic saline, 300-500 cc/h
C. Subcutaneous denosumab, 120 mg now and monthly as needed
D. Intravenous hydrocortisone, 100 mg every 8 hours

15 A 48-year-old man with advanced cirrhosis is found to have a low serum calcium level.

Laboratory test results:
    Serum calcium = 7.0 mg/dL (8.2-10.2 mg/dL)
        (SI: 2.0 mmol/L [2.1-2.6 mmol/L])
    Serum creatinine = 0.9 mg/dL (0.7-1.3 mg/dL)
        (SI: 79.6 µmol/L [61.9-114.9 µmol/L])
    Phosphate = 2.7 mg/dL (2.3-4.7 mg/dL)
        (SI: 0.9 mmol/L [0.7-1.5 mmol/L])

He reports no paresthesias or muscle cramps. On physical examination, he has scleral icterus and jaundice, marked ascites, 2+ pitting pretibial edema, and negative Trousseau and Chvostek signs.

Serum measurement of which of the following would be most useful to explain the laboratory findings?
    A. Intact PTH
    B. 25-Hydroxyvitamin D
    C. 1,25-Dihydroxyvitamin D
    D. Magnesium
    E. Albumin

16 A 50-year-old man is referred to you after results of a DXA. He is generally healthy, but fractured 2 metatarsals recently while stepping into a pothole and twisting his foot. He does not smoke cigarettes, drinks 1 beer nightly, and exercises regularly by running and hiking. He has taken finasteride daily for many years to control male-pattern baldness. His family history is positive for hip fracture in his father when he was age 84 years. The patient's DXA shows the following:

Site	BMD, g/cm²	T-Score
Total hip	0.698	−1.5
Femoral neck	0.658	−1.7
L1-L4	0.983	−0.3

His FRAX 10-year risk is 10% for major osteoporotic fractures and 1.7% for hip fracture.

Laboratory test results:
    Complete blood cell count, normal
    Complete metabolic profile, normal
    TSH, normal
    Vitamin D, normal
    PTH, normal
    24-Hour urinary calcium excretion, normal
    Morning testosterone = 390 ng/dL (300-900 ng/dL)
        (SI: 13.5 nmol/L [10.4-31.2 nmol/L])
    SHBG, normal

Which of the following is the best next step in this patient's management?
    A. Start alendronate
    B. Stop finasteride
    C. Stop finasteride and start alendronate
    D. Continue finasteride and begin transdermal testosterone therapy
    E. Monitor over time without any immediate changes

17 A 65-year-old woman who recently immigrated from a poor Middle Eastern country is referred to you for evaluation of muscle and bone pain, fatigue, weakness, spontaneous fractures, and difficulty walking. After removing her burqa (full outer garment and veil), physical examination reveals diffuse bony tenderness, proximal muscle weakness, and antalgic (waddling) gait.

DXA documents T-scores of −3 to −4 at all sites.

Laboratory test results:
    Electrolytes and renal function = normal
    Calcium (corrected for albumin) = 8.0 mg/dL
        (8.2-10.2 mg/dL) (SI: 2.0 mmol/L [2.1-2.6 mmol/L])
    Phosphate = 2.1 mg/dL (2.3-4.7 mg/dL)
        (SI: 0.7 mmol/L [0.7-1.5 mmol/L])
    Alkaline phosphatase = 325 U/L (50-120 U/L)
        (SI: 5.43 µkat/L [0.84-2.00 µkat/L])
    Intact PTH = 138 pg/mL (10-65 pg/mL)
        (SI: 138 ng/L [10-65 ng/L])
    1,25-Dihydroxyvitamin D = 20 pg/mL
        (16-65 pg/mL) (SI: 52.0 pmol/L
        [41.6-169.0 pmol/L])

Which of the following is the key diagnostic test to order next?
    A. FGF-23 measurement
    B. Total body bone scan (technetium-99m [⁹⁹ᵐTc])
    C. 25-Hydroxyvitamin D measurement
    D. Urinary fractional excretion of phosphate

18 A 25-year-old woman is referred for evaluation of low bone density. Her risk factors include a family history of osteoporosis and a personal history of hypothalamic amenorrhea for 2 years due to excessive exercise. Recently, while training for her third marathon in the past 18 months, she sustained a stress fracture of her right proximal femur and has been unable to run since then. After 6 weeks of inactivity, she regained regular menses, which have continued for the past 2 months. She does not smoke cigarettes, has no eating disorders, and is otherwise in excellent health. Her current DXA reveals Z-scores of −2.7 at the spine and −1.5 at the left femoral neck. A workup for secondary causes of low bone density is negative. Her stress fracture is healing well. Her BMI is 18 kg/m².

In addition to optimal calcium and vitamin D supplementation and counseling about moderating her exercise and improving her nutritional regimen, which of the following would you recommend for this patient's low bone density?

   A. Monitoring only
   B. Teriparatide
   C. Denosumab
   D. Risedronate
   E. Oral contraceptive pill

19 A 22-year-old man presents for evaluation of fragility fractures and low bone density. He had normal childhood and pubertal development but has sustained multiple fractures since adolescence with minimal or no trauma. He notes that he continues to get taller.

On physical examination, his height is 80 in (203 cm), and he is eunuchoid in appearance. He is well virilized with normal male external genitalia and no gynecomastia.

DXA shows Z-scores of −4.4 at the spine and −3.2 at the hip. Bone age is greatly reduced with unfused epiphyses.

Laboratory test results:
   Total testosterone = 1700 ng/dL (300-900 ng/dL)
     (SI: 59.0 nmol/L [10.4-31.2 nmol/L])
   SHBG = 1.2 µg/mL (1.1-6.7 µg/mL)
     (SI: 10.7 nmol/L [10-60 nmol/L])

   LH = 35.0 mIU/mL (1.0-9.0 mIU/mL)
     (SI: 35.0 IU/L [1.0-9.0 IU/L])
   Estradiol, undetectable

Treatment with oral estradiol leads to fusion of epiphyses and marked improvement in bone mass.

Which of the following best explains these findings?

   A. 5α-Reductase deficiency
   B. Inactivating mutation in the gene encoding the estrogen receptor
   C. Complete androgen insensitivity syndrome
   D. Severe aromatase enzyme deficiency
   E. Antiestrogen antibody syndrome

20 A 55-year-old woman seeks your advice because of osteoporosis and fractures. She entered menopause 3 years ago and has not taken hormone therapy. During childhood, she sustained several long-bone fractures that were attributed to her active lifestyle and participation in sports. Her last fracture was at age 15 years. Since menopause, however, she has sustained fractures at the wrist, humerus, and femur in low-trauma falls. Recent DXA reveals T-scores of −3.0 at the spine, −2.8 at the femoral neck, and −2.7 at the total hip. Her mother was diagnosed with osteoporosis at age 65 years.

On physical examination, she is a well-appearing woman without any dysmorphic features. Her height is 65 in (165.1 cm). Sclerae appear slightly greyish. She has no joint deformities or laxity. Her dentition appears normal. She wears bilateral hearing aids.

Laboratory test results:
   Complete blood cell count, normal
   Electrolytes, normal
   Calcium, normal
   Creatinine, normal
   Liver function tests, normal
   Alkaline phosphatase, normal
   TSH, normal
   25-Hydroxyvitamin D, normal
   1,25-Dihydroxyvitamin D, normal
   Intact PTH, normal

Sequencing which of the following genes will establish the diagnosis?

A. Osteoprotegerin gene (*TNFRSF11B*)
B. Type 1 collagen α 1 and 2 genes (*COL1A1/COL1A2*)
C. LDL receptor-related protein 5 (*LRP5*)
D. Vitamin D receptor gene (*VDR*)
E. Sclerostin gene (*SOST*)

21 A 52-year-old man with type 1 diabetes mellitus for 30 years and chronic kidney disease trips while stepping off a curb and fractures his right hip. DXA reveals T-scores of –2.8 at the lumbar spine and –3.0 at the left total hip.

Laboratory test results:
Serum calcium = 8.6 mg/dL (8.2-10.2 mg/dL)
    (SI: 2.2 mmol/L [2.1-2.6 mmol/L])
Albumin = 4.0 g/dL (3.5-5.0 g/dL)
    (SI: 40 g/L [35-50 g/L])
Creatinine = 3.8 mg/dL (0.7-1.3 mg/dL)
    (SI: 335.9 µmol/L [61.9-114.9 µmol/L])
25-Hydroxyvitamin D = 32 ng/mL (30-80 ng/mL
    [optimal]) (SI: 79.9 nmol/L [74.9-199.7 nmol/L])
Hemoglobin A_{1c} = 7.5% (4.0%-5.6%)
    (58 mmol/mol [20-38 mmol/mol])

One month after surgical repair of the hip fracture, you treat him with denosumab, 60 mg subcutaneously in your office.

Which of the following adverse effects is he most likely to experience in the 2 weeks following denosumab administration?

A. Worsening renal function
B. Symptomatic hypocalcemia
C. An acute febrile illness (acute-phase reaction)
D. Symptomatic hypoglycemia
E. Delayed fracture healing

22 A 40-year-old woman is referred to you because of vitamin D deficiency and secondary hyperparathyroidism that were discovered after she fell and broke her wrist. Her medical history is positive for class 3 obesity and hypertension. Lisinopril is her only medication.

On physical examination, her BMI is 48 kg/m² and blood pressure is 120/70 mm Hg. Examination findings are otherwise normal.

Laboratory test results (baseline):
Serum calcium = 8.9 mg/dL (8.2-10.2 mg/dL)
    (SI: 2.2 mmol/L [2.1-2.6 mmol/L])
Albumin = 4.0 g/dL (3.5-5.0 g/dL) (SI: 40 g/L
    [35-50 g/L])
Intact PTH = 88 pg/mL (10-65 pg/mL) (SI: 88 ng/L
    [10-65 ng/L])
25-Hydroxyvitamin D = 8 ng/mL (30-80 ng/mL
    [optimal]) (SI: 20.0 nmol/L [74.9-199.7 nmol/L])
Urinary calcium excretion = 70 mg/24 h
    (100-300 mg/24 h) (SI: 1.8 mmol/d
    [2.5-7.5 mmol/d])
Tissue transglutaminase antibodies, negative

Which of the following treatments would you recommend for this patient?

A. Cholecalciferol, 400 IU daily
B. Cholecalciferol, 1000 IU daily
C. Cholecalciferol, 4000 IU daily
D. Cholecalciferol, 10,000 IU weekly
E. Calcitriol, 0.5 mcg daily

23 A 73-year-old woman comes to see you for a second opinion regarding her skeletal health. She is currently due for her sixth annual infusion of zoledronic acid for treatment of osteoporosis. She did not tolerate oral bisphosphonates. She has never fractured, but her mother died of complications of a hip fracture. On further questioning, she notes aching in her left thigh and bilateral groin areas, which she attributes to increased weight-bearing exercise. A radionuclide bone scan is shown (*see image*).

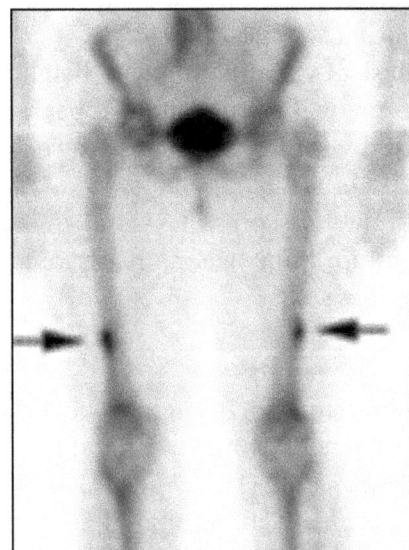

Which of the following is the best next step?
   A. Proceed with the zoledronic acid infusion right away
   B. Proceed with the zoledronic acid infusion but counsel her to limit her weight-bearing exercise for the next 12 weeks
   C. Stop the zoledronic acid infusions and begin abaloparatide
   D. Stop the zoledronic acid infusions and refer to orthopedics
   E. Switch from zoledronic acid to denosumab injections

24 A 68-year-old woman has been taking alendronate, 70 mg weekly, for the past 2 years. She says that she has taken it correctly (except for missing a few doses) and that she has not had any adverse effects. She had a repeated bone density test at the same center as her initial study. The report indicates a significant loss of bone mineral density in the spine and increases in bone mineral density in the femoral neck and total hip. The DXA images and numeric results are shown (*see images and table*).

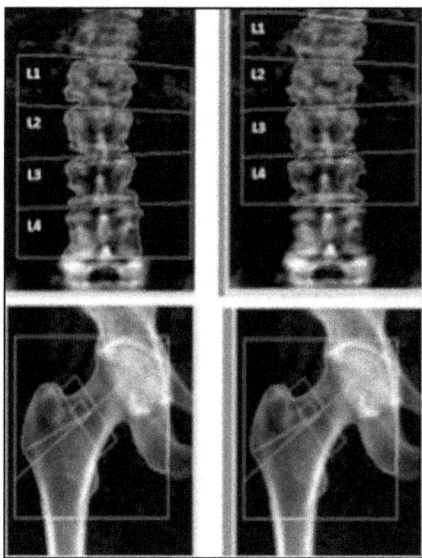

Site	Baseline Bone Mineral Density	Follow-up Bone Mineral Density
L1	0.451	0.423
L2	0.548	0.449
L3	0.593	0.549
L4	0.617	0.591
Total L1-L4	0.557	0.507
Femoral neck	0.480	0.532
Total hip	0.590	0.595

Which of the following would you recommend?
   A. Switch from alendronate to denosumab
   B. Switch from alendronate to zoledronic acid
   C. Evaluate for secondary causes of bone loss
   D. Ask the technician to reanalyze the spine region of interest
   E. Stop alendronate and begin teriparatide

25 A 53-year-old man has had 1 episode of a calcium-containing kidney stone. His workup reveals normal serum calcium and PTH levels, with a 24-hour urinary calcium excretion of 335 mg/24 h (100-300 mg/24 h) (SI: 8.4 mmol/d [2.5-7.5 mmol/d]), but normal 24-hour urinary oxalate, uric acid, sodium, and citrate levels. His urine volume is 1650 mL/24 h. The kidney stone analysis reveals calcium oxalate.

Which of the following recommendations would provide the greatest reduction in his risk of future calcium oxalate stone disease?
   A. Increased fluid intake
   B. Reduced dietary sodium
   C. Reduced dietary oxalate
   D. Potassium citrate
   E. Hydrochlorothiazide

26 You are evaluating a 62-year-old woman who has had several serum calcium measurements in the range of 10.6 to 11.0 mg/dL (2.7 to 2.8 mmol/L) (reference range, 8.2-10.2 mg/dL [SI: 2.1-2.6 mmol/L]). She feels well.

Laboratory test results:
   Serum albumin, normal
   Estimated glomerular filtration rate = 40 mL/min per 1.73 m^2 (>60 mL/min per 1.73 m^2)
   Serum PTH = 90 pg/mL (10-65 pg/mL) (SI: 90 ng/L [10-65 ng/L])
   Urinary calcium = 188 mg/24 h (100-300 mg/24 h) (SI: 4.7 mmol/d [2.5-7.5 mmol/d])

A sestamibi parathyroid scan is reported to be "non-localizing," and neck ultrasonography is negative.

Which of the following is the best next step?
   A. Minimally invasive parathyroidectomy
   B. Parathyroidectomy with identification of all parathyroid glands
   C. Measurement of 1,25-dihydroxyvitamin D
   D. Another sestamibi scan in 6 months
   E. Measurement of serum calcium and creatinine in 6 months

27 You are asked to evaluate a 65-year-old woman who was found to have an elevated serum PTH level of 87 pg/mL (10-65 pg/mL) (SI: 87 ng/L [10-65 ng/L]) as part of an evaluation for osteopenia documented on routine DXA testing (lowest T-scores, –2.1 in the spine and –1.6 in the left femoral neck). Her serum calcium levels have consistently ranged between 9.8 and 10.2 mg/dL (2.4 and 2.6 mmol/L), within the laboratory's reference range, and ionized calcium levels have been normal. Her serum 25-hydroxyvitamin D level is 48 ng/mL (119.8 nmol/L). She has been taking 2000 IU of vitamin D daily for several years. Her dietary calcium intake is 600 mg daily, and she has been taking supplemental calcium, 600 mg daily, for about 1 year.

Additional laboratory test results:
   Urinary creatinine = 0.9 g/24 h (1.0-2.0 g/24 h) (SI: 8.0 mmol/d [8.8-17.7 mmol/d])
   Urinary calcium = 180 mg/24 h (100-300 mg/24 h) (SI: 4.5 mmol/d [2.5-7.5 mmol/d])
   Serum creatinine = 0.8 mg/dL (0.6-1.1 mg/dL) (SI: 70.7 mmol/L [53.0-97.2 mmol/L])
   Phosphate = 2.6 mg/dL (2.3-4.7 mg/dL) (SI: 0.8 mmol/L [0.7-1.5 mmol/L])
   Albumin = 4.3 g/dL (3.5-5.0 g/dL) (SI: 43 g/L [35-50 g/L])

She has no history of kidney stones, fractures, or loss of height and no relevant family history. A repeated PTH measurement is 79 pg/mL (79 ng/L).

Which of the following is the most appropriate next step?
   A. Order DXA of the one-third distal radius
   B. Order sestamibi parathyroid scan
   C. Order renal ultrasonography
   D. Double the calcium supplementation and measure serum calcium and PTH again in 3 months
   E. Measure serum calcium and PTH every 3 months

28 A 53-year old woman presents with a new diagnosis of osteoporosis. She had a hysterectomy 3 years ago for fibroids and developed hot flashes and night sweats last year. The hot flashes interfere with her work during the day and her sleep at night. Last month she fell and broke her wrist. DXA performed at that time revealed T-scores of –2.5 at the spine and –2.3 at the femoral neck. She is otherwise very healthy, up to date on all health care screening, and does not smoke cigarettes. Her BMI is 22 kg/m². Findings from a metabolic workup for secondary causes are negative.

Which of the following would you recommend for this patient?
   A. Paroxetine
   B. Raloxifene
   C. Estradiol patch
   D. Risedronate
   E. Calcitonin

29 A 78-year-old man is found to have a serum alkaline phosphatase level of 185 U/L (50-120 U/L) (SI: 3.09 µkat/L [0.84-2.00 µkat/L]). Nuclear medicine bone scan shows increased activity in the right iliac wing. Radiographs of the area are consistent with Paget disease. He has no symptoms.

Which of the following treatments should you recommend?
   A. Alendronate
   B. Denosumab
   C. Zoledronic acid
   D. Calcitonin
   E. No treatment

30 You are called by an emergency department physician for advice in caring for a 35-year-old woman with a 5-year history of postsurgical hypoparathyroidism, previously well controlled, who has come to the emergency department after having a seizure. She is now conscious but confused. She has been out of town and without her medication for 3 days. Yesterday she told her daughter she was having some problems with tingling and muscle spasms.

Laboratory test results:
    Calcium = 5.8 mg/dL (8.2-10.2 mg/dL)
        (SI: 1.5 mmol/L [2.1-2.6 mmol/L])
    Albumin = 3.8 mg/dL (3.5-5.0 g/dL) (SI: 38 g/L
        [35-50 g/L])
    Phosphate = 5.3 mg/dL (2.3-4.7 mg/dL)
        (SI: 1.7 mmol/L [0.7-1.5 mmol/L])
    Magnesium = 1.9 mg/dL (1.5-2.3 mg/dL)
        (SI: 0.78 mmol/L [0.6-0.9 mmol/L])
    Creatinine = 0.9 mg/dL (0.6-1.1 mg/dL)
        (SI: 79.6 μmol/L [53.0-97.2 μmol/L])

In addition to restarting treatment with oral calcium and calcitriol, which additional treatment would be best?
    A. Intravenous bolus of 100 mg calcium chloride followed by a continuous calcium chloride infusion of 0.5 mg/kg per h
    B. Intravenous bolus of 1 g calcium chloride followed by a continuous calcium chloride infusion of 2 mg/kg per h
    C. Intravenous bolus of 150 mg calcium gluconate followed by a continuous calcium gluconate infusion of 1 mg/kg per h
    D. Intravenous bolus of 500 mg calcium gluconate followed by a continuous calcium gluconate infusion to achieve a total dose of 2000 mg calcium over 24 hours

Obesity/Lipids Board Review

Andrea D. Coviello, MD • Duke University

1 A 36-year-old woman is referred to you for weight loss. Her BMI is 38 kg/m². She has been following a high-fiber, low-fat diet and has been walking 30 to 45 minutes daily. She has lost 20 lb (9 kg) in the last 6 months before hitting a plateau and she is now frustrated with lack of progress. She is interested in trying a weight-loss medication, but she is worried about the potential adverse effects as she is very sensitive to medications.

Which of the following US FDA-approved medications for weight loss would be best in this case, as it has the lowest risk of adverse effects?
- A. Liraglutide, 3 mg daily
- B. Phentermine-topiramate ER, 15 mg/92 mg daily
- C. Lorcaserin, 10 mg twice daily
- D. Bupropion ER-naltrexone ER, 16 mg/180 mg twice daily

2 A 49-year-old man with a history of severe obesity and type 2 diabetes mellitus had a gastric bypass operation 3 years ago. His preoperative BMI was 42 kg/m². After surgery, his diabetes resolved, and his insulin therapy was stopped. His weight decreased and stabilized at a BMI of 29 kg/m². He has not had any follow-up for the last 16 months. Over the past month, he has had several episodes in which he felt shaky, sweaty, and irritable. Family members brought him to the emergency department for confusion that developed after he had a large breakfast at a buffet restaurant. In the emergency department, his glucose concentration was documented to be 35 mg/dL (1.9 mmol/L).

After treating his acute decompensation, which of the following is the most appropriate next treatment?
- A. Dietary modification
- B. Partial pancreatectomy
- C. Octreotide
- D. Acarbose

3 A patient with prediabetes mellitus and hypertension comes to see you for ongoing care. You mention her weight and she becomes frustrated, saying you always focus on her weight but that there is no evidence that she will live longer if she loses weight.

On physical examination, her height is 66 in (167.6 cm) and weight is 234 lb (106.4 kg) (BMI = 37.8 kg/m²). Her blood pressure is 138/76 mm Hg, pulse rate is 86 beats/min, and respiratory rate is 16 breaths/min. Exam findings are otherwise unremarkable.

Laboratory test results:

Hemoglobin A_{1c} = 6.4% (4.0%-5.6%) (46 mmol/mol [20-38 mmol/mol])

Total cholesterol = 220 mg/dL (<200 mg/dL [optimal]) (SI: 5.70 mmol/L [<5.18 mmol/L])

Triglycerides = 380 mg/dL (<150 mg/dL [optimal]) (SI: 4.29 mmol/L [<1.70 mmol/L])

HDL cholesterol = 36 mg/dL (>60 mg/dL [optimal]) (SI: 0.93 mmol/L [>1.55 mmol/L])

LDL cholesterol = 108 mg/dL (<100 mg/dL [optimal]) (SI: 2.80 mmol/L [<2.59 mmol/L])

In which of the following groups has weight loss been shown to reduce mortality in randomized controlled trials?
- A. Persons with obesity who are treated with weight-loss medications
- B. Persons with obesity treated with gastric bypass surgery
- C. Persons with type 2 diabetes treated with lifestyle intervention
- D. Persons with prediabetes treated with lifestyle intervention

4 A 45-year-old woman comes to see you for help losing weight. She has a seizure disorder and was placed on increasing dosages of gabapentin 2 years ago for this problem. She now takes 600 mg of gabapentin 3 times daily. Since starting this medication, she has gained 80 lb (36.4 kg) and now has a BMI of 39 kg/m². She has depression, for which her neurologist prescribed fluoxetine, 20 mg daily. Her hemoglobin A_{1c} level is 6.2% (44 mmol/mol), which is currently not being treated.

Which of the following would be most likely to produce and sustain the most weight loss over the next 12 months in this patient?
   A. Change from fluoxetine to bupropion
   B. Begin a low-carbohydrate diet
   C. Change from gabapentin to topiramate
   D. Initiate treatment with metformin

5 A 36-year-old woman with a peak lifetime BMI of 46 kg/m² had a laparoscopic gastric bypass operation in another state 8 weeks ago. She initially did well, but over the last 3 weeks she began to experience episodes of vomiting. Over the last 5 days, she has been vomiting almost everything she eats. Over the last 2 days, her husband says that she has become increasingly confused, dysarthric, and unsteady on her feet. On neurologic examination, she is clearly confused, has nystagmus, is unsteady on standing, has decreased sensation on her lower extremities, and has a right third nerve palsy.

This patient most likely has a deficiency of which of the following?
   A. Vitamin B_{12}
   B. Folate
   C. Thiamine
   D. Zinc

6 A 28-year-old woman comes to see you after experiencing a 10-lb (4.5-kg) weight gain over the last year. She says that her job has been very stressful and that she has uncontrollable cravings for ice cream and chocolate. The more sweets she eats, the more she craves.

Which brain region(s) is (are) most likely responsible for the rewarding characteristics of highly palatable food in this woman?
   A. Prefrontal cortex
   B. Ventral tegmentum and the nucleus accumbens
   C. Brodmann area 17 in the occipital lobe
   D. Arcuate nucleus
   E. Nucleus of the tractus solitarius and the dorsal vagal nucleus

7 A 53-year-old woman with a 10-year history of poorly controlled type 2 diabetes had a laparoscopic banding procedure 20 months ago. She attended all of her follow-up adjustment visits and lost 21% of her baseline weight. Her diabetes improved, but she still requires glucose-lowering medications. She has a varied diet but does not take any vitamin supplements. You find that she has normal strength and normal muscle bulk and tone but she has moderate distal symmetric peripheral neuropathy.

Which of the following is the most likely cause of her neuropathy?
   A. Vitamin A deficiency
   B. Thiamine deficiency
   C. Diabetes mellitus
   D. B_{12} deficiency
   E. Zinc deficiency

8 A patient asks you about weight-loss medications. She is worried about her weight and thinks that lifestyle changes alone have not helped her achieve her goal. However, she is concerned about potential adverse effects of weight-loss drugs given their history of problems.

Which of the following adverse effects of US FDA–approved weight-loss medications is significant enough to have prompted the adoption a Risk Evaluation and Mitigation Strategy (REMS)?
   A. Lorcaserin for valvular heart disease
   B. Phentermine-topiramate for potential birth defects
   C. Phentermine alone for psychiatric complications including psychosis
   D. Orlistat for fat-soluble vitamin deficiencies
   E. Liraglutide for cholecystitis

9 A 38-year-old man with a BMI of 39 kg/m² asks about weight-loss medications. He is frustrated with his weight and wants the "most effective medication." He is not concerned about adverse effects.

Which of the following would be predicted to provide the greatest weight loss for him?
    A. Lorcaserin, 10 mg twice daily
    B. Phentermine-topiramate ER, 15 mg/92 mg daily
    C. Phentermine, 37.5 mg daily
    D. Liraglutide, 3 mg daily
    E. Orlistat, 120 mg with meals

10 A 51-year-old woman underwent placement of an adjustable gastric band 4 months ago. She has been losing weight gradually and has had no problems. Last night, she was at a restaurant and developed abdominal pain and began vomiting. She is unable to even keep water down. She calls the practice for advice.

Which of the following is the most likely diagnosis?
    A. Anastomotic ulcer causing obstruction
    B. Band erosion
    C. Food impaction
    D. Anastomotic leak
    E. Band slippage

11 A 33-year-old woman with polycystic ovary syndrome comes to see you asking for a weight-loss medication. Her BMI is 33 kg/m². She has a history of multiple deep vein thromboses treated with warfarin and a seizure disorder that is controlled on phenytoin. Due to her deep vein thrombosis risk, she and her partner use only barrier contraception.

Which of the following US FDA–approved weight-loss medications would be the best choice for this patient?
    A. Orlistat, 120 mg 3 times daily
    B. Liraglutide, 3 mg daily
    C. Phentermine-topiramate ER, titrated to 15/92 mg daily
    D. Naltrexone-bupropion, titrated to 32 mg/360 mg daily

12 A 45-year-old man is referred to you from the liver transplant clinic for weight loss. He has gained weight slowly through his adult life and is currently at his peak weight with a BMI of 54 kg/m². He also has obstructive sleep apnea and uses continuous positive airway pressure nightly. He has hypertriglyceridemia and nonalcoholic fatty liver disease (NAFLD) (biopsy-proven with inflammation, some bridging fibrosis but not cirrhosis). He has no known heart disease.

In addition to lifestyle changes, including a reduced-calorie diet and an increase in physical activity, you recommend which of the following weight-loss medications:
    A. Liraglutide, 3 mg daily
    B. Phentermine-topiramate ER, titrated to 15 mg/92 mg daily
    C. Naltrexone-bupropion, titrated to 32 mg/360 mg daily
    D. Lorcaserin, 10 mg twice daily
    E. Phentermine immediate-release, titrated to 8 mg 3 times daily

13 A 45-year-old woman is referred to you for weight loss. Her BMI is 56 kg/m² and she has multiple comorbidities, including degenerative arthritis, hyperlipidemia, fatty liver disease, and oligomenorrhea. She has successfully lost weight in the past but has always gained it back. She needs knee replacement but was told she must first lose 40 lb (18.2 kg). She would like to pursue bariatric surgery with a sleeve gastrectomy and would like to discuss the potential postoperative complications.

Which of the following is the most common adverse effect of sleeve gastrectomy?
    A. Hypertriglyceridemia
    B. Amenorrhea
    C. Hyperglycemia
    D. Kidney stones
    E. Onycholysis

14 Current US FDA–approved medications for weight loss include one hormone receptor antagonist (the GLP-1 receptor antagonist liraglutide), but many hormones have a role in appetite and weight regulation.

Which of the following hormones would be a good target for a hormone receptor antagonist to stimulate weight loss?

- A. Ghrelin
- B. GLP-1
- C. Cholecystokinin
- D. Peptide YY

15 A 30-year-old woman comes to see you for assistance with weight loss. Her height is 62 in (157.5 cm), and weight is 174 lb (79.1 kg) (BMI = 31.8 kg/m²). She is otherwise healthy and takes no medications. She has recently started going to the gym 3 times a week for a combination of aerobic exercise and resistance training. Many people at the gym are following a ketogenic diet and she would like to know what to expect if she tries this diet.

Which of the following is a potential adverse effect of a ketogenic diet?

- A. Cataract formation
- B. Kidney stones
- C. Eruptive xanthoma
- D. Glucosuria

16 A 39-year-old man comes to see you for help treating elevated cholesterol. His father died of a myocardial infarction at age 29 years and his brother developed angina at age 32 years. He has intermittent chest pain that is consistent with angina but has not had any diagnostic testing. He is taking atorvastatin, 80 mg daily, and on this medication his fasting LDL-cholesterol level is 245 mg/dL (6.35 mmol/L).

On physical examination, he has thickened Achilles tendons and nodules on the extensor tendons of his hands.

Which of the following would be the best next step?

- A. Add ezetimibe
- B. Add fenofibrate
- C. Add evolocumab
- D. Add niacin
- E. Change to rosuvastatin 40 mg daily

17 You are evaluating a 57-year-old man who has type 2 diabetes and an American Heart Association 10-year risk of cardiovascular disease of 15%. He also has a history of hepatitis C infection and a mild, chronic elevation of transaminases (<2 times the upper normal limit). He has heard that statins can cause liver injury and he is worried about taking them. His LDL-cholesterol level is 156 mg/dL (4.04 mmol/L), and his fasting triglyceride level is 220 mg/dL (4.49 mmol/L).

Which of the following treatment is the best approach in this patient's management?

- A. A statin
- B. Diet alone until he completes treatment for hepatitis C
- C. A fibrate
- D. Ezetimibe
- E. Niacin

18 A 28-year-old woman has lipid levels drawn at a health fair. She is found to have a triglyceride level of 525 mg/dL (5.93 mmol/L) and an HDL-cholesterol level of 82 mg/dL (2.12 mmol/L). Her LDL-cholesterol level could not be calculated. She is asymptomatic and has no personal or family history of coronary disease, pancreatitis, or known lipid disorders. She is currently taking oral contraceptives.

Which of the following is the most likely explanation for her lipid levels?

- A. Lipoprotein lipase deficiency
- B. Apolipoprotein C2 deficiency
- C. Oral contraceptive use
- D. Cholesterol ester transfer protein deficiency

19 A 54-year-old man with a 10-year history of type 2 diabetes had a myocardial infarction 1 year ago. He was prescribed simvastatin, 20 mg daily, upon hospital discharge and his LDL-cholesterol level on this medication is now 110 mg/dL (2.85 mmol/L).

Which of the following is the most appropriate next step?
   A. Maintain the current treatment
   B. Increase the simvastatin dosage to 40 mg daily
   C. Add ezetimibe, 10 mg daily
   D. Change simvastatin to atorvastatin, 20 mg daily
   E. Change simvastatin to atorvastatin, 80 mg daily

20 A 30-year-old woman without diabetes mellitus has acute pancreatitis and a triglyceride level greater than 5000 mg/dL (>56.50 mmol/L). She is admitted to the hospital and is treated with supportive care as is recommended for all patients of pancreatitis.

Which of the following is an additional therapy that could be used as a method to reduce liver production of triglycerides in this patient?
   A. Insulin and glucose
   B. Fenofibrate
   C. Heparin
   D. Tamoxifen
   E. Metformin

21 You are referred a 38-year-old man with a 12-year history of coronary artery disease and multiple hospitalizations for coronary artery stent placements. The patient's family has a strong history of heart disease: his father and 2 paternal uncles died before age 50 years. The patient takes atorvastatin, 80 mg daily.

Laboratory test results:
   Total cholesterol = 210 mg/dL (<200 mg/dL
      [optimal]) (SI: 5.44 mmol/L [<5.18 mmol/L])
   LDL cholesterol = 150 mg/dL (<100 mg/dL
      [optimal]) (SI: 3.89 mmol/L [<2.59 mmol/L])
   HDL cholesterol = 40 mg/dL (>60 mg/dL
      [optimal]) (SI: 1.04 mmol/L [>1.55 mmol/L])
   Triglycerides = 100 mg/dL (<150 mg/dL [optimal])
      (SI: 1.13 mmol/L [<1.70 mmol/L])

On physical examination, you should look for which of the following findings?
   A. Lipemia retinalis
   B. Corneal arcus
   C. Eruptive xanthomas
   D. Palmar xanthomas
   E. Arthropathy

22 A 55-year-old man is referred for management of hyperlipidemia with intolerance to high-intensity statins. He has type 2 diabetes (hemoglobin A_{1c} = 6.6% [49 mmol/mol]), hypertension, and coronary heart disease with a non–ST-elevation myocardial infarction 2 years ago. He most likely has heterozygous familial hyperlipidemia given his peak total cholesterol concentration of 382 mg/dL (9.89 mmol/L) and LDL-cholesterol of 293 mg/dL (7.59 mmol/L). He had myalgias while taking atorvastatin, rosuvastatin, and simvastatin. He is currently tolerating pravastatin, 20 mg daily; ezetimibe, 10 mg daily; and niacin, 500 mg daily. He is very concerned about preventing a second cardiovascular disease event.

Laboratory test results:
   Total cholesterol = 284 mg/dL (<200 mg/dL
      [optimal]) (SI: 7.36 mmol/L [<5.18 mmol/L])
   LDL cholesterol = 200 mg/dL (<100 mg/dL
      [optimal]) (SI: 5.18 mmol/L [<2.59 mmol/L])
   HDL cholesterol = 55 mg/dL (>60 mg/dL
      [optimal]) (SI: 1.42 mmol/L [>1.55 mmol/L])
   Triglycerides = 145 mg/dL (<150 mg/dL [optimal])
      (SI: 1.64 mmol/L [<1.70 mmol/L])

Which of the following should you recommend as the best next step in this patient's management?
   A. Increase the niacin dosage to 1 g daily
   B. Add alirocumab
   C. Add fenofibrate
   D. Perform lipopheresis

23 You are referred a 30-year-old woman with systemic lupus erythematosus. Her current medications include prednisone, 20 mg daily; hydrochlorothiazide; lisinopril and metoprolol for hypertension; and infliximab.

Laboratory test results:
   Total cholesterol = 300 mg/dL (<200 mg/dL
      [optimal]) (SI: 7.77 mmol/L [<5.18 mmol/L])
   HDL cholesterol = 30 mg/dL (>60 mg/dL
      [optimal]) (SI: 0.78 mmol/L [>1.55 mmol/L])
   Triglycerides = 760 mg/dL (<150 mg/dL [optimal])
      (SI: 8.59 mmol/L [<1.70 mmol/L])
   LDL cholesterol cannot be estimated

You are concerned that medications could be contributing to her dyslipidemia. Which of the following adjustments should you recommend?

   A. Switch prednisone to dexamethasone

   B. Switch metoprolol to amlodipine

   C. Switch hydrochlorothiazide to chlorthalidone

   D. Discontinue lisinopril

24 You are referred a patient with HIV infection who is currently treated with a protease inhibitor and antiviral medications. He has developed mild lipoatrophy and his lipid panel is as follows:

   Total cholesterol = 280 mg/dL (<200 mg/dL [optimal]) (SI: 7.25 mmol/L [<5.18 mmol/L])

   LDL cholesterol = 180 mg/dL (<100 mg/dL [optimal]) (SI: 4.66 mmol/L [<2.59 mmol/L])

   HDL cholesterol = 30 mg/dL (>60 mg/dL [optimal]) (SI: 0.78 mmol/L [>1.55 mmol/L])

   Triglycerides = 350 mg/dL (<150 mg/dL [optimal]) (SI: 3.96 mmol/L [<1.70 mmol/L])

You start treatment with atorvastatin, 10 mg daily, and his LDL-cholesterol level decreases to 120 mg/dL (3.11 mmol/L).

Which of the following is most likely to occur and prevent the use of a higher statin dosage in this patient?

   A. Diabetes mellitus

   B. Myositis

   C. Inhibition of antiviral agents

   D. Interaction with antibiotics

   E. Hepatitis

25 A 58-year-old man with hyperlipidemia is referred to you for further evaluation. He has a history of hypertension, hyperlipidemia, and use to be a heavy cigarette smoker. After a myocardial infarction at age 54 years, he stopped smoking, started exercising, and started a high-intensity statin (atorvastatin, 80 mg daily). His LDL-cholesterol level decreased to less than 100 mg/dL (<2.59 mmol/L). Despite aggressive risk factor modification, he had a second heart attack 3 months ago. His father also has hyperlipidemia and despite statin therapy, he had a myocardial infarction at age 56 years.

On physical examination, his blood pressure is 128/74 mm Hg, pulse rate is 66 beats/min, and BMI is 24 kg/m².

Lipid profile:

   Total cholesterol = 165 mg/dL (<200 mg/dL [optimal]) (SI: 4.27 mmol/L [<5.18 mmol/L])

   LDL cholesterol = 94 mg/dL (<100 mg/dL [optimal]) (SI: 2.43 mmol/L [<2.59 mmol/L])

   HDL cholesterol = 46 mg/dL (>60 mg/dL [optimal]) (SI: 1.19 mmol/L [>1.55 mmol/L])

   Triglycerides = 124 mg/dL (<150 mg/dL [optimal]) (SI: 1.40 mmol/L [<1.70 mmol/L])

   Hemoglobin A_{1c} = 5.4% (4.0%-5.6%) (36 mmol/mol [20-38 mmol/mol])

Elevation of which of the following most likely explains his high cardiovascular disease risk despite good response to statin therapy?

   A. Apolipoprotein B

   B. Lipoprotein (a)

   C. High-sensitivity C-reactive protein

   D. Non-HDL cholesterol

26 A 68-year-old woman is referred to you for further treatment of hypercholesterolemia. She had a myocardial infarction one year ago and was discharged on atorvastatin, 80 mg daily, which was decreased to 40 mg daily 3 months later due to myalgias. She subsequently tried varying dosages of rosuvastatin, simvastatin, and lovastatin, all of which caused myalgias. She is currently taking ezetimibe, 10 mg daily, and her cardiologist wants to add the PCSK9 inhibitor evolocumab to reduce her cardiovascular risk, but she is concerned about potential adverse effects.

Which of the following is the most likely adverse effect she would experience with PCSK9 inhibitor therapy?

   A. Cognitive dysfunction

   B. Elevation of liver function tests

   C. Myalgias

   D. Skin irritation/rash

27 A 70-year-old woman is referred to you for lipid management. She has moderately well-controlled type 2 diabetes with a hemoglobin A_{1c} level of 7.8% (62 mmol/mol). She has a history of several episodes of pancreatitis, as well as a myocardial infarction at age 68 years. After her heart attack, she started atorvastatin, 40 mg daily, which brought her LDL cholesterol down from 158 mg/dL (4.09 mmol/L) to 88 mg/dL (2.28 mmol/L) but her fasting triglycerides are persistently elevated at 760 mg/dL (8.59 mmol/L). She had been prescribed gemfibrozil but has not yet started it.

Which of the following is the best next step in managing her cholesterol?
- A. Stop atorvastatin and start gemfibrozil
- B. Continue atorvastatin and add gemfibrozil
- C. Stop atorvastatin and start fenofibrate
- D. Continue atorvastatin and add fenofibrate
- E. Continue atorvastatin and add niacin

28 A 45-year-old woman with rheumatoid arthritis is referred for hypercholesterolemia and statin-induced myalgias. Creatinine kinase has never been documented to be elevated. Her physician has tried treating her with daily simvastatin, atorvastatin, and rosuvastatin.

Which of the following is the best next step in this patient's care?
- A. Start atorvastatin plus coenzyme Q10
- B. Start rosuvastatin once weekly
- C. Start red yeast rice
- D. Start fish oil
- E. Assess for statin antibodies

29 A 55-year-old man is anxious about his cardiovascular risk. He exercises regularly, has a blood pressure of 115/65 mm Hg, and avoids high-fat, high-cholesterol foods. His father was a World War II veteran who smoked 2 packs of cigarettes daily until having a myocardial infarction at age 62 years.

Laboratory test results:
Total cholesterol = 190 mg/dL (<200 mg/dL [optimal]) (SI: 4.92 mmol/L [<5.18 mmol/L])
LDL cholesterol = 105 mg/dL (<100 mg/dL [optimal]) (SI: 2.72 mmol/L [<2.59 mmol/L])

HDL cholesterol = 70 mg/dL (>60 mg/dL [optimal]) (SI: 1.81 mmol/L [>1.55 mmol/L])
Triglycerides = 75 mg/dL (<150 mg/dL [optimal]) (SI: 0.85 mmol/L [<1.70 mmol/L])

Which additional test could you order to best assess this man's cardiovascular disease risk?
- A. Coronary calcium score
- B. LDL particle size distribution
- C. Apolipoprotein B
- D. Antioxidant levels
- E. Serum palmitate measurement

30 A 43-year-old man seeks help to address high cholesterol. After experiencing an episode of angina, he had a positive treadmill stress test.

On physical examination, he has a firm papulonodular rash on both elbows and orange-yellow linear xanthomas of his palmar creases.

Fasting lipid panel:
Total cholesterol = 325 mg/dL (<200 mg/dL [optimal]) (SI: 8.42 mmol/L [<5.18 mmol/L])
LDL cholesterol = 227 mg/dL (<100 mg/dL [optimal]) (SI: 5.88 mmol/L [<2.59 mmol/L])
HDL cholesterol = 30 mg/dL (>60 mg/dL [optimal]) (SI: 0.78 mmol/L [>1.55 mmol/L])
Triglycerides = 340 mg/dL (<150 mg/dL [optimal]) (SI: 3.84 mmol/L [<1.70 mmol/L])

Which of the following abnormalities does this man most likely have?
- A. ABCA1 deficiency
- B. LDL-receptor deficiency
- C. Apolipoprotein E2/E2
- D. Apolipoprotein C2 deficiency
- E. Overproduction of apolipoprotein B

Pituitary Board Review

Laurence Katznelson, MD • Stanford University

1 A 31-year-old woman with a history of prolactinoma is now in her 37th week of pregnancy. Two years ago, a 14-mm prolactinoma was identified. Her initial prolactin level was 320 ng/mL (4-30 ng/mL) (SI: 13.9 nmol/L [0.17-1.30 nmol/L]), and there was suprasellar extension on MRI, chiasmal compression, and a small visual field defect. With bromocriptine, 2.5 mg nightly, her prolactin normalized, her galactorrhea and amenorrhea resolved, her visual field normalized, and her tumor decreased in size to 5 mm. She stopped bromocriptine when she learned she was pregnant. She now reports increasing headaches that are quite severe. Goldmann visual field testing is normal.

Which of the following is the best next step in this patient's management?
- A. Restart the bromocriptine now
- B. Deliver the baby
- C. Proceed with transsphenoidal surgical tumor removal
- D. Perform a pituitary-directed MRI
- E. Measure serum prolactin

2 Acromegaly is diagnosed in a 63-year-old woman. Initial MRI shows a 1.3-cm pituitary tumor with minimal extension superiorly and laterally. After transsphenoidal surgery, she still has some residual tumor in the left cavernous sinus. Her postoperative GH level is 3.0 ng/mL (3.0 μg/L) and it does not suppress with hyperglycemia after a glucose load. Her IGF-1 level is 290 ng/mL (72-207 ng/mL) (SI: 38.0 nmol/L [9.4-27.1 nmol/L]).

Which of the following treatment options would you recommend now?
- A. Stereotactic radiosurgery of the residual tumor
- B. Lanreotide depot monthly
- C. Another transsphenoidal surgery
- D. Pegvisomant weekly

3 An 18-year-old girl develops severe headaches. Head MRI shows a 2.8 × 2.8 × 2.2-cm cystic sellar and suprasellar mass with calcifications (*see image*). In retrospect, she has been tired, and her menses, which began at age 12 years, stopped 1 year ago. On physical examination, her vision is normal, as are the rest of the examination findings.

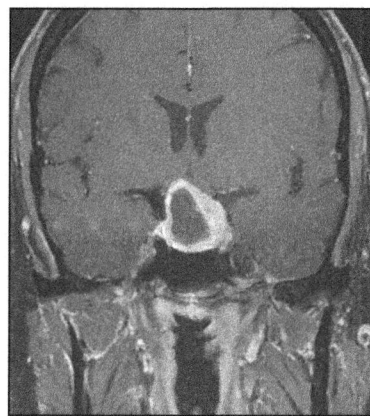

Laboratory test results:
Free T$_4$ = 0.9 ng/dL (0.8-1.8 ng/dL)
  (SI: 11.6 pmol/L [10.30-23.17 pmol/L])
Cortisol (8 AM) = 7.1 μg/dL (5-25 μg/dL)
  (SI: 195.9 nmol/L [137.9-689.7 nmol/L])
Estradiol = 22 pg/mL (27-123 pg/mL)
  (SI: 81 pmol/L [99-452 pmol/L])
Prolactin = 355 ng/mL (4-30 ng/mL)
  (SI: 15.4 nmol/L [0.17-1.30 nmol/L])
IGF-1 = 122 ng/mL (162-541 ng/mL)
  (SI: 16.0 nmol/L [21.2-70.9 nmol/L])

On the basis of the presented information, which of the following treatments should you recommend?
- A. Dopamine agonist
- B. Transcranial surgery
- C. Transsphenoidal surgery
- D. Conventional fractionated irradiation
- E. Stereotactic radiosurgery

4 A 77-year-old woman presents with increasing angina and is found to have hyperthyroidism with a large, multinodular goiter. Atrial fibrillation and heart failure are diagnosed.

Laboratory test results:
  Free T_4 = 2.8 ng/dL (0.8-1.8 ng/dL)
    (SI: 36.0 pmol/L [10.3-23.2 pmol/L])
  Total T_3 = 413 ng/dL (70-200 ng/dL)
    (SI: 6.4 nmol/L [1.08-3.08 nmol/L])
  TSH = 1.9 mU/L (0.5-5.0 mIU/L)

She has a history of extensive coronary artery disease. A radioiodine scan shows a 1.3-cm, nonfunctioning thyroid nodule, and FNAB documents papillary thyroid cancer. MRI reveals a 2.1-cm pituitary adenoma invading the cavernous sinus.

Which of the following is the best next step in this patient's management?
  A. Cabergoline
  B. Saturated solution of potassium iodide
  C. Radioactive iodine
  D. Lanreotide depot
  E. Subtotal thyroidectomy

5 Cushing disease is diagnosed in a 48-year-old woman. Her preoperative morning cortisol level is 26.7 µg/dL (5-25 µg/dL) (SI: 736.6 nmol/L [137.9-689.7 nmol/L]), and her morning ACTH level is 109 pg/mL (10-60 pg/mL) (SI: 24.0 pmol/L [2.2-13.2 pmol/L]). MRI shows a 4-mm pituitary lesion. Glucocorticoids are withheld after surgery. Twenty-four hours after transsphenoidal surgery, her morning cortisol level is 11 µg/dL (303.5 nmol/L). Seventy-two hours after surgery, her morning cortisol level is 10.2 µg/dL (281.4 nmol/L), and she is to be discharged home. One week postoperatively, her morning cortisol level is 13 µg/dL (358.6 nmol/L).

Which of the following is the best management recommendation?
  A. Another transsphenoidal operation performed by an experienced pituitary surgeon
  B. Maintenance hydrocortisone daily, as well as stress dosing for close to a year
  C. Initiation of medical therapy for persistent Cushing disease
  D. Stereotactic radiotherapy
  E. ACTH stimulation test to determine whether maintenance hydrocortisone treatment is needed

6 A 19-year-old man is referred for gigantism. His height is 82 in (208.3 cm) and his weight is 273 lb (123.6 kg), both of which are greater than the 97th percentile. His hands and feet are enlarged, and he has prognathism. A maternal uncle was thought to have had a pituitary adenoma of uncertain type. There is no known family history of calcium disorders or kidney stones. A GH level of 90 ng/mL (90 µg/L) does not suppress adequately during an oral glucose tolerance test.

Other laboratory test results:
  Serum IGF-1 = 1233 ng/mL (147-527 ng/mL)
    (SI: 161.5 nmol/L [19.3-69.0 nmol/L])
  Prolactin = 26 ng/mL (4-23 ng/mL) (SI: 1.1 nmol/L
    [0.17-1.00 nmol/L])
  Thyroid and adrenal axes, normal
  Serum calcium, normal

He has a bitemporal visual field defect. MRI of the brain shows a 4.3 × 3.2 × 2.8-cm pituitary adenoma with suprasellar extension.

A germline mutation in which of the following genes is most likely responsible for the findings in this patient?
  A. *GNAS* (GNAS complex locus)
  B. *TBX19* (T-box 19) (previously *TPIT*)
  C. *PROP1* (PROP paired-like homeobox 1)
  D. *AIP* (aryl hydrocarbon receptor interacting protein)
  E. *MEN1* (menin)

7 An 81-year-old man is referred because a head CT performed after he fell and struck his head showed a pituitary mass. On MRI, this appears to be a 1.2-cm pituitary adenoma with minimal left parasellar extension. He has been feeling well, but in general he thinks he has been slowing down. He has no headaches or vision symptoms. He had a myocardial infarction 10 years ago and currently takes a statin, lisinopril for hypertension, and a baby aspirin. On physical examination, his blood pressure is 136/70 mm Hg and pulse rate is 74 beats/min. His skin has normal texture, and his reflexes are normal.

Laboratory test results:
Testosterone = 218 ng/dL (300-900 ng/dL)
    (SI: 7.6 nmol/L [10.4-31.2 nmol/L])
LH = 2.3 mIU/mL (1.0-9.0 mIU/L)
    (SI: 2.3 IU/L [1.0-9.0 IU/L])
FSH = 1.4 mIU/mL (1.0-13.0 mIU/L)
    (SI: 1.4 IU/L [1.0-13.0 IU/L])
Cortisol (8 AM) = 15.7 μg/dL (5-25 μg/dL)
    (SI: 433.1 nmol/L [137.9-689.7 nmol/L])
Prolactin = 5.7 ng/mL (4-23 ng/mL)
    (SI: 0.2 nmol/L [0.17-1.00 nmol/L])
Free T$_4$ = 1.2 ng/dL (0.8-1.8 ng/dL)
    (SI: 15.4 pmol/L [10.3-23.2 pmol/L])

Which of the following is the most appropriate management for this patient?
  A. Visual field testing
  B. Referral to an experienced pituitary surgeon
  C. Another MRI in 6 months
  D. Stereotactic radiosurgery
  E. Conventional irradiation

8 A 30-year-old woman develops progressive, severe headaches; nausea; vomiting; and fatigue during her 33rd week of pregnancy. She has no notable medical history and was able to become pregnant within 2 months of trying. Her pregnancy course had been smooth until now. Physical examination findings are normal for 33 weeks' gestation. Her obstetrician persuades the radiologist to perform a noncontrast MRI of her head, and the patient is found to have a diffusely enlarged pituitary, measuring 16 mm in height, without abutment of the optic chiasm.

Laboratory test results:
Total T$_4$ = 13 μg/dL (5.5-12.5 μg/dL)
    (SI: 167.3 nmol/L [70.8-160.9 nmol/L])
TSH = 1.3 mIU/L (0.5-5.0 mIU/L)
Cortisol (8 AM) = 9.0 μg/dL (5-25 μg/dL)
    (SI: 248.3 nmol/L [137.9-689.7 nmol/L])
Prolactin = 137 ng/mL (4-30 ng/mL)
    (SI: 6.0 nmol/L [0.17-1.30 nmol/L])

Which of the following is the best next step in this patient's management?
  A. Start bromocriptine
  B. Start cabergoline
  C. Refer for transsphenoidal decompression
  D. Start hydrocortisone
  E. Arrange for an urgent cesarean delivery

9 A 29-year-old man is referred because a head CT performed in the emergency department after an automobile crash showed an empty sella. A subsequent MRI shows an enlarged sella, minimal tissue along the floor of the sella, with the hypothalamic-pituitary stalk reaching the floor of the sella. He was generally well before the accident. However, he states that he received GH injections for many years as a child and stopped when he completed growth at age 18 years. He has also taken thyroid hormone since age 12 years.

Which of the following is the most likely cause of his empty sella?
  A. Trauma-induced pituitary infarction
  B. *PROP1* mutation
  C. Burnt-out hypothalamic/pituitary sarcoidosis
  D. Langerhans cell histiocytosis
  E. Hemochromatosis

10 A 19-year-old woman is known to have hypopituitarism and diabetes insipidus due to Langerhans cell histiocytosis involving her hypothalamus and pituitary stalk. She was just admitted to the hospital following head trauma from a motor vehicle crash and is now in a drug-induced coma. She is being treated with stress-dose steroids and has continued desmopressin, as well as D5W (5% dextrose in water) at a rate of 100 mL/h. You are called to see her when her morning serum sodium concentration is documented to be 112 mEq/L (112 mmol/L).

In addition to holding the desmopressin, which of the following is the best treatment plan?

A. Change the D5W to normal saline and measure serum sodium in 2 to 4 hours
B. Change the D5W to normal saline and measure serum sodium in 12 hours
C. Change the D5W to half-normal saline and measure serum sodium every 2 to 4 hours
D. Give hypertonic saline to raise the serum sodium by 6 mEq/L (6 mmol/L) over 6 hours

11 A 37-year-old woman with amenorrhea and galactorrhea is found to have a prolactin level of 1593 ng/mL (69.3 nmol/L) and a 2.6-cm pituitary macroadenoma. With cabergoline, 0.5 mg twice weekly, prolactin levels normalize and the tumor size decreases to 7 mm. Over the next 18 months (while taking her medication regularly), her prolactin level increases to 284 ng/mL (12.3 nmol/L) and her tumor grows to 1.4 cm. Despite a gradual increase in the cabergoline dosage to 2 mg daily over the next year, her prolactin level rises to 4513 ng/mL (196.2 nmol/L) and her tumor grows to 3.2 cm. She subsequently undergoes a 2-stage transsphenoidal/transcranial near-total resection and stereotactic radiosurgery. Over the ensuing 2 years, the tumor has continued to grow and she is losing vision.

Which of the following treatments is the best choice now?

A. Conventional radiotherapy
B. Another craniotomy
C. Temozolomide
D. Pasireotide

12 A 68-year-old man with metastatic melanoma being treated with chemotherapy is admitted to the hospital with lethargy, altered mental status, and hypotension. He takes levothyroxine for hypothyroidism (thyroidectomy was performed to treat thyroid cancer many years ago).

Laboratory test results:
Random cortisol = 0.9 μg/dL (2-14 μg/dL) (SI: 24.8 nmol/L [55.2-386.2 nmol/L])
ACTH = <5 pg/mL (10-60 pg/mL) (<1.1 pmol/L [2.2-13.2 pmol/L])

Testosterone = 2 ng/dL (300-900 ng/dL) (SI: 0.07 nmol/L [10.4-31.2 nmol/L])
LH = 0.3 mIU/mL (1.0-9.0 mIU/L) (SI: 0.3 IU/L [1.0-9.0 IU/L])
FSH = 2.0 mIU/mL (1.0-13.0 mIU/L) (SI: 2.0 IU/L [1.0-13.0 IU/L])
IGF-1 = 35 ng/mL (67-195 ng/mL) (SI: 4.6 nmol/L [8.8-25.5 nmol/L])
Prolactin = 0.8 ng/mL (4-23 ng/mL) (SI: 0.03 nmol/L [0.17-1.00 nmol/L])
TSH = 0.2 mIU/L (0.5-5.0 mIU/L)

MRI shows homogeneous enlargement of the pituitary and stalk, which was not present on MRI 2 months prior.

Which of the following medications is the most likely cause of these pituitary abnormalities?

A. Prednisone
B. Ipilimumab
C. Temozolomide
D. Sunitinib

13 A 42-year-old man reports fatigue, weight gain, decreased libido, and some difficulty maintaining an erection over the past year. He had been well all his life until these symptoms started, except for a severe headache that lasted for a day about 18 months ago. The headache never recurred. He attributes his symptoms to aging, but his wife urged him to be evaluated. On physical examination, no abnormalities are noted aside from being overweight. The patient is well virilized.

Laboratory test results:
Complete blood cell count, normal
Fasting blood glucose = 123 mg/dL (70-99 mg/dL) (SI: 6.8 mmol/L [3.9-5.5 mmol/L])
TSH = 0.3 mIU/L (0.5-5.0 mIU/L)
Free T$_4$ = 0.5 ng/dL (0.8-1.8 ng/dL) (SI: 6.4 pmol/L [10.30-23.17 pmol/L])
Cortisol (8 AM) = 16 μg/dL (5-25 μg/dL) (SI: 441.1 nmol/L [137.9-689.7 nmol/L])
Total testosterone (8 AM) = 121 ng/dL (300-900 ng/dL) (SI: 4.2 nmol/L [10.4-31.2 nmol/L])
LH = 2.1 mIU/mL (1.0-9.0 mIU/L) (SI: 2.1 IU/L [1.0-9.0 IU/L])

FSH = 1.7 mIU/mL (1.0-13.0 mIU/L)
 (SI: 1.7 IU/L [1.0-13.0 IU/L])
Prolactin = 11.7 ng/mL (4-23 ng/mL)
 (SI: 0.5 nmol/L [0.17-1.00 nmol/L])

MRI shows a partially empty sella.

Which of the following tests should be done to determine whether he is GH deficient?
 A. Arginine stimulation test with measurement of GH
 B. Glucagon stimulation test with measurement of GH
 C. IGF-1 measurement
 D. No test is necessary

14 A 67-year-old woman fell on the ice, striking her head, and she developed a persistent headache. In the emergency department, no intracranial bleed is found, but a 1.5-cm sellar mass is noted. In retrospect, she has had poor energy, frequent urination, increased thirst, and a 10-lb (4.5-kg) weight loss over the past 4 to 5 months. Testing reveals partial hypopituitarism and diabetes insipidus. After starting hormone replacement, she feels better, but because of persistent headaches, an MRI is performed (4 months after the initial imaging) and it shows that the sellar mass has grown to 2 cm.

Which of the following is the most likely diagnosis?
 A. Gonadotroph adenoma
 B. Prolactinoma
 C. Craniopharyngioma
 D. Metastasis

15 A 42-year-old man is found to have a 2.4-cm sellar mass on CT done in the emergency department following minor head trauma. His physical examination findings are normal as are his laboratory test results, aside from a mild prolactin elevation of 31 ng/dL (1.3 nmol/L). Following surgery for what turns out to be a gonadotroph adenoma, his pituitary function is normal, but the 3-month postoperative MRI clearly shows residual tumor present along the sellar floor. The patient is very concerned about the persistence of the tumor.

Which of the following treatments is most likely to prevent further growth of the residual gonadotroph pituitary adenoma?
 A. Radiotherapy
 B. Octreotide LAR
 C. Cabergoline
 D. GnRH antagonist

16 A 75-year-old man is referred because a pituitary incidentaloma was identified on CT performed after he fell on the ice and struck his head. Subsequent MRI confirmed a 1.4-cm mass that appeared to be a pituitary adenoma, with no suprasellar extension. He states that he has been feeling well, but generally has been slowing down. He attributes this to aging. He has no headaches or vision symptoms. He had a myocardial infarction 10 years ago and a subsequent 3-vessel coronary bypass surgery. His only medications are a statin and a daily baby aspirin.

On physical examination, he appears his stated age. His blood pressure is 136/70 mm Hg, and pulse rate is 74 beats/min. His skin has normal texture, and his reflexes are normal. Testes are 10 mL bilaterally.

Laboratory test results (sample drawn at 8 AM):
 LH = 2.3 mIU/mL (1.0-9.0 mIU/L) (SI: 2.3 IU/L [1.0-9.0 IU/L])
 FSH = 1.4 mIU/mL (1.0-13.0 mIU/L) (SI: 1.4 IU/L [1.0-13.0 IU/L])
 Cortisol = 17 µg/dL (5-25 µg/dL) (SI: 469.0 nmol/L [137.9-689.7 nmol/L])
 Testosterone = 210 ng/dL (300-900 ng/dL) (SI: 7.3 nmol/L [10.4-31.2 nmol/L])
 Free T$_4$ = 1.1 ng/dL (0.8-1.8 ng/dL) (SI: 14.2 pmol/L [10.30-23.17 pmol/L])
 Prolactin = 35 ng/mL (4-23 ng/mL) (SI: 1.5 nmol/L [0.17-1.00 nmol/L])

Which of the following is the best next step in this patient's management?
 A. Perform visual field testing
 B. Refer to an experienced pituitary surgeon
 C. Refer for stereotactic radiosurgery
 D. Start dopamine agonist
 E. Repeat the MRI in 6 months

17 A 51-year-old man presents with new-onset atrial fibrillation and a 10-lb (4.5-kg) weight loss. In retrospect, he has noticed some fatigue, a mild tremor, and heat intolerance for several months. His sister has hypothyroidism. He is a biology researcher and works in an animal lab.

On physical examination, his blood pressure is 139/67 mm Hg, pulse rate is 92 beats/min (irregular), and BMI is 24.1 kg/m². He has no proptosis but does have slight lid-lag. His thyroid gland is about 2-fold diffusely enlarged and is soft. He has brisk reflexes and a fine tremor of his outstretched hands.

Laboratory test results:
Free T_4 = 4.5 ng/dL (0.8-1.8 ng/dL)
   (SI: 57.9 pmol/L [10.30-23.17 pmol/L])
Total T_3 = 482 ng/dL (70-200 ng/dL)
   (SI: 7.4 nmol/L [1.08-3.08 nmol/L])
TSH = 9.47 mIU/L (0.5-5.0 mIU/L)
Thyroid-stimulating immunoglobulin index = 1.4
   (<1.3)

Results from repeated tests are similar. MRI of the pituitary gland is normal.

Which of the following tests would be the most helpful in determining the etiology of his hyperthyroidism?
   A. Measurement of HAMA (human anti-mouse antibodies)
   B. T_3 suppression test
   C. Measurement of β-subunit
   D. Petrosal sinus sampling for TSH measurements

18 A 45-year-old woman is referred after a 2.2 × 1.8-cm hypodense right adrenal nodule is found during a staging CT for recently diagnosed breast cancer. She is asymptomatic and has no clinical signs of Cushing syndrome.

Laboratory test results:
DHEA-S, normal
Androstenedione, normal
Testosterone, normal
Urinary free cortisol, normal
Cortisol (AM) = 13.1 µg/dL (361.4 nmol/L)
   (fails to suppress with dexamethasone)

With a diagnosis of an incidental adenoma causing subclinical Cushing syndrome rather than an adrenal metastasis, she undergoes surgery and irradiation for breast cancer. Four months after completion of these treatments, she reports some facial rounding and erythema, peripheral edema, and worsening hirsutism. On physical examination, she has increased hair growth and appears mildly cushingoid.

Urinary free cortisol excretion is 228 µg/24 h (629.3 nmol/d).

Which of the following should be the next step in this patient's management?
   A. Perform an ACTH stimulation test with measurement of 17-hydroxyprogesterone
   B. Refer for laparoscopic right adrenalectomy
   C. Perform petrosal sinus sampling for ACTH
   D. Perform bilateral adrenal venous sampling for cortisol
   E. Measure 8-AM cortisol and ACTH levels

19 A 43-year-old woman with acromegaly has a GH concentration of 11.7 ng/mL (0.01-0.97 ng/mL) (SI: 11.7 µg/L [0.01-0.97 µg/L]) and an IGF-1 level of 890 ng/mL (98-261 ng/mL) (SI: 116.6 nmol/L [12.8-34.2 nmol/L]) after surgery. She is started on octreotide LAR with a dosage increase to 30 mg intramuscular monthly. On this dosage, her IGF-1 level is 625 ng/mL (81.9 nmol/L). She has persistent arthralgias and sweating and modest hyperglycemia with a hemoglobin A_{1c} level of 7.3% [56 mmol/mol]). Brain MRI reveals 0.5-cm residual left cavernous sinus disease.

Which of the following options would be most effective in controlling her acromegaly within the next 6 months?
   A. Change octreotide LAR dosing to every 21 days
   B. Stop the octreotide LAR and switch to cabergoline
   C. Add pegvisomant
   D. Radiation therapy
   E. Switch to pasireotide

20 A 33-year-old woman has developed Cushing syndrome during her 16th week of pregnancy. She has hypertension, diabetes mellitus, hirsutism, and wide, purple striae on her abdomen.

Laboratory test results:
Serum cortisol (8 AM) = 37 μg/dL (5-25 μg/dL)
   (SI: 1020.8 nmol/L [137.9-689.7 nmol/L])
ACTH = 129 pg/mL (10-60 pg/mL)
   (SI: 28.4 pmol/L [2.2-13.2 pmol/L])
Urinary free cortisol = 475 μg/24 h (4-50 μg/24 h)
   (SI: 1311 nmol/d [11-138 nmol/d])

MRI shows a 6-mm pituitary adenoma.

Which of the following treatment options is the most appropriate step to control her Cushing disease?
   A. Ketoconazole
   B. Mifepristone
   C. Transsphenoidal surgery
   D. Pasireotide
   E. Cabergoline

21 A 34-year-old woman has been diagnosed with a 2.5-cm clinically nonfunctioning pituitary macroadenoma that has caused chiasmal compression. Her preoperative evaluation reveals no evidence of acromegaly, Cushing disease, or salt and water imbalance. She undergoes transsphenoidal surgery, which is uneventful. Twenty-eight hours after surgery, she develops marked increase in thirst, as well as polyuria.

Laboratory test results:
Serum sodium = 152 mEq/L (136-142 mEq/L)
   (SI: 152 mmol/L [136-142 mmol/L])
Urine osmolality = 110 mOsm/kg
   (150-1150 mOsm/kg) (SI: 110 mmol/kg
   [150-1150 mmol/kg])

Which of the following treatment options should be initiated?
   A. DDAVP, 0.1 mg orally as needed for polyuria and hypernatremia
   B. Intravenous infusion of normal saline
   C. 1 L fluid restriction
   D. DDAVP, scheduled dosing 1 spray intranasally twice daily

22 A 32-year-old woman with a clinically nonfunctioning pituitary macroadenoma underwent transsphenoidal surgery 8 days ago. Her preoperative testing showed normal pituitary function. She was in the hospital for 2 days, had an uneventful course, and was discharged home on no medications. Today, she noted nausea, vomiting, and fatigue. She went to the local emergency department where the following laboratory test results were obtained:
Liver function, normal
Serum sodium = 121 mEq/L (136-142 mEq/L)
   (SI: 121 mmol/L [136-142 mmol/L])
Urinary sodium = 14 mEq/L (40-217 mEq/24 h)
   (SI: 14 mEq/L [40-217 mmol/d])
Urine osmolality = 373 mOsm/kg
   (150-1150 mOsm/kg) (SI: 373 mmol/kg
   [150-1150 mmol/kg])

Which of the following is the most appropriate treatment for this patient?
   A. Restrict free water intake to less than 1500 mL/24 h
   B. Start demeclocycline
   C. Start tolvaptan
   D. Start a furosemide intravenous drip

23 A 32-year-old man is referred for fatigue and weakness. Nine months ago, he was in a motor vehicle crash and had severe brain injury, resulting in cerebral hemorrhage and edema. He was in a coma for 10 days, followed by prolonged inpatient and then outpatient rehabilitation. Over the past 2 months, he has had progressive fatigue, as well as reduction in muscle mass. He is frustrated by the lack of successful rehabilitation despite physical therapy. He has gained 12 lb (5.5 kg) over the past 3 months.

On physical examination, he has reduced skeletal muscle mass and increased abdominal girth.

Random cortisol = 6.2 μg/dL (2-14 μg/dL)
   (SI: 171.0 nmol/L [55.2-386.2 nmol/L])
ACTH = 9 pg/mL (10-60 pg/mL) (SI: 2.0 pmol/L
   [2.2-13.2 pmol/L])
LH = 5.3 mIU/mL (1.0-9.0 mIU/L) (SI: 5.3 IU/L
   [1.0-9.0 IU/L])
FSH = 4.0 mIU/mL (1.0-13.0 mIU/L) (SI: 4.0 IU/L
   [1.0-13.0 IU/L])

Testosterone = 275 ng/dL (300-900 ng/dL)
  (SI: 9.5 nmol/L [10.4-31.2 nmol/L])
IGF-1 = 35 ng/mL (113-297 ng/mL)
  (SI: 4.6 nmol/L [14.8-38.9 nmol/L])
Prolactin = 1.8 ng/mL (4-23 ng/mL)
  (SI: 0.08 nmol/L [0.17-1.00 nmol/L])
Free T$_4$ = 1.2 ng/dL (0.8-1.8 ng/dL)
  (SI: 15.4 pmol/L [10.30-23.17 pmol/L])
TSH = 0.9 mIU/L (0.5-5.0 mIU/L)

Which of the following is the most likely cause of his progressive fatigue?
  A. Testosterone deficiency
  B. GH deficiency
  C. Adrenal insufficiency
  D. Hypothyroidism
  E. Hypoprolactinemia

24 A 33-year-old woman seeks evaluation for an 18-month history of galactorrhea and a 12-month history of amenorrhea. Her prolactin level is 138 ng/mL (6.0 nmol/L), and MRI shows a 7-mm pituitary microadenoma. Bromocriptine is started at a dosage of 5 mg orally daily, and her prolactin level after 1 month of therapy is 114 ng/mL (5.0 nmol/L). Her regimen is switched to cabergoline, and at a dosage of 1.0 mg twice weekly there is no further change in her serum prolactin level. She has never been pregnant and is interested in fertility.

Which of the following is the best next step in this patient's management?
  A. Increase the cabergoline dosage to 2 mg twice weekly
  B. Recommend radiation therapy
  C. Refer for transsphenoidal surgery
  D. Start clomiphene

25 A 35-year-old woman is found to have acromegaly with a 1.8-cm pituitary adenoma and cavernous sinus involvement. She undergoes surgery, and she is left with a residual tumor in her cavernous sinus. Her IGF-1 level remains elevated at 460 ng/mL (113-297 ng/mL) (SI: 60.3 nmol/L 14.8-38.9 nmol/L) and her prolactin level is 148 ng/mL (4-30 ng/mL) (SI: 6.4 nmol/L [0.17-1.30 nmol/L]). She has had amenorrhea for 1.5 years. Lanreotide depot, 90 mg monthly, is initiated, and this normalizes her IGF-1 Her menstrual cycles resume. She wishes to conceive, and she is counseled to hold lanreotide depot. She conceives in 3 months, and she is now 14 weeks pregnant. She has developed headaches and notes more joint pains and sweating.

Which of the following is the best next step in this patient's management?
  A. Perform pituitary MRI
  B. Initiate subcutaneous, short-acting octreotide titrated to headaches
  C. Administer daily pegvisomant
  D. Measure GH and IGF-1 levels

Diabetes Mellitus, Section 2 Board Review

Michelle F. Magee, MD ● Georgetown University

31 A 57-year-old man with type 2 diabetes mellitus and hypertension is admitted to the hospital with a new diagnosis of congestive heart failure (ejection fraction <10%). His cardiac status is now stabilized with inotropic support. He is being evaluated for advanced heart failure therapies, and he will most likely be in the hospital for another 5 to 7 days. You are consulted for glycemic management. He is eating well and does not report any gastrointestinal disturbances. Your hospital target for blood glucose in patients in medicine units is 140 to 180 mg/dL (7.8 to 10.0 mmol/L).

His point-of-care blood glucose values over the past 24 hours are as follows:

Blood glucose	Time	Insulin Lispro Administered
244 mg/dL (13.5 mmol/L)	12:09 PM	4 units
166 mg/dL (9.2 mmol/L)	07:18 AM	–
212 mg/dL (11.8 mmol/L)	10:05 PM	4 units
203 mg/dL (11.3 mmol/L)	05:18 PM	4 units

Which of the following evidence-based therapies should you recommend as an addition to his hospital glycemic control regimen?

- A. Sitagliptin
- B. Metformin
- C. Pioglitazone
- D. Canagliflozin

32 A 58-year-old woman with type 2 diabetes mellitus had Roux-en-Y gastric bypass 18 months ago. She is admitted to the hospital following a seizure. Her son called 911 when he found her confused. The fingerstick blood glucose done by the emergency medical technicians was 23 mg/dL (1.3 mmol/L), and she responded to treatment with D50.

After her gastric bypass operation, she lost 50 lb (22.7 kg), but she was not able to stop insulin therapy. Her home treatment regimen before this hospital admission was 30 units of insulin glargine daily and 15 units of insulin aspart with each meal. For about 2 months, she has been feeling "funny" and not thinking clearly for approximately 2 hours after meals, particularly after meals with more carbohydrates than usual. Juice relieves these symptoms. She checks fingerstick blood glucose infrequently.

You initiate a continuous glucose monitor, and the results are shown (*see image*):

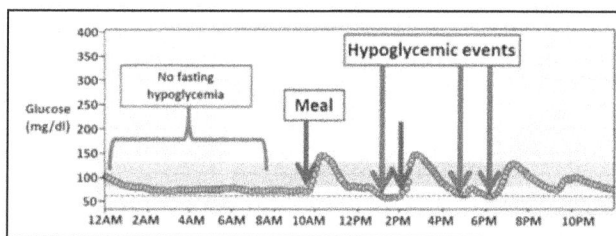

These patterns are typical of glycemic excursions in the setting of postbariatric hypoglycemia.

In conjunction with a controlled portion, low–glycemic index carbohydrate diet (<30 g/meal, 15 g per snack), which addition to her diabetes medication regimen would you consider as a next step for hypoglycemia management?

- A. Octreotide
- B. Diazoxide
- C. Acarbose
- D. Liraglutide

33 A 56-year-old man with longstanding diabetes secondary to chronic pancreatitis has advanced bilateral peripheral neuropathy and blunted glycemic awareness. He is admitted to the hospital following an episode of unconscious hypoglycemia (blood glucose = 34 mg/dL [1.9 mmol/L]). His hemoglobin A_{1c} level was 12.8%

(116 mmol/mol) one month ago. Home blood glucose values range from the 40s to 500 mg/dL (2.2 to 27.8 mmol/L). He takes pancreatic enzymes with each meal and administers insulin glargine, 15 units daily, plus 4 units of rapid-acting insulin with each meal and a low correction dose insulin scale.

He is given his usual dose of insulin glargine and 4 units of insulin lispro with his evening meal. At midnight, he is made nothing-by-mouth status for a procedure the next morning. He has been in the hospital for 2 days.

His blood glucose values over the past 24 hours are shown (*see table*).

Time of Day	Blood Glucose
5:31 PM evening meal (4 units lispro + 15 units glargine)	91 mg/dL (5.1 mmol/L)
11:18 PM nothing-by-mouth status	217 mg/dL (12.0 mmol/L)
7:48 AM	54 mg/dL (3.0 mmol/L)
9:18 AM	107 mg/dL (5.9 mmol/L)
12:22 PM	104 mg/dL (5.8 mmol/L)

Which of the following insulin dosing recommendations would appropriate for this patient?
  A. Hold insulin glargine the next time he is made nothing-by-mouth status
  B. Give 25% of his usual insulin glargine dose if he is to be made nothing-by-mouth status again
  C. Reduce his daily insulin glargine dose
  D. Start an insulin drip if he has another blood glucose value greater than 200 mg/dL (>11.1 mmol/L)

34 A 67-year-old man with an 8-year history of type 2 diabetes has been admitted to the hospital after presenting with an isolated complaint of new-onset double vision and feeling unsteady when walking since this morning. He notes occasional blurry vision after large meals, some tingling in his feet, and decreased libido. He has no symptoms suggestive of thyroid disease or adrenal insufficiency.

On neurologic examination, he is awake and responsive and oriented to person, place, and time. His right eye is deviated "down and out." Left eye movements are normal. The rest of the cranial nerves are intact. There is no ptosis or nystagmus, and pupils are equal and reactive to light. He has mild reduction of sensation bilaterally in the feet.

Laboratory test results (blood drawn at admission):
  Blood glucose = 203 mg/dL (70-99 mg/dL)
    (SI: 11.3 mmol/L [3.9-5.5 mmol/L])
  Hemoglobin A_{1c} = 8.5% (4.0%-5.6%)
    (69 mmol/mol [20-38 mmol/mol])

You are asked to see him after a head CT reveals no evidence of hemorrhage or infarct, but shows an enhancing suprasellar mass involving the superior pituitary stalk. You order an MRI with sellar and suprasellar cuts, which confirms the presence of a pituitary mass with suprasellar extension, but does not show evidence of optic or oculomotor nerve impingement. The diplopia is still present on the third hospital day.

Which of the following is the most likely explanation for his diplopia?
  A. Unilateral endocrine ophthalmopathy
  B. Pituitary macroadenoma with cavernous sinus invasion
  C. Diabetes-related mononeuritis affecting the third cranial nerve
  D. Reversible ischemic neurologic deficit

35 A 58-year-old woman with a history of "mild" diabetes (treated with diet and exercise), hypertension, hyperlipidemia, and hepatitis C virus infection with cirrhosis presents in cardiogenic shock due to sepsis. Her blood glucose concentration is greater than 1000 mg/dL (>55.5 mmol/L), and she has a mixed-pattern acidosis. An insulin drip is started.

The endocrine service is consulted for transition to subcutaneous insulin. She is currently on continuous enteral feedings and an insulin drip. Several days ago, she had required 16 to 18 units/h to maintain her blood glucose values less than 180 mg/dL (<10.0 mmol/L). The drip rate is now 6 units/h, for an extrapolated total daily insulin dose of 144 units/24 h. Her blood glucose values are in the low 200s.

Which of the following subcutaneous insulin regimens would you order for this patient?

A. Rapid-acting insulin every 6 hours
B. Insulin glargine, 70 units twice daily, with supplemental/correction insulin doses when blood glucose is greater than 200 mg/dL (>11.1 mmol/L)
C. Sliding-scale regular insulin every 4 hours
D. Insulin detemir, 30 units twice daily plus 18 units regular insulin every 6 hours

36 A 38-year-old obese woman with type 2 diabetes mellitus is taking metformin, 1000 mg twice daily. Her hemoglobin A_{1c} level is 7.9% (63 mmol/mol), and she reports significant postprandial hyperglycemia.

Which GLP-1 receptor agonist would be the best choice for improving her prandial coverage?

A. Exenatide twice daily
B. Exenatide LAR
C. Liraglutide
D. Dulaglutide

37 A 42-year-old man with type 2 diabetes mellitus is failing therapy with triple oral agents, and you discuss the possibility of starting insulin therapy. His technology company has strict rules about syringe storage, so he is reluctant to bring insulin to work regardless of whether it is a syringe or pen. He is willing to start once-daily basal insulin. His job will soon require travel across time zones, and he wonders when he should time the basal insulin injections when he travels to Europe or Asia. He is concerned about the risk of hypoglycemia while traveling.

Formulary issues aside, which of the following regimens would you recommend for this patient?

A. NPH insulin at bedtime; give it at the same time when traveling
B. Insulin detemir at bedtime; decrease the insulin dose by half when traveling
C. U300 insulin glargine; give it at the same time as he would at home
D. Insulin degludec; give it at his convenience once daily

38 A 29-year-old G2P1 woman with known type 1 diabetes who is at 17 weeks' gestation presents to the emergency department with a 2-day history of vomiting and abdominal pain. She has had ongoing hyperemesis. She takes insulin detemir, 40 units once daily, and insulin aspart, 15 units before meals. Diabetic ketoacidosis is diagnosed, and she is admitted to the intensive care unit and treated with intravenous hydration and an insulin drip.

Twenty-four hours later, she has improved clinically. However, she vomited an hour ago and has some residual abdominal pain.

Laboratory test results:
Sodium = 135 mEq/L (136-142 mEq/L) (SI: 135 mmol/L [136-142 mmol/L])
Chloride = 105 mEq/L (96-106 mEq/L) (SI: 105 mmol/L [96-106 mmol/L])
Potassium = 4.5 mEq/L (3.5-5.0 mEq/L) (SI: 4.5 mmol/L [3.5-5.0 mmol/L])
Carbon dioxide = 21 mEq/L (22-28 mEq/L) (SI: 21 mmol/L [22-28 mmol/L])
Creatinine = 1.0 mg/dL (0.6-1.1 mg/dL) (SI: 88.4 μmol/L [53.0-97.2 μmol/L]
Anion gap = 9
Albumin = 1.8 g/dL (3.5-5.0 g/dL) (SI: 18 g/L [35-50 g/L])
Serum glucose = 132 mg/dL (70-99 mg/dL) (SI: 7.3 mmol/L [3.9-5.5 mmol/L])
Serum β-hydroxybutyrate, negative

The intensive care unit team calls you for advice on transitioning the patient's regimen to subcutaneous insulin. For the last 6 hours, the hourly rate of her insulin drip has been 4 units/h.

Which of the following is your best advice now?

A. Transition to insulin glargine, 38 units daily, after overlapping the insulin drip for 2 hours and start insulin lispro, 12 units with meals

B. Transition to insulin detemir, 38 units daily, after overlapping the insulin drip for 2 hours and start insulin lispro, 12 units with meals

C. Transition to insulin degludec, 38 units daily, after overlapping the insulin drip for 2 hours and start insulin lispro, 12 units with meals

D. Continue the intravenous insulin drip, allow the patient to eat, start insulin aspart with meals, and re-check a basic metabolic panel in 4 hours

E. Continue the intravenous insulin drip, keep her on nothing-mouth-status, and re-check a basic metabolic panel in 4 hours

39 An otherwise healthy 78-year-old man has had type 2 diabetes mellitus for 30 years. He has successfully kept his hemoglobin A_{1c} level in the range of 6.5% to 7.0% (48 to 53 mmol/mol) and has no microvascular or macrovascular complications. Recently, a coworker has been giving him candy or juice when he seems to be thinking less clearly, which is several times daily. You are asked to review his diabetes relative to his ability to continue serving in his current job.

He is alert and oriented and knows the details of his medical history. He took insulin glargine, 40 units daily, with a sliding-scale regimen of insulin aspart with each meal until 2 months ago when his endocrinologist reduced the glargine dosage to 20 units after documenting a hemoglobin A_{1c} level of 6.2% (44 mmol/mol). He does not write down his meal insulin doses and cannot tell you the sliding scale, but he may take up to 15 units of insulin aspart with a meal.

Laboratory test results:
    Hemoglobin A_{1c} = 7.3% (4.0%-5.6%)
        (56 mmol/mol [20-38 mmol/mol])
    Fructosamine = 330 μmol/L (200-285 μmol/L)
    C-peptide = <0.1 ng/mL (0.9-4.3 ng/mL)
        (SI: 0.03 nmol/L [0.30-1.42 nmol/L])

An ACTH stimulation test reveals a baseline cortisol value of 18.0 μg/dL (496.6 mmol/L) and a 30-minute value of 22.8 μg/dL (629.0 mmol/L).

You order diagnostic continuous glucose monitor testing, the results of which are shown (*see image*).

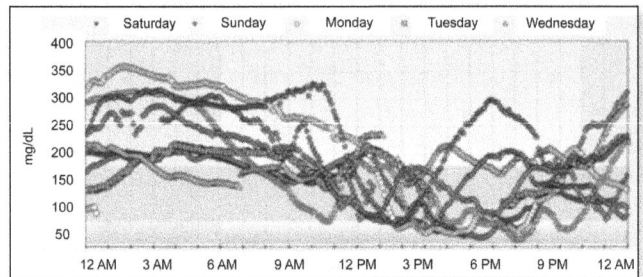

Which of the following simplification strategies would you recommend to adjust the insulin regimen for this patient?

A. Replace the sliding scale with a fixed and reduced dose of insulin with each meal

B. Replace the meal-time insulin with once-daily noninsulin agents to control postprandial glycemia

C. Move basal insulin to the morning and titrate the dose up to control fasting hyperglycemia

D. Coordinate with his wife and coworkers to assist the patient when he seems to be thinking less clearly

40 A 71-year-old white female participant in the National Institutes of Health Diabetes Prevention Program Observational Study (DPP-OS) was diagnosed with diabetes mellitus 17 years ago. Her condition is now managed with insulin alone. She has proliferative retinopathy and stage 3 chronic kidney disease. Her glycemic control has been variable for the last few years, with hemoglobin A_{1c} values ranging from 5.0% to 9.9% (31 to 85 mmol/mol). Her most recent hemoglobin A_{1c} measurement is 8.4% (68 mmol/mol).

She and her husband are wondering whether her hemoglobin A_{1c} is accurate because it has varied so much and her current blood glucose values are so variable.

Laboratory test results:
    Serum creatinine = 1.5 mg/dL (0.6-1.1 mg/dL)
        (SI: 132.6 μmol/L [53.0-97.2 μmol/L])
    Estimated glomerular filtration rate = 46 mL/min
        per 1.73 m² (>60 mL/min per 1.73 m²)
    Hemoglobin, normal
    Hematocrit, normal

Triglycerides = 374 mg/dL (<150 mg/dL [optimal])
(SI: 4.23 mmol/L [<1.70 mmol/L])
Fructosamine = 570 μmol/L (200-285 μmol/L)
(correlates with an hemoglobin A$_{1c}$ >14%
[>130 mmol/mol])

Which of the following is most likely responsible for the falsely low hemoglobin A$_{1c}$ level in this woman?
  A. Uremia
  B. Race
  C. Hereditary spherocytosis
  D. Hypertriglyceridemia

41 A 48-year-old man with longstanding type 1 diabetes mellitus and peripheral neuropathy presents for a follow-up visit. He has had a right plantar ulcer in the past. His hemoglobin A$_{1c}$ level is 7.6% (60 mmol/mol). On foot examination, he has absent sensation to 10-g monofilament, absent ankle reflexes, callus formation on the plantar aspect of the second and third metatarsal heads, and absent pedal pulses.

Which of the following is the strongest predictor of the development of future foot ulcers in this patient?
  A. History of previous ulceration
  B. Absent pedal pulses
  C. Absent knee reflexes
  D. Abnormal monofilament testing

42 A 24-year-old man with cystic fibrosis presents to you for consultation and management of newly diagnosed cystic fibrosis–related diabetes. He asks about the use of oral agents vs insulin therapy.

Based on current guidelines, which of the following would be the recommended treatment for his new cystic fibrosis–related diabetes?
  A. Pioglitazone
  B. Insulin
  C. Sulfonylurea
  D. GLP-1 receptor agonist

43 A 47-year-old woman with type 2 diabetes mellitus presents for follow-up. She recently began walking to work and is eager to safely take on a more vigorous exercise regimen. Her type 2 diabetes is managed with insulin glargine. Her hemoglobin A$_{1c}$ has ranged from 7.0% to 8.0% (53 to 64 mmol/mol) in the past year and she rarely has hypoglycemia. Her family history is positive for type 2 diabetes and hypertension and is negative for premature coronary heart disease.

On physical examination, her BMI is 27 kg/m^2 and blood pressure is 130/88 mm Hg.

Laboratory test results:
  Hemoglobin A$_{1c}$ = 7.4% (4.0%-5.6%)
  (57 mmol/mol [20-38 mmol/mol])
  LDL cholesterol = 122 mg/dL (<100 mg/dL
  [optimal]) (SI: 3.16 mmol/L [<2.59 mmol/L])
  HDL cholesterol = 39 mg/dL (>60 mg/dL
  [optimal]) (SI: 1.01 mmol/L [>1.55 mmol/L])

Renal function and electrocardiography are normal.

Which of the following should you recommend regarding her exercise plans?
  A. Perform an exercise tolerance test before starting more vigorous exercise
  B. Perform a stress echocardiography test before starting more vigorous exercise
  C. Progressively initiate more vigorous regular exercise
  D. Enroll in a cardiac rehabilitation program to initiate more vigorous exercise

44 A 34-year-old woman delivered a baby 2 years ago. During that pregnancy, she was treated for gestational diabetes. Three months postpartum, her 2-hour plasma glucose value during a follow-up oral glucose tolerance test was documented to be 136 mg/dL (7.5 mmol/L). She now presents for a visit (6 months postpartum). Her last menstrual period was 6 weeks ago, and she has a positive pregnancy test confirmed by her obstetrician. She currently has no symptoms of diabetes.

Which of the following approaches is the most sensitive way to evaluate this woman's glycemic status?
- A. Do not screen for type 2 diabetes now, but screen for gestational diabetes with 50-g oral glucose tolerance testing at 24 to 28 weeks' gestation
- B. Screen for type 2 diabetes now with hemoglobin A_{1c} measurement; screen for gestational diabetes with 100-g oral glucose tolerance testing at 24 to 28 weeks' gestation
- C. Screen for type 2 diabetes now with 75-g oral glucose tolerance testing; screen for gestational diabetes with 75-g oral glucose tolerance testing at 24 to 28 weeks' gestation
- D. Screen for type 2 diabetes now with fasting plasma glucose measurement; screen for gestational diabetes with 75-g oral glucose tolerance testing at 24 to 28 weeks' gestation

45 A 52-year-old woman has had poorly controlled type 2 diabetes mellitus for 21 years. She was recently found to have decreased visual acuity ascribed to diffuse proliferative diabetic retinopathy and ischemia on retinal examination.

Which of the following treatments should she undergo?
- A. Focal laser photocoagulation
- B. Panretinal laser photocoagulation
- C. Ranibizumab injections
- D. Vitrectomy

46 A 64-year-old woman with poorly controlled type 2 diabetes mellitus presents to the emergency department with a 1-week history of left-sided flank pain. She has no fever, chills, dysuria, nausea, postprandial pain, or change in bowel habit. Her medical history is notable for retinopathy requiring laser photocoagulation and distal somatosensory neuropathy. She has had 2 toe amputations, coronary artery bypass surgery, and right femoral popliteal bypass surgery.

On physical examination, she is afebrile. The left flank and left upper quadrant are exquisitely tender to even superficial palpation. Muscle strength in the legs is normal; sensation is reduced below the knees and absent in the feet. There is no rash.

Laboratory test results:
   Fecal occult blood screening, negative
   Urinalysis, 2+ protein
   White blood cell count = 7200/μL with normal differential
   Chemistry panel, normal
   Liver function tests, normal
   Amylase and lipase, normal

Abdominal CT is negative for urinary or biliary calcification, and there are no abnormalities of the pancreas, intestine, or kidneys.

Which of the following is the most likely cause of her pain?
- A. Diabetic autonomic neuropathy
- B. Herpes zoster
- C. Pancreatitis
- D. Diabetic radiculopathy

47 A 69-year-old man with interstitial pulmonary fibrosis is hospitalized with pneumonia and respiratory failure requiring ventilator support in the intensive care unit. There is no history of diabetes. At presentation, his random blood glucose level is 183 mg/dL (10.2 mmol/L). After treatment with methylprednisolone, his blood glucose climbs to 402 mg/dL (22.3 mmol/L) and remains in the upper 300s.

Which of the following is the best approach to manage this patient's hyperglycemia?
- A. Human regular insulin subcutaneously every 4 hours, adjusted to maintain blood glucose greater than 180 mg/dL (>10.0 mmol/L)
- B. Intravenous human regular insulin infusion titrated to maintain blood glucose between 140 and 180 mg/dL (7.8 and 10.0 mmol/L)
- C. Intravenous human regular insulin infusion titrated to maintain blood glucose between 80 and 110 mg/dL (4.4 and 6.1 mmol/L)
- D. Daily insulin glargine plus insulin aspart subcutaneously every 6 hours, adjusted to maintain blood glucose between 140 and 180 mg/dL (7.8 and 10.0 mmol/L)

48 A 23-year-old woman with a 15-year history of type 1 diabetes mellitus presents with a new skin lesion. She reports a nonpainful sore on her anterior left lower extremity that has enlarged over the past 3 months.

On physical examination, you observe this lesion (*see image*).

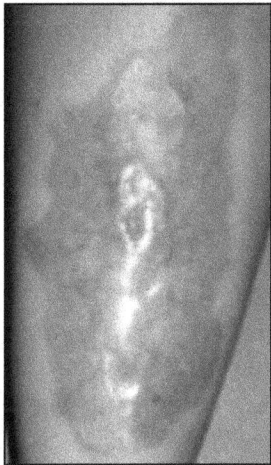

You diagnose diabetes-related necrobiosis lipoidica with early ulceration.

Which of the following approaches is most likely to result in complete resolution of this patient's skin lesion?
- A. Kidney transplant without a pancreas transplant
- B. Dipyridamole
- C. Pancreas transplant with or without a kidney transplant
- D. Intralesional corticosteroids

49 A motivated 25-year-old woman with a 16-year history of type 1 diabetes mellitus asks if she would benefit from the use of a continuous glucose sensor. She is currently treated with multiple daily insulin injections. She travels frequently for work and she has difficulty monitoring her blood glucose as often as she should. She has been having frequent hypoglycemic episodes and does not always have warning symptoms. Her current hemoglobin A_{1c} level is 8.0% (64 mmol/mol).

In counseling this patient, you should tell her that continuous glucose sensor systems:
- A. Provide less accurate results than standard patient glucose meters, so fingersticks will still always be necessary to support the continuous glucose monitoring data
- B. Are useful when combined with insulin pump therapy only
- C. Measure interstitial glucose concentrations, which lag behind capillary glucose concentrations by about 30 minutes
- D. Result in improved glycemic control if used most days of the week, particularly in adults

50 A 20-year-old man with a 3-year history of type 1 diabetes mellitus never does self-monitoring of blood glucose and does not adjust his premeal insulin. His hemoglobin A_{1c} level is 9.2% (77 mmol/mol), and it has never been lower than 8.8% (73 mmol/mol). He is beginning to be concerned about his risk for developing diabetes-related complications, especially blindness, and he wants to know if this can be prevented.

What will you tell him is the adjusted mean risk for developing retinopathy based on Diabetes Control and Complications Trial (DCCT) data for the intensively treated group?
- A. 12%
- B. 24%
- C. 48%
- D. 76%
- E. 98%

51 A 57-year-old woman presents for management of type 2 diabetes mellitus. She is currently taking metformin, 1000 mg twice daily, and once-daily glargine. Her hemoglobin A_{1c} level is 7.2% (55 mmol/mol).

Which of the following is the recommended fasting or premeal glucose target for this patient?
- A. 60-120 mg/dL (3.3-6.7 mmol/L)
- B. 70-130 mg/dL (3.9-7.2 mmol/L)
- C. 80-130 mg/dL (4.4-7.2 mmol/L)
- D. 90-140 mg/dL (5.0-7.8 mmol/L)

52 A woman with type 1 diabetes mellitus who lives in Miami, Florida, went on a ski trip to Park City, Utah. She experienced problems maintaining her usual excellent diabetes control. She documented consistently higher glucose levels not explained by food or activity.

You explain that which of the following factor(s) can affect the accuracy of some blood glucose meter readings?
A. Both temperature and altitude
B. Altitude, but not temperature
C. Temperature, but not altitude
D. Neither temperature nor altitude
E. Low barometric pressure

53 You see a 28-year-old woman with type 1 diabetes mellitus who is 6 weeks pregnant. She has retinopathy, albuminuria, hypertension, and dyslipidemia. She is treated with a basal-bolus insulin regimen. She also takes a statin and lisinopril. Her blood pressure is 128/92 mm Hg.

Her overnight (3 AM) and fasting blood glucose levels range from 110 to 122 mg/dL (6.1 to 6.8 mmol/L), and her peak (1-hour) postprandial glucose levels range from 112 to 129 mg/dL (6.2 to 7.2 mmol/L).

Which of the following recommendations will reduce the risk of congenital malformations and macrosomia in her fetus?
A. Discontinue the statin during the second trimester
B. Replace lisinopril with losartan
C. Increase her meal insulin doses to achieve postprandial blood glucose <110 mg/dL (<6.1 mmol/L)
D. Increase basal insulin to achieve overnight blood glucose levels between 60 and 99 mg/dL (3.3 and 5.5 mmol/L)
E. Monitor hemoglobin A_{1c} every 3 months

54 A 27-year-old man with type 1 diabetes mellitus who uses an insulin pump wants to begin jogging 2 to 3 hours several times weekly. He is concerned about his risk of hypoglycemia and asks for advice on how to minimize this.

In addition to monitoring blood glucose before, during, and after exercise, you advise that:
A. He should consider a brief period of weightlifting before jogging to reduce the chance of hypoglycemia
B. Aerobic activity can cause postexercise hyperglycemia, so he should raise his basal rate during jogging to avoid it
C. Aerobic activity such as jogging will not cause hypoglycemia as long as his glucose level is greater than 150 mg/dL (>8.3 mmol/L) before starting
D. He should avoid aerobic activity to avoid hypoglycemia

55 A 49-year-old man is referred from a walk-in clinic where he was noted to have a blood glucose level of 246 mg/dL (13.7 mmol/L) during evaluation of an acute gastrointestinal syndrome. One week later, his fasting blood glucose is 190 mg/dL (10.5 mmol/L) and the diagnosis of diabetes mellitus is confirmed. He has not had medical care for many years. His blood pressure is 145/92 mm Hg, ophthalmoscopy shows no changes consistent with background retinopathy, and he has no evidence of peripheral neuropathy.

Which of the following would you recommend to assess his risk for diabetic nephropathy?
A. 24-Hour urine collection, estimation of creatinine clearance, and measurement of total protein excretion
B. Estimation of glomerular filtration rate using the CKD-EPI formula (Chronic Kidney Disease Epidemiology Collaboration)
C. Measurement of cystatin C
D. Spot urine collection and measurement of albumin and creatinine

56 A 39-year-old man is referred to you for evaluation of metabolic syndrome. The patient has gained 26 lb (11.8 kg) over the past year and has developed hypertension and dyslipidemia. His medical history is notable for schizoaffective disorder that has required medication. His current antipsychotic medications are olanzapine and trazodone, which he has taken for the past 15 months. He also takes hydrochlorothiazide and a calcium-channel blocker for hypertension.

On physical examination, he has a flat affect. His blood pressure is 128/68 mm Hg. Weight is 238 lb (108.2 kg) (BMI = 34.1 kg/m²), and waist circumference is 41.5 in (105 cm). He has central obesity, and his abdomen has pale striae. Muscle bulk and strength are normal.

Laboratory test results (fasting):
TSH = 1.1 mIU/L (0.5-5.0 mIU/L)
Glucose = 119 mg/dL (70-99 mg/dL)
   (SI: 6.6 mmol/L [3.9-5.5 mmol/L])
Total cholesterol = 224 mg/dL (<200 mg/dL
   [optimal]) (SI: 5.80 mmol/L [<5.18 mmol/L])
Triglycerides = 427 mg/dL (<150 mg/dL [optimal])
   (SI: 4.83 mmol/L [<1.70 mmol/L])
LDL cholesterol = 92 mg/dL (<100 mg/dL
   [optimal]) (SI: 2.38 mmol/L [<2.59 mmol/L])
HDL cholesterol = 38 mg/dL (>60 mg/dL
   [optimal]) (SI: 0.98 mmol/L [>1.55 mmol/L])

Which of the following would you recommend as the best next step in this patient's care?
   A. Change from olanzapine to clozapine
   B. Change from olanzapine to aripiprazole
   C. Start gemfibrozil
   D. Start metformin
   E. Start phentermine-topiramate

57 A 60-year-old woman sees you for follow-up of type 2 diabetes mellitus and is concerned about vision changes. She has had diabetes for 16 years. She has a diagnosis of background retinopathy first noted 18 months ago. For the past month she has had blurred vision, affecting the near and distant vision of both eyes. Her glucose control is stable with hemoglobin A_{1c} values ranging from 7.6% to 8.2% (60 to 66 mmol/mol) over the past 2 years. Her blood pressure is 132/78 mm Hg. Visual fields are intact to confrontation, tests of extraocular muscle movements are normal, and your nondilated fundoscopic examination shows some microaneurysms and cotton wool spots.

Which of the following is the most likely cause of this woman's vision symptoms?
   A. Retinal detachment
   B. Macular edema
   C. Vitreous hemorrhage
   D. Cataracts
   E. Mononeuritis of the third cranial nerve

58 A 71-year-old woman is referred with newly diagnosed type 2 diabetes mellitus. She has longstanding hypertension, one hospital admission for heart failure 5 years ago, and a hip fracture with surgical treatment 2 years ago. Before her visit with you, 2 fasting glucose measurements were documented to be 172 and 190 mg/dL (9.5 and 10.5 mmol/L), and her hemoglobin A_{1c} level was 8.2% (66 mmol/mol). She has a BMI of 31 kg/m² and no evidence of neuropathy on examination. A recent metabolic profile revealed a serum creatinine concentration of 1.4 mg/dL (123.8 μmol/L) and her estimated glomerular filtration rate is 54 mL/min per m². You decide to focus on a hemoglobin A_{1c} goal of 7.5% (58 mmol/mol).

Which of the following medications should be prescribed to treat her diabetes?
   A. α-Glucosidase inhibitor
   B. Pioglitazone
   C. DPP-4 inhibitor
   D. GLP-1 receptor agonist
   E. Metformin

59 A 63-year-old man has had type 2 diabetes mellitus for 8 years. His current therapy includes insulin glargine, 65 units in the morning; metformin, 1000 mg twice daily; and repaglinide, 2 mg before meals. Recent laboratory evaluation included a hemoglobin A_{1c} measurement of 8.4% (68 mmol/mol) and a fasting plasma glucose value of 111 mg/dL (6.2 mmol/L). Fingerstick blood glucose monitoring daily before breakfast shows an average of 116 mg/dL (6.4 mmol/L), with a range of 84 to 132 mg/dL (4.7 to 7.3 mmol/L) on 26 readings taken over the past 30 days. Over the past 2 to 3 weeks, he has experienced 2 episodes of nocturnal hypoglycemia.

Which of the following is the best next step in this patient's care?
   A. Measure glycosylated albumin
   B. Start diagnostic continuous glucose monitoring
   C. Measure C-peptide
   D. Measure insulin antibodies

Female Reproduction Board Review

Kathryn A. Martin, MD • Massachusetts General Hospital

1 A 32-year-old woman with polycystic ovary syndrome presents to your office to discuss fatigue. Over the past 3 years, she has gained approximately 40 lb (18.2 kg) (from 160 to 200 lb [73 to 91 kg]). In addition, she has been unusually tired at work and sometimes finds it hard to stay awake in meetings. She had menarche at age 11 years, hirsutism and acne since age 13 years, and has been on a combined estrogen-progestin contraceptive for the past 10 years. She has a family history of hypertension and type 2 diabetes mellitus. A recent hemoglobin A_{1c} measurement was normal.

On physical examination, her blood pressure is 130/90 mm Hg and BMI is 30 kg/m².

Which of the following is the best next step in this patient's evaluation?
A. 24-Hour urinary free cortisol measurement
B. Oral glucose tolerance test
C. Sleep study
D. Serum total testosterone measurement

2 A 26-year-old woman who is 2 weeks postpartum presents to discuss contraceptive options. This was her first pregnancy. Menarche was at age 12 years, and her periods have always been regular. Her BMI is 25 kg/m². She has occasional acne. She is planning to breastfeed until her infant is 9 months old.

Which of the following is the best contraceptive option for this patient?
A. Transdermal patch containing ethinyl estradiol and levonorgestrel
B. Progestin-only pill
C. Combined estrogen-progestin oral contraceptive
D. No contraception is needed if she is breastfeeding

3 A 27-year-old woman presents for further evaluation of amenorrhea. Menarche was at age 14 years. Her periods were irregular for 18 months after menarche, then regular every 28 days. She had mild acne as a teenager but has never had hirsutism. She was on oral contraceptives from age 16 years until age 25 when she conceived. She had a vaginal delivery 11 months ago, but had retained products of conception, requiring a surgical procedure for extraction (complicated by endometritis). Since that time, she has had no menstrual bleeding. She breastfed for 4 months.

Initial evaluation documented negative hCG and a normal TSH value. Since she stopped breastfeeding, she has experienced cyclic (monthly) breast soreness and irritability that lasts several days, most recently about 2 weeks ago. Her BMI is 20 kg/m². You draw blood today for further evaluation.

Which of the following patterns of hormone levels would you expect in this patient?

Answer	FSH	LH	Estradiol	Prolactin
A.	Normal	High	High	Normal
B.	High	High	Low	Normal
C.	Low	Low	Low	Low
D.	Low	Low	Low	High

4 A 28-year-old woman presents with infertility. She had menarche at age 13 years and had regular menses during high school and college except for periods of amenorrhea when she ran cross-country. She took an oral contraceptive pill from age 22 to 27 years but stopped 18 months ago to try and conceive. She has Hashimoto thyroiditis and takes a stable dosage of levothyroxine. She is currently having menses every 24 to 25 days. She exercises 3 times per week for 1.5 hours each session. She has mild acne, no hot flashes, and no galactorrhea. Her BMI is 20 kg/m².

Laboratory test results from blood samples drawn on cycle day 3:

FSH = 12.0 mIU/mL (2.0-12.0 mIU/mL)
(SI: 12.0 IU/L [2.0-12.0 IU/L])

Estradiol = 28 pg/mL (10-180 pg/mL)
(SI: 102.8 pmol/L [36.7-660.8 pmol/L])

Antimullerian hormone = 1.2 ng/mL
(0.9-9.5 ng/mL) (SI: 8.6 pmol/L [6.4-67.9 pmol/L])

TSH = 2.1 mIU/L (0.5-5.0 mIU/L)

Which of the following is the most likely diagnosis?
- A. Polycystic ovary syndrome
- B. FSH-secreting pituitary adenoma
- C. Functional hypothalamic amenorrhea
- D. Primary ovarian insufficiency

5 A 28-year-old patient whose birth-assigned sex was female, but whose gender identity is now male, sees you for gender-affirming hormonal therapy (testosterone). You refer the patient to a mental health provider to confirm the diagnosis of gender dysphoria/gender incongruence and to rule out any coexisting disorders such as depression. Baseline findings on pelvic examination and Pap smear are normal. The patient meets the criteria for gender-affirming hormone therapy. You review treatment options with the patient.

After starting hormone therapy, which of the following monitoring should be done during the first year of treatment?
- A. Measurement of serum total testosterone immediately before a testosterone enanthate/cypionate injection or immediately before application of testosterone gel, every 3 months
- B. Hemoglobin A_{1c} measurement every 6 months
- C. Hematocrit or hemoglobin measurement every 3 months
- D. Measurement of bone density at 1 year
- E. Pap smear at 1 year

6 A 41-year-old woman presents with severe hot flashes and insomnia. She underwent normal menarche and had regular menses until age 40 years, when she noted some irregularity. Leiomyomata were diagnosed, and 6 months ago she underwent total abdominal hysterectomy and bilateral salpingo-oophorectomy. Since her surgery, she has had intractable hot flashes at night,

as well as during the day. Her sleep is poor and she is having trouble functioning at work. She is otherwise in good health, takes no medications, and maintains a healthful diet and lifestyle. Her grandmother had breast cancer at age 78 years, her father has hypertension and hyperlipidemia, and her mother has osteoporosis.

Findings on physical examination are normal, and her BMI is 24 kg/m².

She has been told that she should not take estrogen because it has so many health risks. She comes to see you for a second opinion.

Which of the following do you suggest for her hot flashes?
- A. Oral 17β-estradiol, 2 mg daily
- B. Combined estradiol, 50 mcg/norethindrone acetate, 0.25 mg transdermal patch
- C. Venlafaxine, 75 mg daily
- D. Low-dosage oral contraceptives (ethinyl estradiol, 20 mcg/norethindrone acetate, 1 mg)

7 A 50-year-old woman presents to your office with concerns of hirsutism and scalp hair loss. She had menarche at age 12 years, regular menses and 2 uncomplicated pregnancies. Her final menstrual period was 1 year ago. Over the past 18 months, she has developed facial hair and scalp hair loss that has continued to progress. She has also noticed an increase in libido.

On physical examination, her BMI is 27 kg/m² and blood pressure is 150/90 mm Hg. She is very muscular. She has terminal hairs on her chin in a full-beard distribution, as well as hair on her upper abdomen, lower back, and sternum with a Ferriman-Gallwey score of 12 (>8 considered to be abnormal). Her clitoris measures 11 mm × 5 mm (clitoral index = 55 mm²).

Laboratory test results:

Testosterone = 350 ng/dL (8-60 ng/dL)
(SI: 12.1 nmol/L [0.3-2.1 nmol/L])

DHEA-S = 120 mg/dL (15-200 mg/dL)
(SI: 3.3 mmol/L [0.41-5.42 mmol/L])

FSH = 19 mIU/mL (>30 mIU/mL) (SI: 19 IU/L [>30 IU/L])

LH = 8 mIU/mL (>30 mIU/mL) (SI: 8 IU/L [>30 IU/L])

Which of the following is the best next test to evaluate this patient?
   A. Transvaginal ultrasonography
   B. Dexamethasone suppression test
   C. Combined ovarian-adrenal venous sampling
   D. Adrenal CT

8 A 20-year-old Hispanic woman presents for evaluation of irregular periods and hirsutism. She had early development of pubic hair at age 7 years. Menarche was at age 11 years. Her cycles have been irregular since then, and she has been treated intermittently with oral contraceptives but has been off oral contraceptives for the past year. She is currently having periods every 2 to 3 months. Her last menstrual period was 60 days ago.

On physical examination, her BMI is 29 kg/m². She has hair on her chin, upper lip, neck, midsternum, and upper abdomen. Her Ferriman-Gallwey score is 10. She has no clitoromegaly, acne, or alopecia.

Laboratory test results on day 60 of her menstrual cycle:
   LH = 5.0 mIU/mL (1.0-18.0 mIU/mL) (SI: 5.0 IU/L [1.0-18.0 IU/L])
   FSH = 4.0 mIU/mL (2.0-12.0 mIU/mL) (SI: 4.0 IU/L [2.0-12.0 IU/L])
   Testosterone = 50 ng/dL (8-60 ng/dL) (SI: 1.7 nmol/L [0.3-2.1 nmol/L])
   17-Hydroxyprogesterone = 470 ng/dL (<80 ng/dL) (SI: 14.2 nmol/L [<2.42 nmol/L])
   Prolactin = 18 ng/mL (4-30 ng/mL) (SI: 0.78 nmol/L [0.17-1.30 nmol/L])
   TSH = 2.1 mU/L (0.5-5.0 mIU/L)

Which of the following is the best treatment?
   A. Dexamethasone
   B. Metformin
   C. Oral contraceptive
   D. Spironolactone

9 A 45-year-old woman seeks evaluation for night sweats, hot flashes during the day, and one year of irregular periods. She also wants to know which contraceptive options would be best at her age. She is having menses every 6 to 8 weeks, sometimes with heavy flow. Her symptoms and lack of sleep are interfering with her ability to perform well at work. She is otherwise in good health with no history of cigarette smoking, hypertension, dyslipidemia, venous thromboembolism, or diabetes mellitus. She has no family history of venous thromboembolism or coronary disease. Her BMI is 22 kg/m².

Which of the following treatments would you suggest for this patient?
   A. Transdermal estradiol, 0.025 mg patch, with oral micronized progesterone, 100 mg daily
   B. Combined estrogen-progestin contraceptive (ethinyl estradiol, 20 mcg, with norethindrone, 1 mg, given continuously [ie, no placebos])
   C. Levonorgestrel-releasing intrauterine device and gabapentin, 300 mg orally at bedtime
   D. Medroxyprogesterone acetate, 10 mg for 10 days every other month

10 An 18-year-old woman presents with primary amenorrhea and short stature. Her blood pressure is 140/90 mm Hg. Her height is 56 in (142.2 cm) (BMI = 28 kg/m²). She has absent breast development and scant pubic and axillary hair.

Laboratory test results:
   FSH = 35.0 mIU/mL (2.0-12.0 mIU/mL) (SI: 35.0 IU/L [2.0-12.0 IU/L])
   LH = 28.0 mIU/mL (1.0-18.0 mIU/mL) (SI: 28.0 IU/L [1.0-18.0 IU/L])
   Estradiol = <10 pg/mL (10-180 pg/mL) (SI: <36.7 pmol/L [36.7-660.8 pmol/L])
   Karyotype: 45,X

Which of the following studies would you order next?
   A. Transvaginal ultrasonography
   B. Hemoglobin A$_{1c}$ measurement
   C. Thyroid ultrasonography
   D. Cardiac MRI

11 A 28-year-old patient whose birth-assigned sex was female, but whose gender identity is now male, sees you for gender-affirming hormonal therapy (testosterone). You refer the patient to a mental health provider to confirm the diagnosis of gender dysphoria/gender incongruence and to rule out any coexisting disorders such as depression. The patient meets the criteria for gender-affirming hormone therapy. You review treatment options with the patient.

Which of the following options is the best therapy to achieve this patient's goals for transition to the male phenotype?

A. Medroxyprogesterone, 150 mg intramuscularly every month, and DHEA, 100 mg orally daily

B. GnRH analogue intramuscularly monthly and testosterone gel, 1.6% 25 mg daily

C. DHEA, 100 mg twice daily, and spironolactone, 100 mg daily

D. Testosterone cypionate, 200 mg intramuscularly every 2 weeks

12 A 17-year-old girl presents with primary amenorrhea. She is otherwise healthy, and there is no family history of reproductive disorders. She has sparse axillary and pubic hair but normal Tanner stage 5 breast development. Her pelvic examination reveals a blind vaginal vault, and no uterus is seen on transvaginal ultrasonography.

Initial laboratory test results:
hCG = <3.0 mIU/L (<3.0 mIU/mL) (SI: <3.0 IU/L [<3.0 IU/L])
FSH = 7.0 mIU/mL (2.0-12.0 mIU/mL) (SI: 7.0 IU/L [2.0-12.0 IU/L])
LH = 18.0 mIU/mL (1.0-18.0 mIU/mL) (SI: 18.0 IU/L [1.0-18.0 IU/L])
Prolactin = 17 ng/mL (4-30 ng/mL) (SI: 0.7 nmol/L [0.17-1.30 nmol/L])

In addition to performing karyotype analysis, which of the following should be measured to diagnose her pubertal disorder?

A. Serum total testosterone

B. Serum estradiol

C. Serum 17-hydroxyprogesterone

D. Serum dihydrotestosterone

13 A 25-year-old woman with polycystic ovary syndrome presents to discuss treatment options. Menarche was at age 11 years, and her menses have always been irregular. She had onset of hirsutism and acne at age 12 years. She was on oral contraceptives briefly as a teenager. Six months ago, she started metformin, 500 mg twice daily, for her hirsutism and to regularize her

menstrual cycles. Her cycles have become more regular, but she feels as if her hirsutism has not improved.

On physical examination, her BMI is 27 kg/m² and blood pressure is 110/70 mm Hg.

She wants to modify her regimen to improve her hirsutism. She is currently using barrier methods for contraception.

Which of the following treatment options would be best for this patient?

A. Levonorgestrel-releasing intrauterine device and a higher metformin dosage

B. Addition of spironolactone

C. Oral contraceptive containing norethindrone

D. Addition of finasteride

14 A 20-year-old college student presents with a 4-month history of amenorrhea. She has fatigue and mild acne, but no hirsutism. She has no headaches or vision symptoms. Menarche was at age 14 years. She played sports in high school and occasionally missed a period. During college, her menses have been every 30 to 35 days. She attributes this to stress related to her schoolwork. Her physical examination findings are normal.

Laboratory test results:
FSH = 1.0 mIU/mL (2.0-12.0 mIU/mL) (SI: 1.0 IU/L [2.0-12.0 IU/L])
LH = 2.0 mIU/L (1.0-18.0 mIU/mL) (SI: 2.0 IU/L [1.0-18.0 IU/L])
Estradiol = 520 pg/mL (10-180 pg/mL) (SI: 1909 pmol/L [36.7-660.8 pmol/L])
Prolactin = 68 ng/mL (4-30 ng/mL) (SI: 3.0 nmol/L [0.17-1.30 nmol/L])

Which of the following is the most likely diagnosis in this patient?

A. Polycystic ovary syndrome

B. Pregnancy

C. Prolactinoma

D. Primary ovarian insufficiency

15 A 23-year-old woman presents with a history of irregular menses and then amenorrhea. Menarche was at age 14 years; her periods were irregular for 18 months, then regular every 28 days. She had a miscarriage 6 months ago when she was 12 weeks pregnant, which required a dilatation and curettage. Since that time, she has had no menstrual bleeding. She runs 5 miles 3 times a week. Her BMI is 20 kg/m^2.

Laboratory test results:
hCG = <3.0 mIU/mL (<3.0 mIU/mL)
   (SI: <3.0 IU/L [<3.0 IU/L])
LH = 4.0 mIU/mL (1.0-18.0 mIU/mL)
   (SI: 4.0 IU/L [1.0-18.0 IU/L])
FSH = 5.0 mIU/mL (2.0-12.0 mIU/mL)
   (SI: 5.0 IU/L [2.0-12.0 IU/L])
Estradiol = 70 pg/mL (10-180 pg/mL)
   (SI: 257.0 pmol/L [36.7-660.8 pmol/L])
Prolactin = 17 ng/mL (4-30 ng/mL) (SI: 0.7 nmol/L
   [0.17-1.30 nmol/L])

Which of the following is the most likely cause of her amenorrhea?
   A. Prolactinoma
   B. Functional hypothalamic amenorrhea
   C. Intrauterine adhesions (Asherman syndrome)
   D. Primary ovarian insufficiency

16 A 46-year-old perimenopausal woman presents to your office with persistent symptoms despite taking menopausal hormone therapy. Two years ago, she developed severe hot flashes, night sweats, and irritability. She also described "not feeling like herself." She was prescribed transdermal estradiol, 25 mcg twice weekly. She had a levonorgestrel-releasing intrauterine device inserted 2 years ago, so she does not need additional progestin therapy. Her hot flashes improved dramatically when her estradiol dosage was increased to 37.5 mcg twice weekly. However, other bothersome symptoms persist (eg, lack of energy and not feeling like herself). A recent TSH measurement was normal. She is otherwise in excellent health.

On physical examination, her blood pressure is 105/70 mm Hg and BMI is 21 kg/m^2.

Which of the following do you suggest next in this patient's management?
   A. Increase the estrogen dosage to a 50-mcg patch
   B. Start escitalopram, 10 mg daily
   C. Switch to a low-dosage estrogen-progestin oral contraceptive
   D. Refer for cognitive behavioral therapy

17 A 46-year-old woman seeks evaluation for irregular menses. Since menarche at age 12 years, she had regular 28- to 30-day cycles until about 6 months ago when her intermenstrual interval shortened to 24 to 25 days. Now her cycles are unpredictable (anywhere from every 24 to 90 days). She exercises daily for 30 minutes. She has no hot flashes, but she is not sleeping well and has been experiencing mild aches and pains (without swelling) since her periods became irregular. She has no galactorrhea or headaches. A recent TSH measurement was normal and hCG was negative. She would like to know what is causing her irregular periods.

On physical examination, her blood pressure is 90/65 mm Hg and BMI is 19.5 kg/m^2.

Which of the following tests should you order to determine the cause of this patient's problem?
   A. Transvaginal ultrasonography
   B. FSH measurement
   C. Antimullerian hormone measurement
   D. No testing required

18 A 70-year-old woman sees you for a second opinion for recent-onset hirsutism, alopecia, and vaginal bleeding. Six months ago, she noticed that her scalp hair was thinning and that she was developing hair on her chin, neck, upper lip, and stomach. She has been experiencing intrusive sexual thoughts, but has not noticed a change in her voice. She is otherwise in good health and is at low surgical risk.

On physical examination, her blood pressure is 130/85 mm Hg and BMI is 26 kg/m^2. She has frontal hair recession and diffuse thinning scalp hair. She has dark hair on her neck, chin, upper lip, midsternum, upper abdomen, and upper and lower back (Ferriman-Gallwey score = 12). There is no acne or galactorrhea. She has clitoromegaly, with a clitoral measurement of 10 mm × 5 mm.

Laboratory test results:
Serum total testosterone = 650 ng/dL (repeat value 700 ng/dL) (8-60 ng/dL) (SI: 22.6 nmol/L [0.3-2.1 nmol/L])
LH = 12.0 mIU/mL (>30 mIU/mL) (SI: 12.0 IU/L [>30 IU/L])
FSH = 16.0 mIU/mL (>30 mIU/mL) (SI: 16.0 IU/L [>30 IU/L])
Estradiol = 290 pg/mL (<20 pg/mL) (SI: 1065 pmol/L [<73.4 pmol/L])
DHEA-S = 220 µg/dL (15-157 µg/dL) (SI: 6.0 µmol/L [0.41-4.25 µmol/L])
TSH = 2.8 mIU/L (0.5-5.0 mIU/L)
Prolactin = 17 ng/mL (4-30 ng/mL) (SI: 0.74 nmol/L [0.17-1.30 nmol/L])

Transvaginal ultrasonography shows an endometrial thickness of 11 mm (normal thickness in a postmenopausal woman is less than 4 to 5 mm), normal-sized ovaries for age, and no masses or cysts. Endometrial biopsy reveals endometrial hyperplasia. No masses are identified on adrenal CT.

Which of the following should you recommend now?
A. Repeated imaging studies in 3 months
B. Hysterectomy with bilateral oophorectomy
C. Ovarian-adrenal venous sampling to determine the source of the androgen excess
D. Measurement of serum free testosterone

19 A 22-year-old woman with a 4-year history of functional hypothalamic amenorrhea comes to see you for follow-up. She has a history of excessive exercise, and she was a restricted eater. Her BMI at her initial visit with you was 17 kg/m², and she had low bone mineral density (T-score at femoral neck = –2.2). She understands that her low bone mineral density is related to her nutrition and excessive exercise, as evaluation for secondary causes has been negative. Eighteen months ago, she decided to implement lifestyle changes; she has moderated her exercise and improved her nutrition. Her weight has increased, and her BMI is now 18.5 kg/m². She is pleased that she has been able to make these changes but is disappointed that her periods have not returned. She wonders whether something else is wrong.

Laboratory test results:
hCG = <3.0 mIU/mL (<3.0 mIU/mL) (SI: <3.0 IU/L [<3.0 IU/L])
TSH = 1.9 mIU/L (0.5-5.0 mIU/L)
Prolactin = 15 ng/mL (4-30 ng/mL) (SI: 0.65 nmol/L [0.17-1.30 nmol/L])
Estradiol = 110 pg/mL (10-180 pg/mL) (SI: 403.8 pmol/L [36.7-660.8 pmol/L])
LH = 6.0 mIU/mL (1.0-18.0 mIU/mL) (SI: 6.0 IU/L [1.0-18.0 IU/L])
FSH = 8.0 mIU/mL (2.0-12.0 mIU/mL) (SI: 8.0 IU/L [2.0-12.0 IU/L])
Progesterone = 7.0 ng/mL (≤1.0 ng/mL) (SI: 22.3 nmol/L [≤3.2 nmol/L])

Which of the following should you recommend now?
A. Start transdermal 17β-estradiol patch with cyclic micronized progesterone
B. Start alendronate, 70 mg weekly
C. Start low-dosage combined estrogen-progestin oral contraceptive
D. No treatment necessary

20 A 23-year-old woman with a diagnosis of functional hypothalamic amenorrhea sees you to discuss her recent DXA. Her bone mineral density continues to decline, and her femoral neck T-score is now –2.6, decreased from –2.2 two years ago. She has no history of fractures. She runs 80 miles per week and is a restricted eater. Her BMI is 17 kg/m².

Which of the following is the best management strategy for improving her bone density?
A. ETransdermal estradiol, 100 mcg twice weekly, with oral micronized progesterone, 200 mg (first 12 days of the month)
B. Improved nutrition and weight gain
C. Combined oral estrogen-progestin contraceptive (20 mcg ethinyl estradiol with norethindrone acetate 1 mg)
D. Alendronate, 70 mg orally once weekly

Male Reproduction Board Review

Frances J. Hayes, MD • Massachusetts General Hospital

1 A 65-year-old man is referred by his primary care physician for management of hypogonadism. At the time of diagnosis, he described decreased energy and libido and was found to have 2 morning testosterone values in the hypogonadal range (190 and 215 ng/dL [6.6 and 7.5 nmol/L]) and a hematocrit measurement of 50% (0.50). He has been on treatment with intramuscular injections of testosterone enanthate, 200 mg every 2 weeks, for the past 6 months. His libido has improved on this regimen, but he continues to feel tired and sometimes takes an afternoon nap. He does not smoke cigarettes.

On physical examination, his BMI is 36 kg/m². He is well virilized, he has a normal testicular exam, and his lungs are clear to auscultation. His trough testosterone level drawn before his next injection is 325 ng/dL (11.3 nmol/L) and his hematocrit is now 54% (0.54).

Which of the following is the best next step in this patient's management?
   A. Arrange for a sleep study
   B. Switch from testosterone enanthate to cypionate at the current dosage
   C. Continue his current testosterone regimen but arrange for him to have monthly phlebotomy
   D. Increase the testosterone dosage to 250 mg every 2 weeks

2 A 60-year-old man is referred by his primary care physician to discuss testosterone replacement therapy. During workup for decreased libido and erectile dysfunction, hypogonadism was diagnosed and he is eager to start therapy. He has no lower urinary tract symptoms. He has a history of obstructive sleep apnea for which he uses continuous positive airway pressure and reports no daytime somnolence. He had a myocardial infarction 10 years earlier and is taking an extended-release formulation of isosorbide mononitrate on which he has no angina. His family history is notable for prostate cancer in his father.

On physical examination, his BMI is 32 kg/m² and blood pressure is 125/80 mm Hg. He is well virilized and has normal testes. His prostate feels slightly enlarged but no nodules are palpable.

Laboratory test results:
   Testosterone (8 AM) = 190 ng/dL (300-900 ng/dL) (SI: 6.6 nmol/L [10.4-31.2 nmol/L]) (repeated value 195 ng/dL [6.8 nmol/L])
   LH = 7.9 mIU/mL (1.0-9.0 mIU/mL) (SI: 7.9 IU/L [1.0-9.0 IU/L])
   FSH = 9.0 mIU/mL (1.0-13.0 mIU/mL) (SI: 9.0 IU/L [1.0-13.0 IU/L])
   Hematocrit = 47% (41%-50%) (SI: 0.47 [0.41-0.50])
   PSA = 3.3 ng/mL (<3.8 ng/mL) (SI: 3.3 µg/L [<3.8 µg/L]) (repeated value 3.1 ng/mL [3.1 µg/L])

Which of the following is the best next step in this patient's management?
   A. Start a phosphodiesterase inhibitor
   B. Start testosterone replacement therapy
   C. Arrange for a sleep study
   D. Refer him to a urologist

3 A 70-year-old man returns to clinic for follow-up 12 months after starting testosterone therapy. At the time of diagnosis, his morning total testosterone level was 200 ng/dL (6.9 nmol/L) and his PSA level was 1.3 ng/mL (1.3 µg/L). His prostate was symmetrically enlarged without nodules. He was started on a 1% testosterone gel, 5 g daily on which his testosterone level increased to 451 ng/dL (15.6 nmol/L). The patient reports improved sexual function and energy on treatment and has no lower urinary tract symptoms.

On physical examination at today's appointment, his prostate is unchanged.

His PSA is now 3.3 ng/mL (3.3 μg/L). A repeat measurement is 3.0 ng/mL (3.0 μg/L).

Which of the following is the best next step in this patient's management?
- A. Discontinue testosterone therapy
- B. Refer him to a urologist
- C. Provide reassurance and schedule a follow-up appointment in 12 months
- D. Start a 5α-reductase inhibitor

4 A 25-year-old man is referred to you for evaluation of hypogonadism 2 months after sustaining a head injury after being knocked off his motorcycle. Brain imaging done at the time revealed no hypothalamic, pituitary stalk, or pituitary abnormalities. He has made good progress since his accident, but still has some problems with short-term memory and strength. His libido, which had been quite low after being discharged from hospital, is now beginning to improve and he can get and sustain an erection adequate for intercourse. He is married and would like to start a family in the next 1 to 2 years.

On physical examination, his BMI is 24 kg/m². He has normal secondary sexual characteristics and normal testicular size. His neurologic examination reveals no focal deficits.

Laboratory test results:
　　Total testosterone = 150 ng/dL (5.2 nmol/L)
　　　(reference range, 300-900 ng/dL
　　　[10.4-31.2 nmol/L])
　　LH = 3.5 mIU/mL (3.5 IU/L)

Which of the following is the most appropriate next step in this patient's management?
- A. Start treatment with hCG
- B. Start testosterone replacement
- C. Reevaluate his hypothalamic-pituitary-gonadal axis in 6 to 12 months
- D. Start a phosphodiesterase inhibitor

5 A 30-year-old man presents with decreased libido and erectile dysfunction. Ulcerative colitis was diagnosed 6 months ago after he presented with bloody diarrhea. His symptoms persisted on sulfasalazine and his regimen was switched to prednisone, 60 mg daily, on which his symptoms improved.

On physical examination, his BMI is 30 kg/m². He has cushingoid facies and several ecchymoses on his arms. His testes are 15 mL bilaterally.

He has 2 morning testosterone values documented: 150 and 180 ng/dL (5.2 and 6.2 nmol/L).

Which of the following hormone profiles is most likely to characterize this patient's hypogonadism?

Answer	LH	FSH	Testosterone	SHBG
A.	2.3 mIU/mL (2.3 IU/L)	5.0 mIU/mL (5.0 IU/L)	150 ng/dL (5.2 nmol/L)	7.9 μg/mL (70 nmol/L)
B.	2.3 mIU/mL (2.3 IU/L)	5.0 mIU/mL (5.0 IU/L)	150 ng/dL (5.2 nmol/L)	1.3 μg/mL (12 nmol/L)
C.	18.1 mIU/mL (18.1 IU/L)	12.3 mIU/mL (12.3 IU/L)	150 ng/dL (5.2 nmol/L)	1.3 μg/mL (12 nmol/L)
D.	18.1 mIU/mL (18.1 IU/L)	12.3 mIU/mL (12.3 IU/L)	150 ng/dL (5.2 nmol/L)	7.9 μg/mL (70 nmol/L)

6 A 49-year-old man presents with a 2-year history of increasing fatigue, loss of libido, and erectile dysfunction. He underwent normal puberty and has 2 biologic children. His medical history includes hepatitis C infection but no head or testicular trauma. He states that he does not use androgens.

On physical examination, the patient is normally virilized. His BMI is 26.5 kg/m². He has bilateral gynecomastia. His phallus is normal. Testes are 15 mL bilaterally.

Laboratory test results:
　　Total testosterone (8 AM) (by liquid chromatography
　　　tandem mass spectrometry) = 810 ng/dL
　　　(300-900 ng/dL) (SI: 28.1 nmol/L
　　　[10.4-31.2 nmol/L]) (repeated measurement
　　　750 ng/dL [26.0 nmol/L])
　　LH = 8.7 mIU/mL (1.0-9.0 mIU/mL) (SI: 8.7 IU/L
　　　[1.0-9.0 IU/L])
　　FSH = 7.0 mIU/mL (1.0-13.0 mIU/mL)
　　　(SI: 7.0 IU/L [1.0-13.0 IU/L])
　　TSH = 2.2 mIU/L (0.5-5.0 mIU/L)

Free T_4 = 1.1 ng/dL (0.8-1.8 ng/dL)
  (SI: 14.2 pmol/L [10.30-23.17 pmol/L])
Cortisol (10 AM) = 19.8 µg/dL (5-25 µg/dL)
  (SI: 546.2 nmol/L [137.9-689.7 nmol/L])

Which of the following is the best next diagnostic step in this patient's evaluation?
A. Measure free testosterone
B. Determine urinary testosterone-to-epitestosterone ratio
C. Screen for mutations in the androgen receptor gene
D. Refer to evaluate for depression

7 A 20-year-old man is transferred to you by his pediatrician for ongoing management of idiopathic hypogonadotropic hypogonadism. The diagnosis was made at age 18 years during workup for delayed puberty, when he was found to have a serum testosterone level of 55 ng/dL (1.9 nmol/L) and low gonadotropin levels (LH = 0.8 mIU/mL [0.8 IU/L], FSH = 1.1 mIU/mL [1.1 IU/L]). Results of the rest of his pituitary function testing were normal, as was sellar imaging. He has been treated with testosterone from age 18 years, and his levels are normal on treatment. He has a normal sense of smell and normal sexual function but reports fatigue and occasional dizziness.

On physical examination, his height is 75 in (190.5 cm). His blood pressure is 95/60 mm Hg lying down and 80/55 mm Hg standing. He is well virilized and has no gynecomastia. He has pigmentation of buccal mucosa and palmar creases. Testes are 4 mL bilaterally.

Laboratory test results:
Baseline cortisol = 1.0 µg/dL (5-25 mg/dL)
  (SI: 27.6 nmol/L [137.9-689.7 nmol/L])
Plasma ACTH = 310 pg/mL (10-80 pg/mL)
  (SI: 68.2 pmol/L [2.2-17.6 pmol/L])
1 hour after stimulation with 250 mcg of intravenous cosyntropin, cortisol = 5.0 µg/dL (SI: 137.9 nmol/L)

Which of the following is the most likely diagnosis?
A. Partial hypopituitarism
B. Autoimmune polyglandular endocrine deficiency syndrome type 1
C. Adrenal hypoplasia congenita
D. Kallmann syndrome

8 A 36-year-old man is referred for evaluation of a low serum testosterone level identified during workup of decreasing libido and low energy levels. He is otherwise well and has a 6-year-old daughter. He is taking no medications.

On physical examination, his BMI is 24 kg/m^2 and blood pressure is 120/80 mm Hg. He has normal secondary sexual characteristics and no gynecomastia. He has no acne or striae. His testicular volume is 15 mL bilaterally. Muscle strength is normal and he is able to do squats without using his arms to assist.

Laboratory test results:
Total testosterone = 150 ng/dL (300-900 ng/dL)
  (SI: 5.2 nmol/L [10.4-31.2 nmol/L])
Calculated free testosterone = 3.5 ng/dL
  (9.0-30.0 ng/dL) (SI: [0.31-1.04 nmol/L])
LH = 2.0 mIU/mL (1.0-9.0 mIU/mL) (SI: 2.0 IU/L
  [1.0-9.0 IU/L])
FSH = 3.0 mIU/mL (1.0-13.0 mIU/mL)
  (SI: 3.0 IU/L [1.0-13.0 IU/L])

Pituitary MRI is normal.

Which of the following is the most appropriate next test?
A. 24-Hour urinary free cortisol measurement
B. Karyotype analysis
C. Urine epitestosterone measurement
D. Serum prolactin measurement

9 An 18-year-old man is referred because he failed to go through puberty. He grew normally in childhood but never experienced a growth spurt. He has a normal sense of smell. He does not take any medications and does not abuse drugs. He has no family history of anosmia, delayed puberty, or hypogonadism.

On physical examination, his height is 67 in (170 cm), arm span is 70 in (177.8 cm), and BMI is 21 kg/m^2. He has slight axillary hair and Tanner stage 2 pubic hair but no facial or chest hair. He has no gynecomastia. His testes measure 2 mL bilaterally. Neurologic examination reveals that his visual fields are full to confrontation and that he does not have mirror movements.

Laboratory test results (morning):
  Total testosterone = 47 ng/dL (300-900 ng/dL)
    (SI: 1.6 nmol/L [10.4-31.2 nmol/L])
  Free T$_4$ = 1.3 ng/dL (0.8-1.8 ng/dL)
    (SI: 16.7 pmol/L [10.30-23.17 pmol/L])
  TSH = 1.41 mIU/L (0.5-5.0 mIU/L)
  LH = <0.2 mIU/mL (1.0-9.0 mIU/mL)
    (SI: <0.2 IU/L [1.0-9.0 IU/L])
  FSH = 0.3 mIU/mL (1.0-13.0 mIU/mL)
    (SI: 0.3 IU/L [1.0-13.0 IU/L])
  Prolactin = 17 ng/mL (4-23 ng/mL) (SI: 0.7 nmol/L
    [0.17-1.00 nmol/L])
  Cortisol (8 AM) = 18.0 µg/dL (5-25 µg/dL)
    (SI: 496.6 nmol/L [137.9-689.7 nmol/L])
  IGF-1, low-normal

Which of the following is the most appropriate diagnostic test to perform next?
  A. A. Genetic testing for a mutation in *KAL1*
  B. GnRH stimulation test
  C. MRI of the sella
  D. Measurement of free testosterone

10 A 36-year-old pharmacist is referred for evaluation of a low serum testosterone level. He reports decreased libido and energy. On review of systems, his only other complaint is pain in the small joints of his hands. He takes no medications. He has a 5-year-old biologic daughter.

On physical examination, his BMI is 24 kg/m² and blood pressure is 115/70 mm Hg. He has normal secondary sexual characteristics and no gynecomastia. He has no striae or bruises and has no difficulty rising from a squatting position. Testicular volume is 15 mL bilaterally.

Laboratory test results:
  Total testosterone = 150 ng/dL (300-900 ng/dL)
    (SI: 5.2 nmol/L [10.4-31.2 nmol/L])
  Serum prolactin = 15 ng/mL (4-23 ng/mL)
    (SI: 0.9 nmol [0.17-1.00 nmol/L])
  FSH = 3.0 mIU/mL (1.0-13.0 mIU/mL)
    (SI: 3.0 IU/L [1.0-13.0 IU/L])
  LH = 3.0 mIU/mL (1.0-9.0 mIU/mL) (SI: 3.0 IU/L
    [1.0-9.0 IU/L])
  Plasma glucose (fasting) = 101 mg/dL
    (70-99 mg/dL) (SI: 5.6 mmol/L [3.9-5.5 mmol/L])

X-ray of the hands reveals chondrocalcinosis of the small joints bilaterally. Sellar MRI reveals no pituitary mass.

Which of the following tests is most likely to lead to this patient's specific diagnosis?
  A. Measurement of transferrin saturation
  B. Urine toxicology screen for opioids
  C. Dexamethasone suppression test
  D. Measurement of serum prolactin after serial dilution

11 A 63-year-old man is referred to you for evaluation of hypogonadism because he has been experiencing low mood, decreased energy levels, and decreased libido. He had been discharged from the hospital 3 weeks earlier following treatment of an exacerbation of chronic obstructive pulmonary disease. His primary care physician saw him last week and measured a serum testosterone concentration, which was low.

On physical examination, his BMI is 26.5 kg/m². He is well virilized and has no gynecomastia.

His phallus is normal, and tests are 25-mL bilaterally.

Laboratory test results (sample drawn in the early morning):
  Total testosterone = 210 ng/dL (300-900 ng/dL)
    (SI: 7.3 nmol/L [10.4-31.2 nmol/L])
  Repeat testosterone drawn in the early morning of
    today's clinic visit = 235 ng/dL (SI: 8.2 nmol/L)
  Serum LH = 4.0 mIU/mL (1.0-9.0 mIU/mL)
    (SI: 4.0 IU/L [1.0-9.0 IU/L])

Which of the following is the best next diagnostic test to order?
  A. Free testosterone measurement
  B. Serum iron studies
  C. Serum prolactin measurement
  D. Serum total testosterone measurement in 3 months

12 A 30-year-old man presents for evaluation of infertility. He has a history of congenital hypopituitarism, and he was treated with GH and hydrocortisone in childhood. Puberty was induced with testosterone. His current medications are hydrocortisone, 15 mg daily; testosterone gel, 50 mg daily; and levothyroxine, 112 mcg daily. He reports normal libido and erections. His 28-year-old wife has regular menstrual cycles.

On physical examination, he has normal secondary sexual characteristics and a testicular volume of 3 mL bilaterally.

Hormone testing after discontinuing testosterone therapy:

Testosterone = 55 ng/dL (300-900 ng/dL) (SI: 1.9 nmol/L [10.4-31.2 nmol/L])

LH = 1.0 mIU/mL (1.0-9.0 mIU/mL) (SI: 1.0 IU/L [1.0-9.0 IU/L])

FSH = 1.1 mIU/mL (1.0-13.0 mIU/mL) (SI: 1.1 IU/L [1.0-13.0 IU/L])

Semen analysis shows normal semen volume and azoospermia.

Which of the following treatment options is most likely to induce fertility in this patient?

A. Pulsatile GnRH therapy
B. Intracytoplasmic sperm injection
C. hCG injections
D. hCG and FSH injections

13 A 25-year-old man is referred by his oncologist to discuss options for fertility preservation. He has recently been diagnosed with Hodgkin lymphoma, which will require treatment with cyclophosphamide. The patient is currently single but would like to have children in the future.

On physical examination, his testes are 25 mL in volume. His testosterone level is 350 ng/dL (12.1 nmol/L).

A semen analysis documents a sperm concentration of 11 million/mL.

Which of the following should be offered to this patient for fertility preservation?

A. Treatment with an aromatase inhibitor during chemotherapy
B. Treatment with a GnRH agonist during chemotherapy
C. Cryopreservation of spermatogonial stem cells before chemotherapy for future transplantation
D. Sperm cryopreservation before chemotherapy

14 A 25-year-old man is referred to you because he was found to have azoospermia during a workup for infertility. He and his wife have been having unprotected intercourse for the past 3 years without a confirmed pregnancy. The patient underwent normal puberty and reports normal libido and erections. Finding on his wife's workup are normal.

On physical examination, he is a well-built man with normal muscle mass. His BMI is 25.5 kg/m². There is no gynecomastia. His testes are 15 mL bilaterally, and his vas deferens is palpable bilaterally.

Laboratory test results:

Total testosterone = 550 ng/dL (300-900 ng/dL) (SI: 19.1 nmol/L [10.4-31.2 nmol/L])

FSH = 25.5 mIU/mL (1.0-13.0 mIU/mL) (SI: 25.5 IU/L [1.0-13.0 IU/L])

LH = 3.8 mIU/mL (1.0-9.0 mIU/mL) (SI: 3.8 IU/L [1.0-9.0 IU/L])

Inhibin B, undetectable

Karyotype = 46,XY (100 cells counted)

A second semen analysis confirms azoospermia. Semen volume is 3 mL and fructose is positive.

Which of the following genetic abnormalities is this patient most likely to have?

A. Y-Chromosome microdeletion
B. Klinefelter syndrome
C. Mutation in the *KISS1R* gene
D. Mutation in the *CFTR* gene

15 A 34-year-old man seeks a second opinion for management of infertility. He and his wife have had regular unprotected intercourse for 18 months without a documented pregnancy. His wife's workup is normal. He brings the results of his laboratory testing:

Total testosterone = 250 ng/dL (300-900 ng/dL)
  (SI: 8.7 nmol/L [10.4-31.2 nmol/L])
LH = 3.5 mIU/mL (1.0-9.0 mIU/mL) (SI: 3.5 IU/L
  [1.0-9.0 IU/L])
FSH = 4.0 mIU/mL (1.0-13.0 mIU/mL)
  (SI: 4.0 IU/L [1.0-13.0 IU/L])
Prolactin = 12 ng/mL (4-23 ng/mL) (SI: 0.5 nmol/L
  [0.17-1.00 nmol/L])
Transferrin saturation = 35% (14%-50%)

He does not have a copy of his semen analyses, but he was told that they showed no sperm. Adult-onset hypogonadotropic hypogonadism is diagnosed, and hCG injections are initiated. His testosterone level increases to 600 ng/dL (20.8 nmol/L) but he remains azoospermic.

On physical examination, he is an obese, otherwise healthy man who is well virilized. His testes are 20 mL bilaterally, but you have difficulty palpating his vas deferens.

Which of the following is the most appropriate next step?
  A. Add FSH injections
  B. Arrange for transrectal ultrasonography
  C. Increase the hCG dosage
  D. Switch to clomiphene citrate

16 A 20-year-old man presents for evaluation of painless breast enlargement, which has been present since puberty. He reports normal sexual function. He has no history of testicular pain, swelling or trauma. He drinks 4 to 6 beers on the weekends.

On physical examination, his height is 72 in (183 cm), arm span is 71 in (180 cm), and BMI is 23 kg/m². His blood pressure is 110/70 mm Hg. He is well virilized. There is 4-cm bilateral gynecomastia with no galactorrhea. He has a normal phallus with no hypospadias. His testes are small and firm, measuring 6 mL bilaterally.

Laboratory test results:
  Total testosterone = 250 ng/dL (300-900 ng/dL)
    (SI: 8.7 nmol/L [10.4-31.2 nmol/L])
  Estradiol = 52 pg/mL (10-40 pg/mL)
    (SI: 190.9 pmol/L [36.7-146.8 pmol/L])
  FSH = 38.0 mIU/mL (1.0-13.0 mIU/mL)
    (SI: 38 IU/L [1.0-13.0 IU/L])
  LH = 18.0 mIU/mL (1.0-9.0 mIU/mL)
    (SI: 18 IU/L [1.0-9.0 IU/L])

Which of the following is the most likely cause of this patient's presentation?
  A. Inactivating mutation in the gene encoding the FSH receptor
  B. Klinefelter syndrome
  C. Congenital adrenal hyperplasia due to 17α-hydroxylase deficiency
  D. Mumps orchitis

17 An 18-year-old man presents for evaluation of bilateral breast enlargement, which he first noticed 3 years earlier. The breast tissue is no longer growing and the tenderness that he initially experienced has now resolved. However, he is very embarrassed by the cosmetic appearance and has given up swimming. He has no nipple discharge. He takes no medications or herbal products and does not use illicit drugs.

On physical examination, the patient has normal body hair and has facial acne. Palpation of the breasts reveals rubbery, mobile subareolar tissue (3 cm on the left and 3.5 cm on the right). There is no nipple discharge or retraction. Findings on genital examination are age appropriate, with a normal phallus, testes of 15 mL bilaterally, and Tanner stage 5 pubic hair.

Hormonal workup documents normal concentrations of testosterone, estradiol, LH, FSH, and TSH. β-hCG is negative.

Which of the following is the best next step in this patient's care?
  A. Mammography
  B. Reassurance and observation
  C. Referral for surgical consultation
  D. Aromatase inhibitor therapy

18 A 28-year-old man presents for evaluation of a 3-month history of tender gynecomastia. He reports normal energy levels and sexual function. He has no heat intolerance, diaphoresis, or palpitations. His medical history is remarkable for hepatitis C and premature male-pattern balding for which he takes finasteride, 1 mg daily.

On physical examination, his BMI is 22 kg/m² and pulse rate is 72 beats/min. His thyroid gland is normal. He has tender bilateral gynecomastia measuring about 3 cm bilaterally. His phallus is normal, and testes are 15 mL bilaterally with no masses palpable.

Laboratory test results:

Total testosterone = 900 ng/dL (300-900 ng/dL) (SI: 31.2 nmol/L [10.4-31.2 nmol/L])

Free testosterone (calculated) = 31 ng/dL (9.0-30.0 ng/dL) (SI: 1.08 nmol/L [0.31-1.04 nmol/L])

Estradiol = 90 pg/mL (10-40 pg/mL) (SI: 330.4 pmol/L [36.7-146.8 pmol/L])

FSH = 0.5 mIU/mL (1.0-13.0 mIU/mL) (SI: 0.5 IU/L [1.0-13.0 IU/L])

LH = 0.5 mIU/mL (1.0-9.0 mIU/mL) (SI: 0.5 IU/L [1.0-9.0 IU/L])

Which of the following most likely explains his hormone profile?

A. Elevated SHBG due to hepatitis C

B. Estrogen-secreting testicular tumor

C. Decreased 5α-reductase activity due to finasteride

D. Testosterone abuse

19 A primary care doctor asks for your help in interpreting the hormone profile of a patient he suspects is taking anabolic steroids.

Laboratory test results:

Testosterone = 950 ng/dL (300-900 ng/dL) (SI: 33.0 nmol/L [10.4-31.2 nmol/L])

Estradiol = 15 pg/mL (4-40 pg/mL) (SI: 55.1 pmol/L [36.7-146.8 pmol/L])

LH = <1.0 mIU/mL (1.0-9.0 mIU/mL) (SI: <1.0 IU/L [1.0-9.0 IU/L])

FSH = <1.0 mIU/mL (1.0-13.0 mIU/mL) (SI: <1.0 IU/L [1.0-13.0 IU/L])

HDL cholesterol = 5 mg/dL (>60 mg/dL [optimal]) (SI: 0.13 mmol/L [>1.55 mmol/L])

Which of the following regimens best explains this patient's hormone profile?

A. Testosterone plus an aromatase inhibitor

B. Testosterone plus an androgenic anabolic steroid

C. Testosterone plus an androgenic anabolic steroid plus an aromatase inhibitor

D. Androgenic anabolic steroid plus an aromatase inhibitor

20 A 40-year-old transgender woman is admitted to the hospital with abdominal pain and is found to have pancreatitis. She has a strong family history of hyperlipidemia and was diagnosed with hypertriglyceridemia in her late teens. She has been prescribed rosuvastatin and fenofibrate but has not been taking her medications consistently. At age 18 years, she started hormone therapy with conjugated equine estrogens and spironolactone and started living as a woman. In her late 20s, she had breast augmentation and facial surgery. Six months before admission, type 2 diabetes mellitus was diagnosed, and it has since been managed by diet alone.

Laboratory test results:

Triglycerides = 6050 mg/dL (<150 mg/dL) (SI: 68.37 mmol/L [<1.70 mmol/L])

Lipase = 778 U/L (10-73 U/L) (SI: 13.0 μkat/L [0.17-1.22 μkat/L])

Glucose = 255 mg/dL (70-99 mg/dL) (SI: 14.2 mmol/L [3.9-5.5 mmol/L])

She responds well to fluids, insulin, and intensification of her lipid-lowering therapy. Her hormone therapy is held. On review in clinic 6 weeks later, her triglycerides are back to baseline, her blood glucose values are in the range of 100 to 120 mg/dL (5.6 to 6.7 mmol/L), and she is keen to resume hormone therapy.

Which of the following is the most appropriate management option for this patient?

A. Resume the previous regimen of conjugated equine estrogen and spironolactone

B. Start a GnRH agonist with a 0.05-mg estradiol patch

C. Tell the patient that she is not a candidate for any further hormonal intervention

D. Switch her regimen to ethinyl estradiol and spironolactone

Thyroid Board Review

Elizabeth N. Pearce, MD, MSc • Boston University

1 A 36-year-old man presents with a 2.6-cm left-sided thyroid nodule. This was first noted 18 months ago when it was palpated during a routine physical exam. On ultrasonography, the nodule is solid and hypoechoic, with irregular margins. There are no microcalcifications. There is no cervical lymphadenopathy. The right lobe has a normal echotexture, without any discrete nodules. The nodule was initially biopsied 6 months ago, and a repeated FNAB was performed 3 months ago. Both biopsies were performed with ultrasound guidance, and the second time the biopsy was performed with on-site cytopathologic evaluation. In both instances, the cytopathology was interpreted as Bethesda I (nondiagnostic/unsatisfactory), with an inadequate number of cells. The nodule has increased 7 to 9 mm in each dimension since the initial ultrasound 18 months ago. The patient has no compressive symptoms.

Laboratory test result:
Serum TSH = 1.74 mIU/L (0.5-5.0 mIU/L)

Which of the following is the best next step in this patient's management?
   A. Repeat the ultrasound in 6 to 12 months
   B. Repeat ultrasound-guided FNAB with molecular markers
   C. Perform ^{18}F-fluorodeoxyglucose PET/CT imaging
   D. Perform thyroid lobectomy
   E. Measure serum calcitonin

2 A 44-year-old woman is incidentally found to have a right thyroid nodule on cervical spine MRI, which was performed to evaluate posterior neck pain. She had been in good health previously and takes no medications. There is no history of radiation exposure or family history of thyroid cancer.

On physical examination, the nodule is not palpable and no adenopathy is noted. Ultrasonography confirms a 1.0-cm nodule with microcalcifications. FNAB findings are suspicious for cancer, and the patient undergoes a right thyroid lobectomy. A 0.9-cm classic papillary thyroid cancer is documented. No lymph nodes are removed.

Which of the following is the best next step in this patient's management?
   A. Thyroid hormone therapy with a target TSH level between 0.5 and 2.0 mIU/L
   B. Completion thyroidectomy followed by radioiodine remnant ablation
   C. Completion thyroidectomy without radioiodine remnant ablation
   D. Radioiodine ablation of the left lobe of the thyroid

3 A 63-year-old man with refractory atrial fibrillation is prescribed amiodarone. Baseline thyroid function is normal. One month later, the patient is asymptomatic, but is noted to have the following laboratory findings:
Total T_4 = 13.4 µg/dL (5.5-12.5 µg/dL) (SI: 172.5 nmol/L [94.02-213.68 nmol/L])
Free T_4 = 1.91 ng/dL (0.8-1.8 ng/dL) (SI: 24.6 pmol/L [10.30-23.17 pmol/L])
Total T_3 = 65 ng/dL (70-200 ng/dL) (SI: 1.0 nmol/L [1.08-3.08 nmol/L])
TSH = 4.1 mIU/L (0.5-5.0 mIU/L)

Which of the following is the most likely explanation for these findings?
   A. Type 1 amiodarone-induced thyrotoxicosis
   B. Type 2 amiodarone-induced thyrotoxicosis
   C. Expected changes in euthyroid patients on amiodarone
   D. Assay interference by amiodarone metabolites
   E. Euthyroid sick syndrome

4 A 24-year-old woman presents for initial evaluation. She has a history of developmental delay. Her physical examination is notable for round facies and shortened fourth metacarpals. Her height is 59 in (152 cm), and weight is 186 lb (84 kg) (BMI = 37.6 kg/m^2). Her thyroid is soft to palpation, has no nodules, and measures 20 g. She reports that her mother has a history of hypocalcemia, but she is not aware of any details of her mother's diagnosis. The patient currently takes no medications.

Laboratory test results:
  Calcium = 6.9 mg/dL (8.2-10.2 mg/dL)
    (SI: 1.7 mmol/L [2.1-2.6 mmol/L])
  Phosphate = 5.1 mg/dL (2.3-4.7 mg/dL)
    (SI: 1.6 mmol/L [0.7-1.5 mmol/L])
  Albumin = 3.9 mg/dL (3.5-5.0 g/dL) (SI: 39 g/L
    [35-50 g/L])
  PTH = 103 pg/mL (10-65 pg/mL) (SI: 103 ng/L
    [10-65 ng/L])
  TSH = 9.74 mIU/L (0.5-5.0 mIU/L)

Which of the following is the most likely underlying mechanism for this patient's TSH elevation?
  A. Heterophilic antibody interference with the TSH assay
  B. Hashimoto thyroiditis
  C. Resistance to TSH
  D. TSH-secreting pituitary adenoma
  E. Thyroid hormone transporter defect

5 A 42-year-old man is seen for follow-up of a right-sided thyroid nodule. His nodule was first assessed 8 years ago, after being noted incidentally on a chest CT. He has no family history of thyroid cancer and no personal history of head or neck radiation exposure. He underwent FNAB at an outside institution 8 years ago, this was interpreted as Bethesda II (benign). The nodule was biopsied a second time 3 years ago for growth in maximal dimension from 1.9 cm to 3.1 cm. The second biopsy findings were again interpreted as benign. On ultrasonography now, the nodule measures 2.8 cm × 2.4 cm × 3.8 cm (*see image*). There is no cervical lymphadenopathy. He has no compressive symptoms. His serum TSH level is 2.01 mIU/L (0.5-5.0 mIU/L).

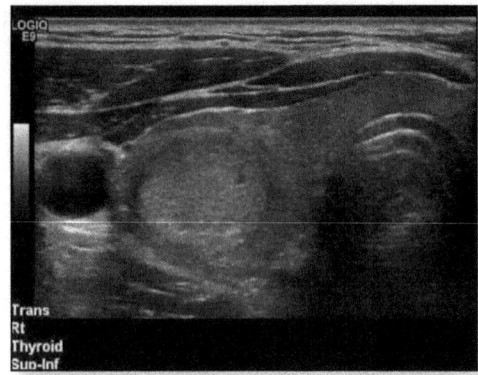

Bahn RS, Castro MR. *J Clin Endocrinol Metab.* 2011;96(5):1202-1212.

Which of the following is the most appropriate next step in the management of this nodule?
  A. Thyroid lobectomy
  B. Another ultrasound-guided FNAB
  C. Ultrasonography again in 6 months
  D. Core biopsy
  E. Continued monitoring for compressive symptoms

6 A 36-year-old woman presents with a new 14-lb (4.5-kg) weight gain, constipation, irregular menses, and cold intolerance. She gets up very early in the morning for her job as a school bus driver and reports that she is exhausted by the early afternoon.

Laboratory test results (sample collected while fasting):
  TSH = 134 mIU/L (0.5-5.0 mIU/L)
  Free T$_4$ = 0.2 ng/dL (0.8-1.8 ng/dL) (SI: 2.6 pmol/L
    [10.30-23.17 pmol/L])
  TPO antibodies = 466 IU/mL (<2.0 IU/mL)
    (SI: 466 kIU/L [<2.0 kIU/L])
  LDL cholesterol = 201 mg/dL (<100 mg/dL
    [optimal]) (SI: 5.21 mmol/L [<2.59 mmol/L])
  Total cholesterol = 300 mg/dL (<200 mg/dL
    [optimal]) (SI: 7.77 mmol/L [<5.18 mmol/L])
  HDL cholesterol = 52 mg/dL (>60 mg/dL
    [optimal]) (SI: 1.35 mmol/L [>1.55 mmol/L])
  Triglycerides = 195 mg/dL (<150 mg/dL [optimal])
    (SI: 2.20 mmol/L [<1.70 mmol/L])
  Homocysteine = 2.97 mg/L (≤1.76 mg/L)
    (SI: 22 µmol/L [≤13 µmol/L])

Levothyroxine is started.

Once she is euthyroid, which of the following effects should the patient anticipate as a result of levothyroxine therapy?

A. Significant loss of fat mass
B. Decreased total cholesterol and increased HDL cholesterol
C. Increased serum homocysteine
D. Restoration of ovulatory menstrual cycles

7 A 52-year-old woman presents with enlargement of her anterior neck over the last 6 months. Her TSH level is 0.96 mIU/L (0.5-5.0 mIU/L). Ultrasonography shows a 4.2-cm simple cyst in the left lobe extending into the isthmus. After aspiration of 10 cc of dark brown fluid, the nodule decreases in size to 3.1 cm. Cytopathologic results are interpreted as Bethesda I (nondiagnostic). Three months after her initial visit and cyst aspiration, repeat ultrasonography shows that the cyst fluid has completely reaccumulated. She describes a constant pressure sensation in her anterior neck and discomfort when she lies flat. The patient strongly wishes to avoid surgery.

Which of the following is the best option for control of compressive symptoms?

A. Reaspiration of the cyst
B. Ethanol injection of the cyst
C. Radiofrequency ablation
D. Laser ablation
E. Radioactive iodine treatment

8 A 25-year-old woman is newly diagnosed with Graves hyperthyroidism and has recently started methimazole, 30 mg daily. She has no eye disease. She and her husband are planning a first pregnancy within the next 1 to 2 years, and she is very concerned about the risks her Graves disease will pose for a potential fetus. Her menses are regular and she has no other medical history.

Which of the following is the best strategy to reduce the risk of fetal malformations?

A. Recommend radioactive iodine treatment at least 6 months before pregnancy with normalization of TSH on levothyroxine before conception
B. Change from methimazole to propylthiouracil before conception
C. Change from methimazole to propylthiouracil as soon as pregnancy is diagnosed
D. Decrease the methimazole dosage to the lowest possible to maintain free T_4 just above the upper normal limit once pregnancy is diagnosed

9 A 59-year-old man presented 5 months ago with a palpable left-sided thyroid nodule. Thyroid ultrasonography demonstrated a solitary hypoechoic nodule with regular margins. FNAB of the nodule was interpreted as Bethesda III (atypia of uncertain significance/follicular lesion of uncertain significance) and he subsequently underwent left thyroid lobectomy 6 weeks ago. Surgical pathology revealed a 3.2-cm fully encapsulated tumor. This had a follicular growth pattern with less than 1% papillae and no psammoma bodies. No vascular or capsular invasion was detected after complete examination of the capsule. Nuclear enlargement, overlapping, and grooves were noted. There was no tumor necrosis.

Laboratory test results:
Serum TSH = 1.04 mIU/L (0.5-53.0 mIU/L)
Thyroglobulin antibodies = <4.0 IU/mL (≤4.0 IU/mL) (SI: <4.0 kIU/L [≤4.0 kIU/L])
Thyroglobulin = 6 ng/mL (3-42 ng/mL) (SI: 6 μg/L [3-42 μg/L])

He returns today to discuss the surgical pathology and next steps for management.

Which of the following is the best next step in this patient's management?

    A. Completion thyroidectomy

    B. Completion thyroidectomy followed by radioiodine remnant ablation

    C. Levothyroxine therapy to keep TSH suppressed to less than 0.1 mIU/L

    D. Levothyroxine therapy with a goal TSH between 0.5 and 2.0 mIU/L

10 A 52-year-old woman was recently admitted to the hospital with altered mental status. Her family reports worsening dementia, confusion, and somnolence over the last several weeks.

On physical examination, she is afebrile, her pulse rate is 89 beats/min, and blood pressure is 112/66 mm Hg. She has a tremor and diffuse hyperreflexia. There is no periorbital edema.

Nonspecific slowing of background activity is seen on electrocardiography. Findings on brain MRI are normal. Serum electrolytes, creatinine, glucose, calcium, complete blood count, and urinalysis and urine culture are all normal, and toxicology screening is negative. The cerebrospinal fluid protein concentration is elevated at 96 mg/dL; other cerebrospinal laboratory values, including cultures, are normal.

Laboratory test results:

    TSH = 8.74 mIU/L (0.5-5.0 mIU/L)

    Free T_4 = 1.1 ng/dL(0.8-1.8 ng/dL) (SI: 14.2 pmol/L [10.30-23.17 pmol/L])

    TPO antibodies = 1456 IU/mL(<2.0 IU/mL) (SI: 1456 kIU/L [<2.0 kIU/L])

    Thyroglobulin antibodies = 340 IU/mL (≤4.0 IU/mL) (SI: 340 kIU/L [≤4.0 kIU/L])

Which of the following treatments is most likely to improve her mental status?

    A. Initial intravenous levothyroxine, 200 mcg, and liothyronine, 10 mcg, followed by daily intravenous doses of levothyroxine, 100 mcg, and liothyronine, 5 mcg

    B. Initial intravenous levothyroxine, 300 mcg, followed by daily intravenous doses of 150 mcg

    C. Oral levothyroxine, 75 mcg daily

    D. Oral prednisone, 60 mg daily

    E. SSKI, 5 drops daily

11 A 48-year-old woman with a history of thyrotoxicosis due to a 2.2-cm TSH-producing pituitary macroadenoma invading the cavernous sinus undergoes transsphenoidal surgery. Postoperatively, the patient is noted to have persistent hyperthyroidism.

Thyroid function test results:

    Free T_4 = 4.7 ng/mL (0.8-1.8 ng/mL) (SI: 60.5 pmol/L [10.30-23.17 pmol/L])

    TSH = 4.8 mIU/L (0.5-5.0 mIU/L)

MRI of the sella turcica at 1 month shows a persistent but decreased pituitary mass.

Which of the following is the most appropriate initial intervention now?

    A. Thyroidectomy

    B. Methimazole

    C. Bromocriptine

    D. Triiodothyroacetic acid (TRIAC)

    E. Octreotide

12 A 47-year-old woman who is having difficulty losing weight is referred for abnormal thyroid function test results. She is otherwise asymptomatic and takes no medications. Her mother has hypothyroidism.

On physical examination, her pulse rate is 86 beats/min. Her thyroid is slightly enlarged without nodules or bruit, there is no tremor, and deep tendon reflexes are normal.

Laboratory test results:

    TSH = 0.02 mIU/L (0.5-5.0 mIU/L)

    Free T_4 = 1.7 ng/dL (0.8-1.8 ng/mL) (SI: 21.9 pmol/L [10.30-23.17 pmol/L])

    Total T_3 = 154 ng/dL (70-200 ng/dL) (SI: 2.4 nmol/L [1.08-3.08 nmol/L])

    Thyroid-stimulating immunoglobulin = 124% (normal ≤120%)

Which of the following is the best next step in this patient's management?

    A. Start methimazole, 20 mg daily

    B. Start atenolol, 50 mg daily

    C. Treat with radioiodine therapy

    D. Repeat laboratory tests in 3 months

13 A 54-year-old woman with longstanding nontoxic multinodular goiter reports taking high doses of a nutritional supplement marketed for thyroid health for the last 4 months. Two months ago, she developed palpitations, tremor, heat intolerance, and weight loss.

Laboratory test results:

TSH = <0.01 mIU/L (0.5-5.0 mIU/L)

Total T_3 = 287 ng/dL (70-200 ng/dL)
  (SI: 4.4 nmol/L [1.08-3.08 nmol/L])

Free T_4 = 3.9 ng/dL (0.8-1.8 ng/dL)
  (SI: 50.2 pmol/L [10.30-23.17 pmol/L])

TPO antibodies = <2.0 IU/mL (<2.0 IU/mL)
  (SI: <2.0 kIU/L [<2.0 kIU/L])

Serum thyroglobulin = 79 ng/mL (3-42 ng/mL)
  (SI: 79 µg/L [3-42 µg/L])

Which of the following is most likely to be present in the supplements?
  A. Selenium
  B. Iodine
  C. Thyroid hormone extract
  D. Perchlorate
  E. Biotin

14 A 72-year-old woman has a history of papillary thyroid cancer. Five years ago, she underwent total thyroidectomy for a 4.2-cm papillary cancer with extrathyroidal invasion. She was subsequently treated with 100 mCi radioactive iodine. On her initial posttreatment scan, there was uptake only in the thyroid bed. Three years ago, she underwent repeated radioactive iodine treatment with 100 mCi for persistent thyroglobulin elevation, with no uptake on her posttreatment scan and no subsequent change in her serum thyroglobulin levels. She feels well. She is currently taking levothyroxine, 137 mcg daily.

On physical examination, her blood pressure is 128/72 mm Hg and pulse rate is 84 beats/min. There is no palpable thyroid tissue or cervical lymphadenopathy.

Laboratory test results:

TSH = 0.2 mIU/L (0.5-5.0 mIU/L)

Thyroglobulin antibodies = <4.0 IU/mL
  (≤4.0 IU/mL) (SI: <4.0 kIU/L [≤4.0 kIU/L])

Thyroglobulin = 11 ng/mL (3-42 ng/mL)
  (SI: 11 µg/L [3-42 µg/L])

Her serum thyroglobulin has been stable for the last 3 years. Neck ultrasonography shows no sign of tumor recurrence. No tumor foci are observed on PET/CT imaging. On a recent DXA, her T-score was –2.7 at the spine and –1.9 at the hip. She has not fractured.

Which of the following management strategies is most appropriate for this patient?
  A. Continue current levothyroxine
  B. Increase levothyroxine for goal TSH less than 0.01 mIU/L
  C. Treat with sorafenib
  D. Treat with radioactive iodine

15 A 44-year-old man with a remote history of Graves disease is referred for evaluation. Three years earlier, he developed ocular pain, chemosis, and eyelid swelling after receiving radioiodine therapy. Currently he has persistent diplopia and inability to fully close his eyes while sleeping.

On physical examination, he has pain with eye movement, but no conjunctival erythema or edema and no lid swelling. Proptosis measures 26 mm on the right side and 28 mm on the left side, with dysconjugate gaze (*see image*). He takes levothyroxine, and his current TSH concentration is 1.2 mIU/L (0.5-5.0 mIU/L).

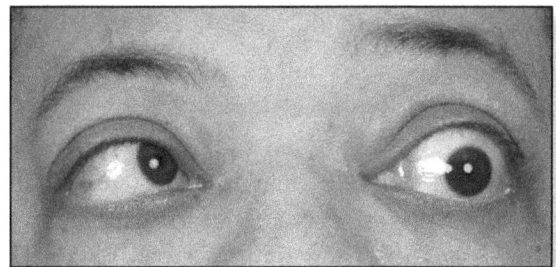

Which of the following should be recommended for this patient?
  A. Orbital radiotherapy
  B. Rituximab therapy
  C. Pulse corticosteroid therapy
  D. Orbital decompression followed by strabismus surgery
  E. Strabismus surgery alone

16 A 44-year-old woman with surgical hypo-thyroidism and type 2 diabetes mellitus is referred for a progressively increasing levothyroxine dosage requirement over the past 12 months. Other medications include metformin, lisinopril, and aspirin. She reports strict adherence to her therapeutic regimen and takes no over-the-counter preparations.

On physical examination, her blood pressure is 140/88 mm Hg. She has a small goiter, normal deep-tendon reflexes, and moderate lower-extremity edema.

Laboratory test results:
Serum TSH = 8.7 mIU/L (0.5-5.0 mIU/L)
Free T_4 = 1.2 ng/dL (0.8-1.8 ng/dL)
  (SI: 15.4 pmol/L [10.30-23.17 pmol/L])
Total cholesterol = 305 mg/dL (<200 mg/dL
  [optimal]) (SI: 7.90 mmol/L [<5.18 mmol/L])
Triglycerides = 880 mg/dL (<150 mg/dL [optimal])
  (SI: 9.94 mmol/L [<1.70 mmol/L])
Serum albumin = 2.6 g/dL (3.5-5.0 g/dL)
  (SI: 26 g/L [35-50 g/L])
Hemoglobin A_{1c} = 7.1% (4.0%-5.6%)
  (54 mmol/mol [20-38 mmol/mol])
Urinalysis, positive for protein (2.2 g/g creatinine)

Which of the following is the most likely cause of this patient's increasing levothyroxine dosage requirement?
  A. Metformin therapy
  B. Medication nonadherence
  C. Celiac disease
  D. Euthyroid sick syndrome
  E. Nephrotic syndrome

17 A 63-year-old man is being treated for a nonthyroid cancer. Before treatment initiation, his TSH concentration was 1.94 mIU/L (0.5-5.0 mIU/L) and his free T_4 concentration was 1.3 ng/dL (0.8-1.8 ng/dL) (SI: 16.7 pmol/L [10.30-23.17 pmol/L]). Ten weeks after starting the cancer therapy, he reports fatigue, constipation, and cold intolerance. Results from repeated thyroid function tests document a TSH concentration of 47 mIU/L and a free T_4 concentration of 0.5 ng/dL (SI: 6.4 pmol/L).

Which of the following medications is the most likely cause of his thyroid dysfunction?
  A. Sunitinib
  B. Denileukin diftitox
  C. Bexarotene
  D. Ipilimumab

18 A 62-year-old woman with weight gain and fatigue is found by her primary care physician to have an elevated serum TSH level. Levothyroxine is prescribed. She is referred to you for assistance in managing levothyroxine replacement therapy. In addition to levothyroxine, she takes calcium and multivitamins with iron.

On physical examination, her pulse rate is 80 beats/min, she has no goiter or thyroidectomy scar, and her deep tendon reflexes are normal. Serial thyroid function test results and levothyroxine dosing are shown (*see table*).

Date	TSH (reference range, 0.5-5.0 mIU/L)	Free T_4 (reference range, 0.8-1.8 ng/dL [10.30-23.17 pmol/L])	Levothyroxine Dosage
January	11.9 mIU/L	1.3 ng/dL (16.7 pmol/L)	None
March	10.2 mIU/L	1.8 ng/dL (23.2 pmol/L)	75 mcg daily
May	10.7 mIU/L	2.1 ng/dL (27.0 pmol/L)	112 mcg daily

Which of the following is the most likely explanation for these findings?
  A. Poor absorption of levothyroxine
  B. Resistance to thyroid hormone
  C. TSH-secreting pituitary adenoma
  D. Poor adherence to therapy
  E. Heterophilic antibody interference with the TSH assay

19 A 75-year-old woman with longstanding subclinical hyperthyroidism takes methimazole, 5 mg daily, and is concerned about fatigue.

On physical examination, her pulse rate is 64 beats/min and her thyroid is enlarged and nodular.

Laboratory test results:
TSH = 8.9 mIU/L (0.5-5.0 mIU/L)
Free T_4 = 0.75 ng/dL (0.8-1.8 ng/dL)
  (SI: 9.7 pmol/L [10.30-23.17 pmol/L])

Thyroid scan from 2 years earlier is shown (*see image*).

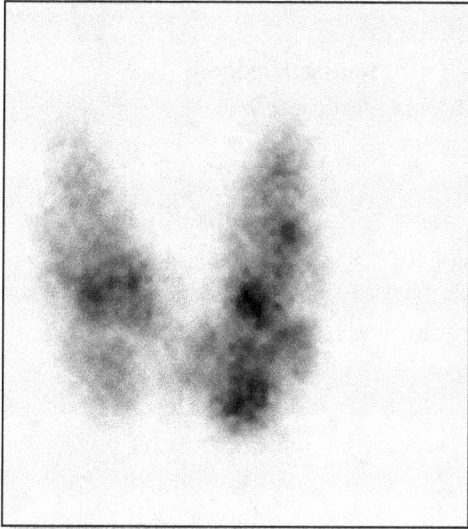

Which of the following is the most important next step in this patient's management?
A. Perform the thyroid scan again with radioactive iodine uptake
B. Reduce the methimazole dosage
C. Discontinue methimazole and start levothyroxine therapy
D. Discontinue methimazole

20 A 27-year-old man is noted to have a goiter and is referred for further evaluation. The patient's medical history is otherwise unremarkable. On physical examination, the patient's pulse rate is 90 beats/min. He has a diffuse goiter, twice normal size, without nodule or bruit. Deep tendon reflexes are normal and he has no tremor.

Laboratory test results:
   Free T_4 = 2.7 ng/dL(0.8-1.8 ng/dL) (SI: 34.8 pmol/L [10.30-23.17 pmol/L])
   Total T_3 = 300 ng/dL (70-200 ng/dL) (SI: 4.6 nmol/L [1.08-3.08 nmol/L])
   TSH = 3.8 mIU/L (0.5-5.0 mIU/L)
   α-subunit = 0.3 ng/mL (<1.2 ng/mL)

MRI of the pituitary is normal. There is a linear pattern of TSH values with serial dilution.

Which of the following is the most likely explanation?
A. Thyroid hormone resistance
B. A TSH-producing pituitary adenoma
C. Heterophilic antibody interference with the TSH assay
D. T_4 antibody interference with the free T_4 assay
E. Surreptitious use of thyroid hormone

21 Which of the following nodules is most likely to have an FNAB result suggestive of thyroid cancer?

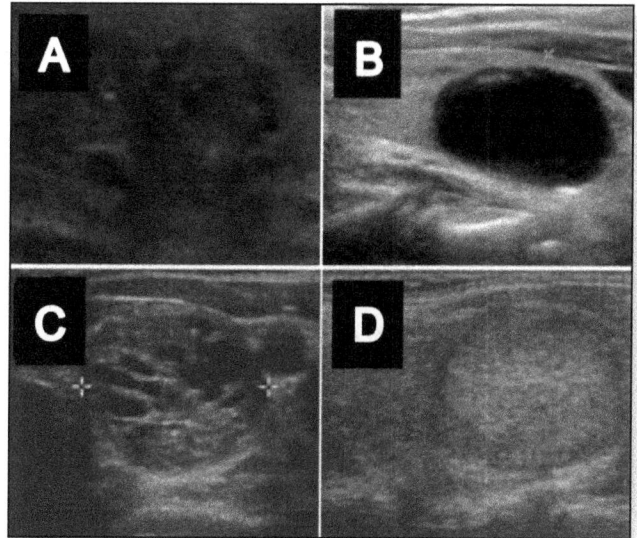

A. Figure A
B. Figure B
C. Figure C
D. Figure D

22 A 39-year-old woman presents with a 2.0-cm nodule at the lower pole of the left thyroid lobe (*see image*). FNAB reveals watery, clear, colorless fluid.

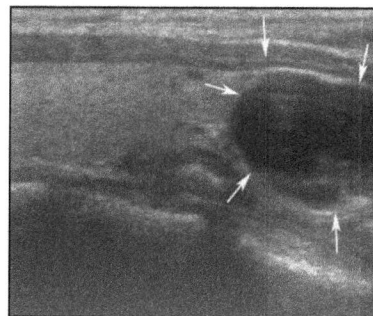

Which of the following is the most likely diagnosis?
   A. Branchial cleft cyst
   B. Follicular thyroid carcinoma
   C. Thyroglossal duct cyst
   D. Aberrant salivary gland cyst
   E. Parathyroid cyst

23 A 37-year-old woman is noted to have a 3.2-cm right thyroid nodule. She is in good health and takes no medications. Family history is negative for thyroid cancer.

On physical examination, her blood pressure is 118/78 mm Hg and pulse rate is 80 beats/min. She has no palpable lymph nodes in the neck.

Findings on FNAB are suggestive of medullary thyroid cancer.

Laboratory test results:
   Serum calcitonin = 420 pg/mL (<8 pg/mL)
     (SI: 122.6 pmol/L [<2.34 pmol/L])
   Serum calcium = 8.9 mg/dL (8.2-10.2 mg/dL)
     (SI: 2.2 mmol/L [2.1-2.6 mmol/L])
   PTH = 33 pg/mL (10-65 pg/mL) (SI: 33 ng/L
     [10-65 ng/L])
   Plasma metanephrines, normal

This patient should not undergo thyroidectomy until she has had which of the following assessments?
   A. Fluorodeoxyglucose PET scan
   B. Adrenal CT
   C. Neck ultrasonography
   D. Sestamibi scan

24 A 49-year-old woman has just undergone total thyroidectomy for a 3-cm nodule interpreted as Bethesda VI (malignant) on cytopathology. Surgical pathology showed a 3.2-cm unifocal classic variant of papillary thyroid cancer. Two of 6 resected lymph nodes were positive for tumor (with tumor foci measuring <0.2 cm in largest dimension). Surgical margins were negative, tumor capsule invasion was absent, venous/lymphatic invasion was absent, and perineural invasion was not identified. She comes to you to discuss radioactive iodine ablation.

Which of the following is the best next step in this patient's management?
   A. No radioactive iodine
   B. 30 mCi radioactive iodine
   C. 75 mCi radioactive iodine
   D. 100 mCi radioactive iodine

25 A 19-year-old college student describes intermittent inability to move his legs in the early morning. He has had several such episodes over the past 3 months, usually occurring after drinking alcohol the evening before. Episodes have resolved spontaneously within 1 to 2 hours. His last episode was 1 week ago. He has lost 10 lb (4.5 kg) during the past 6 months.

On physical examination, his pulse rate is 90 beats/min and he has a slight goiter. A fine tremor is noted and deep tendon reflexes are brisk, but findings on neurologic examination are otherwise normal.

Laboratory test results:
   Serum free T_4 = 2.5 ng/dL (0.8-1.8 ng/dL)
     (SI: 32.2 pmol/L [10.30-23.17 pmol/L])
   TSH = <0.01 mIU/L (0.5-5.0 mIU/L)
   Serum potassium = 4.1 mEq/L (3.5-5.0 mEq/L)
     (SI: 4.1 mmol/L [3.5-5.0 mmol/L])
   Calcium = 9.5 mg/dL (8.2-10.2 mg/dL)
     (SI: 2.4 mmol/L [2.1-2.6 mmol/L])
   Albumin = 4.1 g/dL (3.5-5.0 g/dL) (SI: 41 g/L
     [35-50 g/L])
   Magnesium = 2.2 mg/dL (1.5-2.3 mg/dL)
     (SI: 0.9 mmol/L [0.6-0.9 mmol/L])

Which of the following should be initiated as the most rapid means to prevent additional episodes?
   A. Methimazole
   B. Propranolol
   C. A daily potassium supplement
   D. A supervised exercise program
   E. Pyridostigmine

26 A 77-year-old woman with a history of Hashimoto hypothyroidism since age 42 years presents with rapid thyroid enlargement over the course of several weeks. While on levothyroxine, her serum TSH concentration is 1.34 mIU/L and her TPO antibody level is 462 IU/mL (462 kIU/L). Ultrasonography shows a markedly heterogeneous gland with a 5.4-cm left-sided nodule. FNAB of the nodule is performed (*see image*).

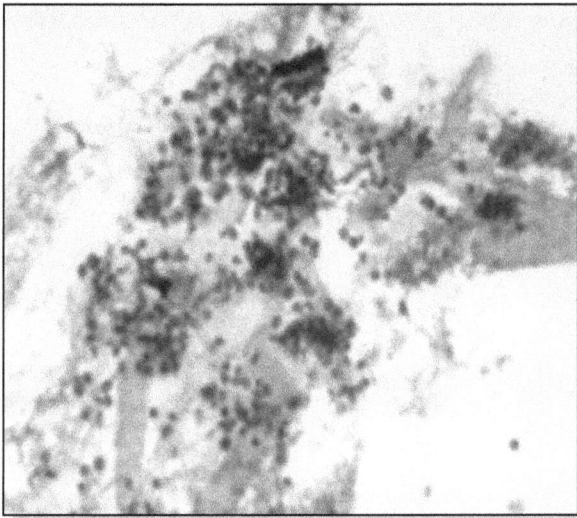

Which of the following is the best next step in this patient's management?

A. ^{123}I scan
B. Total thyroidectomy
C. Repeated FNAB with gene classifier testing
D. Repeated FNAB with flow cytometry

27 A 56-year-old woman with widely metastatic papillary thyroid carcinoma returns for follow-up. She underwent total thyroidectomy 8 years ago. She has subsequently been treated 3 times with radioactive iodine (cumulative dose 370 mCi). There was no uptake on her posttreatment scans after her second and third treatments. On recent PET/CT imaging, she had diffuse lung metastases throughout both lobes and widespread mediastinal lymphadenopathy. She has no brain lesions.

On physical examination, her blood pressure is 122/74 mm Hg, and pulse rate is 74 beats/min. Her weight is 142 lb (64.5 kg). She has been experiencing rapidly worsening exertional dyspnea.

Laboratory test results:
    Serum TSH = 0.1 mIU/L (0.5-5.0 mIU/L)
    Serum thyroglobulin = 1245 ng/mL (3-42 ng/mL)
      (SI: 1245 µg/L [3-42 µg/L]) (substantially increased from her last measurement 6 months ago)
    Thyroglobulin antibodies, negative

Which of the following is the best next step in her treatment?

A. Cytotoxic chemotherapy with doxorubicin and cisplatin
B. Lenvatinib
C. Ipilimumab
D. Palbociclib
E. No treatment

28 A 26-year-old woman is noted to have a 1.2-cm right thyroid nodule during the ninth week of pregnancy. The patient has no relevant medical history and her family history is negative for thyroid cancer. Ultrasonography reveals no suspicious features and FNAB is deferred. At 18 weeks' gestation, the nodule is noted to have a maximal diameter of 2.4 cm and is solid on ultrasonography.

On physical examination, in addition to the nodule, a 2-cm ipsilateral central compartment lymph node is noted. FNAB confirms papillary thyroid cancer in both the nodule and lymph node. Her serum TSH concentration is 0.9 mIU/L (0.5-5.0 mIU/L).

Which of the following is the best next step in this patient's management?

A. Start levothyroxine suppressive therapy
B. Refer for immediate total thyroidectomy with neck dissection
C. Defer surgery until the third trimester
D. Recommend no intervention until after delivery

29 A 47-year-old man is begun on a regimen of interferon alfa for chronic hepatitis C. Three months later, he reports palpitations and a 5-lb (2.3-kg) weight loss. He has no vision problems or neck pain.

On physical examination, his pulse rate is 95 beats/min, and his thyroid is 25 g without tenderness, nodules, or bruit.

Laboratory test results:
    TSH = <0.01 mIU/L (0.5-5.0 mIU/L)
    Free T$_4$ = 2.4 ng/dL (0.8-1.8 ng/dL)
      (SI: 29.6 pmol/L [10.30-23.17 pmol/L])
    TPO antibody titer = 230 IU/mL (<2.0 IU/mL)
      (SI: 180 kIU/L [<2.0 kIU/L])
    Radioactive iodine uptake at 24 hours = 0.4%

His hepatologist stops the interferon alfa.

Which of the following should you recommend now?
   A. Methimazole
   B. Prednisone
   C. Intravenous immunoglobulin
   D. Atenolol

30 A 56-year-old woman is found to have a thyroid nodule by her gynecologist. She has been in excellent health and takes no medications. Her family history is negative for thyroid cancer. Her serum TSH concentration is 1.8 mIU/L (0.5-5.0 mIU/L). The patient undergoes thyroid FNAB with findings of a predominance of normal-appearing groups of follicular cells and colloid, as well as occasional focal groups of cells with enlarged nuclei and nuclear grooves.

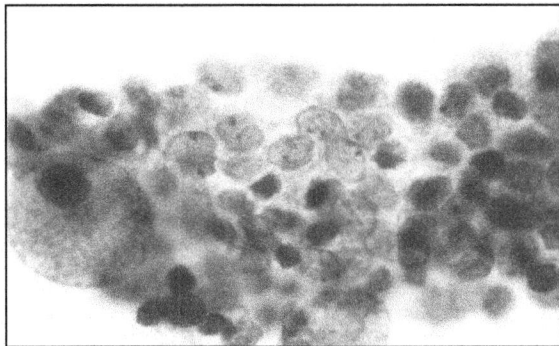

According to the Bethesda System for Reporting Thyroid Cytopathology, which of the following is the correct classification for this FNAB result?
   A. Nondiagnostic
   B. Benign
   C. Atypia of undetermined significance
   D. Suspicious for malignancy
   E. Malignant

ENDOCRINE
BOARD
REVIEW

Diabetes Mellitus, Section 1 Board Review

Serge A. Jabbour, MD • Thomas Jefferson University

1 ANSWER: A) Now

According to the American Diabetes Association guidelines, screening for diabetes should begin at age 45 years regardless of other factors such as ethnicity, family history, BMI, blood pressure, and dyslipidemia. Thus, this patient should be screened for diabetes now (Answer A). The US Preventive Services Task Force, the Centers for disease Control and Prevention, the Canadian Task Force on Preventive Health Care, and the International Diabetes Federation all recommend that screening start at age 40 to 45 years in asymptomatic patients.

In asymptomatic adults, diabetes screening should be considered in patients who are overweight or obese who have 1 or more of the following risk factors: first-degree relative with diabetes, high-risk race/ethnicity, history of cardiovascular disease, hypertension, HDL-cholesterol level <35 mg/dL (<0.90 mmol/L) and/or triglyceride level >250 mg/dL (>2.82 mmol/L), polycystic ovary syndrome (in women), and physical inactivity. Patients with prediabetes should have annual testing, and women diagnosed with gestational diabetes should have testing at least every 3 years.

EDUCATIONAL OBJECTIVE
Recommend when to screen for diabetes mellitus in an asymptomatic adult.

REFERENCE(S)
American Diabetes Association. Standards of medical care in diabetes-2018. *Diabetes Care.* 2018;41(Suppl 1):S1-S153.

Pottie K, Jaramillo A, Lewin G, et al; Canadian Task Force on Preventive Health Care. Recommendations on screening for type 2 diabetes in adults [published correction appears in *CMAJ.* 2012;184(16):1815]. *CMAJ.* 2012;184(15):1687-1696. PMID: 23073674

Siu AI; US Preventive Services Task Force. Screening for abnormal blood glucose and type 2 diabetes mellitus: U.S. Preventive Services Task Force Recommendation Statement. *Ann Intern Med.* 2015;163(11):861-868. PMID: 26501513

2 ANSWER: E) Eye examination

In a 2-year trial (SUSTAIN-6) involving patients with type 2 diabetes and high cardiovascular risk, more events of diabetic retinopathy complications occurred in patients treated with semaglutide (3.0%) compared with placebo (1.8%). The difference was seen very early in the trial (in the first 2 to 8 weeks). The absolute risk increase for diabetic retinopathy complications was larger among patients with a history of diabetic retinopathy at baseline (semaglutide, 8.2%; placebo, 5.2%) than among patients without a known history of diabetic retinopathy (semaglutide, 0.7%; placebo, 0.4%). Rapid improvement in glucose control has been associated with a temporary worsening of diabetic retinopathy. The applicability of such an association to semaglutide and retinopathy is unclear, and a direct effect of semaglutide cannot be ruled out. The effect of long-term glycemic control with semaglutide on diabetic retinopathy complications has not been studied. Patients with a history of diabetic retinopathy should be monitored for progression. Thus, this patient should have an eye examination (Answer E) at his follow-up visit.

GLP-1 receptor agonists have a boxed warning regarding the risk of C-cell tumors observed in rodents and a warning regarding acute pancreatitis. However, measuring calcitonin (Answer B) is not recommended unless there is a suspicion for medullary thyroid carcinoma (based on thyroid biopsy, family history, or presence of multiple endocrine neoplasia type 2). Similarly, it is not recommended to measure serum amylase and lipase (Answer A) unless the patient has gastrointestinal symptoms suggestive of acute pancreatitis.

GLP-1 receptor agonists have a warning regarding renal impairment/acute kidney injury, but this is in the setting of a patient with baseline kidney dysfunction and severe gastrointestinal symptoms (diarrhea, vomiting) leading to dehydration with subsequent worsening of the renal impairment. Thus, creatinine measurement (Answer D) is not necessary now.

GLP-1 receptor agonists have not been associated with foot injuries such as amputations (as opposed to certain SGLT-2 inhibitors). Thus, monofilament testing (Answer C) is not required now.

EDUCATIONAL OBJECTIVE
Monitor for progression of diabetic retinopathy in a patient with diabetes mellitus taking a GLP-1 receptor agonist.

REFERENCE(S)
Marso SP, Bain SC, Consoli A, et al; SUSTAIN-6 Investigators. Semaglutide and cardiovascular outcomes in patients with type 2 diabetes. *N Engl J Med.* 2016;375(19):1834-1844. PMID: 27633186

Semaglutide [package insert]. Plainsboro, NJ: Novo Nordisk; 2017.

Drab SR. Glucagon-like peptide-1 receptor agonists for type 2 diabetes: a clinical update of safety and efficacy. *Curr Diabetes Rev.* 2016;12(4):403-413. PMID: 26694823

3 ANSWER: D) Liraglutide

Of the agents listed as answer options, only liraglutide (Answer D) has been shown to significantly lower the 3-point major adverse cardiovascular events (MACE) in the LEADER trial. MACE includes the first occurrence of death of cardiovascular causes, nonfatal myocardial infarction, or nonfatal stroke. The other drugs (lixisenatide [Answer A], once-weekly exenatide [Answer B], sitagliptin [Answer C], alogliptin [Answer E]) were neutral regarding MACE in their respective trials (ELIXA, EXSCEL, TECOS, EXAMINE).

In the LEADER trial, the primary outcome (3-point MACE) occurred in significantly fewer patients in the liraglutide group (608 of 4668 patients [13.0%]) than in the placebo group (694 of 4672 patients [14.9%]) (hazard ratio, 0.87; 95% confidence interval, 0.78 to 0.97; *P* < .001 for non-inferiority; *P* = .01 for superiority). Because of the LEADER trial results, an additional indication was added to liraglutide prescribing information, which reads as follows:

Liraglutide is a GLP-1 receptor agonist indicated:

- As an adjunct to diet and exercise to improve glycemic control in adults with type 2 diabetes mellitus.
- To reduce the risk of major adverse cardiovascular events in adults with type 2 diabetes mellitus and established cardiovascular disease.

EDUCATIONAL OBJECTIVE
In patients with type 2 diabetes and established cardiovascular disease, recommend an agent to decrease hemoglobin A_{1c} and reduce the risk of major adverse cardiovascular events.

REFERENCE(S)
Marso SP, Daniels GH, Brown-Frandsen K, et al; LEADER Trial Investigators. Liraglutide and cardiovascular outcomes in type 2 diabetes. *N Engl J Med.* 2016;375(4):311-322. PMID: 27295427

Liraglutide [package insert]. Plainsboro, NJ: Novo Nordisk; 2017.

Semaglutide [package insert]. Plainsboro, NJ: Novo Nordisk; 2017.

Cefalu WT, Kaul S, Gerstein HC, et al. Cardiovascular outcomes trials in type 2 diabetes: where do we go from here? Reflections from a Diabetes Care Editors' Expert Forum. *Diabetes Care.* 2018;41(1):14-31. PMID: 29263194

4 ANSWER: E) Lixisenatide

Lixisenatide (Answer E), a once-daily GLP-1 receptor agonist, is the best option in this case, as the other drugs are not indicated.

Dapagliflozin (Answer A) and ertugliflozin (Answer D) are not indicated in patients with an estimated glomerular filtration rate less than 60 mL/min per 1.73 m². Dapagliflozin should not be used in patients with active bladder cancer. An imbalance in bladder cancers was observed in clinical trials (0.17% with dapagliflozin vs 0.03% with placebo/comparator). There were too few cases to determine whether the emergence of these events is related to dapagliflozin, and there were insufficient data to determine whether dapagliflozin has an effect on preexisting bladder tumors. Dapagliflozin should not be used in patients with active bladder cancer.

Canagliflozin (Answer B) is not indicated in patients with a history of lower limb amputation. An approximately 2-fold increased risk of lower limb amputations associated with canagliflozin use was observed in CANVAS and CANVAS-R, 2 large, randomized, placebo-controlled trials evaluating patients with type 2 diabetes who had either established cardiovascular disease or were at risk for cardiovascular disease. In CANVAS, canagliflozin-treated patients and placebo-treated patients had 5.9 and 2.8 amputations per 1000 patients per year, respectively. In CANVAS-R, canagliflozin-treated patients and placebo-treated patients had 7.5 and 4.2 amputations per 1000 patients per year, respectively. The risk of lower limb amputations was observed at both the 100 mg and 300 mg once-daily dosage regimens. Lower limb infections, gangrene, and diabetic foot ulcers were the most common precipitating medical events leading to the need for an amputation. The risk of amputation was highest in patients with a baseline history of amputation, peripheral vascular disease, and neuropathy.

In the cardiovascular outcome trial SAVOR-TIMI, 3.5% of patients who received saxagliptin (Answer C) were hospitalized for heart failure vs 2.8% of patients who received placebo. This is the same as 35 of every 1000 patients compared with 28 of every 1000 patients. Risk factors included history of heart failure or kidney impairment, as in the current case.

EDUCATIONAL OBJECTIVE
List contraindications of various oral agents used to treat type 2 diabetes mellitus.

REFERENCE(S)
Neal B, Perkovic V, Mahaffey KW, de Zeeuw D, et al; CANVAS Program Collaborative Group. Canagliflozin and cardiovascular and renal events in type 2 diabetes. *N Engl J Med.* 2017;377(7):644-657. PMID: 28605608

Scirica BM, Bhatt DL, Braunwald E, et al; SAVOR-TIMI 53 Steering Committee and Investigators. Saxagliptin and cardiovascular outcomes in patients with type 2 diabetes mellitus. *N Engl J Med.* 2013;369(14):1317-1326. PMID: 23992601

Dapagliflozin [package insert]. Wilmington, DE: AstraZeneca; 2017.

Ertugliflozin [package insert]. Whitehouse Station, NJ: Merck & Co, Inc; 2017.

Liraglutide [package insert]. Plainsboro, NJ: Novo Nordisk; 2017.

5   ANSWER: D) A3243G mutation in mitochondrial DNA

Maternally inherited diabetes and deafness (MIDD) is a rare form of diabetes first described in 1992. It is a mitochondrial disorder that is characterized by progressive insulinopenia and sensorineural hearing loss, most commonly caused by a genetic mutation at position 3243 (A to G substitution) in the tRNA (Answer D). Mitochondrial DNA is exclusively maternally inherited, so all offspring of an affected mother inherit the genetic defect. Because egg cells, but not sperm cells, contribute mitochondria to the developing embryo, only females pass mitochondrial conditions to their children. Mitochondrial disorders can appear in every generation of a family and can affect both males and females.

There is wide variability in the phenotypic expression of MIDD (*see box*). Onset of the diabetes phenotype usually occurs between ages 15 and 70 years, with a mean age of 32.8 to 38.8 years. The mean duration of diabetes before insulin dependence is only 3.9 years. The mean age of onset of hearing impairment is 33.2 years. Hearing loss is progressive and nearly universal. Impaired renal function and proteinuria from mitochondrial dysfunction is a known phenotype of this genetic disorder. As such, these complications may be misinterpreted as a diabetic microvascular complication. The renal lesions observed in MIDD include focal segmental glomerulosclerosis with hyalinized glomeruli and myocyte necrosis in afferent arterioles and small arteries. Macular pattern dystrophy is a retinal lesion that is commonly seen in MIDD. This has the appearance of linear pigmentation on the retina surrounding the macula and the optic disc. Patients can also have cardiac conduction defects (such as Wolf-Parkinson-White syndrome), myopathy, and exercise intolerance, which improves after coenzyme Q10 supplementation.

Reported clinical manifestations of the A3243G mitochondrial mutation
Diabetes
Sensorineural hearing loss
Cardiac issues
Conduction abnormalities (Wolf-Parkinson-White syndrome, atrial fibrillation, sick sinus syndrome
Cardiomyopathy (dilated and hypertrophic)
Neurologic disorders
Mitochondrial myopathy
Basal ganglia calcifications
Cerebellar ataxia
Oculomotor palsy
Weakness and exercise intolerance
Neuropsychiatric disorders
Mental retardation
Dementia
Depression
Psychosis
Ophthalmic disorders
Macular pattern degeneration
Cataracts
Renal disorders
Focal segmental glomerulosclerosis with hyalinized glomeruli
Myocyte necrosis in afferent arterioles and small arteries
Complications of pregnancy
Placenta accreta
Preterm labor

Zinc transporter 8 (ZnT8) antibodies (Answer A) and glutamic acid decarboxylase antibodies (GAD 65) (Answer B) test for type 1 diabetes/latent autoimmune diabetes in adults. Although she could possibly have type 1 diabetes given her BMI and rapid insulin dependence, the constellation of other findings makes MIDD much more likely. Both *GCK* (glucokinase) gene mutations (Answer B) and *HNF1A* (hepatocyte nuclear factor 1α) gene mutations (Answer E) lead to maturity-onset diabetes of the young, which occurs at an age younger than 25 years and can often be controlled with diet or a secretagogue.

EDUCATIONAL OBJECTIVE
Diagnose maternally inherited diabetes and deafness associated with the A3243G mitochondrial mutation.

REFERENCE(S)
Donovan LE, Severein NE0. Maternally inherited diabetes and deafness in the North American kindred: tips for making the diagnosis and review of unique management issues. *J Clin Endocrinol Metab*. 2006;91(12):4737-4742. PMID: 17018649

Naing A, Kenchaiah M, Krishnan B, et al. Maternally inherited diabetes and deafness (MIDD): diagnosis and management. *J Diabetes Complications*. 2014;28(4):542-546. PMID: 24746802

6 ANSWER: C) Intake of cow milk
It has been proposed that some component of albumin in cow milk (Answer C) (bovine serum albumin), the basis for most infant milk formulas, may trigger an autoimmune response. As an example, epidemiologic data from Finland suggest that there is an increased risk of type 1 diabetes associated with introduction to dairy products at an early age and with high milk consumption during childhood. It has also been suggested that a cell-mediated response to a specific cow milk protein, β-casein, may be involved in the pathogenesis of type 1 diabetes. In one report, 36 patients with recent-onset type 1 diabetes were compared with 36 normal participants. Exposure to bovine β-casein led to proliferation of peripheral blood T cells in 51% of the patients with type 1 diabetes vs in only 1 (3%) of the normal participants. In addition, an epidemiologic study of children from 10 countries revealed a strong correlation between the incidence of type 1 diabetes and the consumption of β-casein.

Although cow milk may be associated with an increased risk for type 1 diabetes, one component, vitamin D, may be protective. Support for this hypothesis comes from a case-control study in 7 European countries that suggests that vitamin D supplementation (Answer A) in early infancy can protect against development of type 1 diabetes. A similar protective effect was noted in a birth-cohort study of more than 10,000 children. The children who regularly took vitamin D (2000 IU daily) had a reduced risk of type 1 diabetes compared with children whose vitamin D intake was less (relative risk, 0.22).

In a case-control study from Norway, children with type 1 diabetes were less likely to be given cod liver oil (containing omega-3 fatty acids [Answer B] and vitamin D) during infancy than children without diabetes. In addition, a longitudinal observational study of children at increased risk for type 1 diabetes reported an inverse association between omega-3 fatty acid intake and development of islet autoimmunity (adjusted hazard ratio, 0.45; 95% confidence interval, 0.21-0.96).

Studies in Colorado and in Yorkshire (United Kingdom) have found that the incidence of type 1 diabetes correlates with the concentration of nitrates in the drinking water. The incidence is approximately 30% higher in areas with nitrate concentrations above 14.8 mg/L compared with areas with concentrations below 3.2 mg/L (Answer D).

A few observations suggest that exposure to enteroviruses or Coxsackie virus can induce β-cell damage and lead to clinical diabetes. However, some data also suggest that viruses might protect against diabetes. Rhinovirus (Answer E) has never been implicated in the pathogenesis of type 1 diabetes.

EDUCATIONAL OBJECTIVE
Identify environmental factors known to increase the risk of type 1 diabetes mellitus.

REFERENCE(S)

Knip M, Virtanen SM, Akerblom HK. Infant feeding and the risk of type 1 diabetes. *Am J Clin Nutr.* 2010;91(5):1506S-1513S. PMID: 20335552

Hyppönen E, Laara E, Reunanen A, Jarvelin MR, Virtanen SM. Intake of vitamin D and risk of type 1 diabetes: a birth-cohort study. *Lancet.* 2001;358(9292):1500-1503. PMID: 11705562

Norris JM, Yin X, Lamb MM, et al. Omega-3 polyunsaturated fatty acid intake and islet autoimmunity in children at increased risk for type 1 diabetes. *JAMA.* 2007;298(12):1420-1428. PMID: 17895458

Filippi CM, von Herrath MG. Viral trigger for type 1 diabetes. *Diabetes.* 2008;57(11):2863-2871. PMID: 18971433

7 **ANSWER: D) Lower the renal threshold for glucose excretion from 220 mg/dL to less than 100 mg/dL**
SGLTs cotransport sodium and glucose into cells using the sodium gradient produced by sodium-potassium ATPase pumps at the basolateral cell membranes. SGLT-2 is expressed in segments S1 and S2 of the proximal convoluted tubules and is responsible for renal reabsorption of glucose. Renal tubular reabsorption is known to undergo adaptations in the setting of uncontrolled diabetes. Particularly relevant in this context is the up-regulation of renal SGLT-2, which is an important adaptation in diabetes to maintain renal tubular glucose reabsorption. SGLT-2 is not present in the S3 segment (thus, Answer A is incorrect) or in the distal tubule (thus, Answer C is incorrect).

SGLT-2 inhibitors reduce filtered glucose reabsorption by epithelial cells of the kidney proximal tubule. The renal threshold for glucose reabsorption in patients with type 2 diabetes mellitus was reported to be between 200 and 250 mg/dL, which is higher than that of normal persons (170-200 mg/dL). SGLT-2 inhibitors, by blocking SGLT-2, lower the threshold from around 220 to 240 mg/dL to less than 100 mg/dL (thus, Answer D is correct and Answer B is incorrect).

EDUCATIONAL OBJECTIVE
Explain the mechanism of action of SGLT-2 inhibitors at the kidney level.

REFERENCE(S)

Nair S, Wilding JP. Sodium glucose cotransporter 2 inhibitors as a new treatment for diabetes mellitus. *J Clin Endocrinol Metab.* 2010;95(1):34-42. PMID: 19892839

Osaki A, Okada S, Saito T, et al. Renal threshold for glucose reabsorption predicts diabetes improvement by sodium glucose cotransporter 2 inhibitor therapy. *J Diabetes Investig.* 2016;7(5):751-754. PMID: 27181936

8 **ANSWER: E) Canagliflozin**
In this case, the patient's blood glucose fingerstick values are consistent with her hemoglobin A_{1c} level of 6.8% (51 mmol/mol). However, her 1,5-anhydroglucitol level is less than 10 µg/mL (which indicates poor glycemic control, mostly postprandially with blood glucose peaks above 180 mg/dL after meals). This discrepancy indicates that there is some interference with 1,5-anhydroglucitol measurement in this patient. Anemia (Answer A), iron supplementation (Answer B), and sickle cell trait/disease (Answer C) can affect hemoglobin A_{1c} measurement. However, we know this patient has an accurate hemoglobin A_{1c},

as it is consistent with the blood glucose finger-stick measurements, but not 1,5-anhydroglucitol. Cinnamon (Answer D) does not interfere with any of these tests.

Measurement of serum 1,5-anhydroglucitol, a naturally occurring dietary polyol (a monosaccharide that is structurally similar to glucose), is another assessment to provide information on daily glycemic variations. When blood glucose levels are well controlled, most circulating 1,5-anhydroglucitol is reabsorbed in the kidneys instead of being excreted in the urine. In healthy individuals, circulating levels of 1,5-anhydroglucitol are high, with median values exceeding 20 µg/mL.

Renal reabsorption of 1,5-anhydroglucitol is competitively inhibited by glucose. Therefore, when blood glucose levels are high (above 180 mg/dL [>9.9 mmol/L]), glucosuria occurs, blocking 1,5-anhydroglucitol reabsorption, and most is excreted in the urine. Individuals with type 2 diabetes and low circulating levels of 1,5-anhydroglucitol (<10 µg/mL) have more frequent and extreme hyperglycemic excursions over the previous 2-week period. An optimal 1,5-anhydroglucitol level in patients with diabetes is greater than 10 µg/mL.

SGLT-2 inhibitors decrease plasma glucose in patients with hyperglycemia by inhibiting renal glucose reabsorption via SGLT-2 (the primary renal transporter responsible for reabsorption of glucose from the urine), thereby increasing urinary glucose excretion, as well as 1,5-anhydroglucitol excretion. Thus, interference with the 1,5-anhydroglucitol assay by SGLT-2 inhibitors (Answer E) may lead to falsely low serum 1,5-anhydroglucitol measurements in patients with improved glycemic control who are treated with this class of agent.

EDUCATIONAL OBJECTIVE
Identify SGLT-2 inhibitors as a factor in falsely low serum 1,5-anhydroglucitol measurements in patients with improved glycemic control.

REFERENCE(S)
Wang Y, Zhang YL, Wang YP, Lei CH, Sun ZL. A study on the association of serum 1,5-anhydroglucitol levels and the hyperglycaemic excursions as measured by continuous glucose monitoring system among people with type 2 diabetes in China. *Diabetes Metab Res Rev.* 2012;28(4):357-362. PMID: 22238204

Dungan KM, Buse JB, Largay J, et al. 1,5-anhydroglucitol and postpriandal hyperglycemia as measured by continuous glucose monitoring system in moderately controlled patients with diabetes. *Diabetes Care.* 2006;29(6):1214-1219. 16731998

Balis DA, Tong C, Meininger G. Effect of canagliflozin, a sodium-glucose cotransporter 2 inhibitor, on measurement of serum 1,5-anhydroglucitol. *J Diabetes.* 2014;6(4):378-381. PMID: 24330128

9 **ANSWER: B) Basal Rate = 0.6 units/h; Carbohydrate Ratio = 1 units/15 g; Sensitivity Factor = 1 unit/55 mg/dL**
Understanding how to convert a regimen of multiple daily injections to continuous subcutaneous insulin infusion is very important. Many articles explain the conversion, all summarized nicely in the 2014 American Association of Clinical Endocrinologists/American College of Endocrinology Consensus Statement. References may vary slightly regarding the conversion numbers. For example, the pump total daily dose (TDD) can be 0.75 to 1 × prepump TDD depending on the patient's glycemic control. The carbohydrate ratio is 450 to 500 divided by the TDD, and the insulin sensitivity factor is 1700 to 1800 divided by the TDD. Thus, the optimal parameters are listed in Answer B.

EDUCATIONAL OBJECTIVE
Convert a regimen of multiple daily insulin injections to insulin pump therapy in a patient with type 1 diabetes mellitus.

REFERENCE(S)

Grunberger C, Abelseth JM, Bailey TS, et al. Consensus statement by the American Association of Clinical Endocrinologists/ American College of Endocrinology Insulin Pump Management Task Force. *Endocr Pract.* 2014;20(5):463-489. PMID: 24816754

Bode BW, Kyllo J, Kaufman ER. *Pumping Protocol: A Guide to Insulin Pump Initiation.* Medical Education Academia. Northridge, CA: Medtronic, 2013.

10 ANSWER: A) Type 1 diabetes mellitus

The lesion in the photograph is necrobiosis lipoidica, which frequently occurs in association with diabetes mellitus (Answer A), thus accounting for the past use of the term *necrobiosis lipoidica diabeticorum* for this condition. Necrobiosis lipoidica usually begins as asymptomatic, well-circumscribed, yellow to pink-brown or red-brown, slightly elevated papules or plaques. Erythema or a violaceous skin color may be present at the periphery. Necrobiosis lipoidica is most often found on the pretibial area, but can involve the scalp, face, trunk, genitals, or upper extremities. Biopsy of the lesion shows collagen degeneration with a granulomatous and inflammatory response, thickening of blood vessel walls, and fat deposition in the dermis.

The other listed conditions can have associated skin manifestations that look different from this patient's lesion. Glucagonoma (Answer C) is associated with necrolytic migratory erythema (biopsy would show superficial necrolysis with separation of the outer layers of the epidermis and perivascular infiltration with lymphocytes and histiocytes). Graves disease (Answer B) is associated with pretibial myxedema (biopsy would show mucinous edema and the fragmentation of collagen fibers with deposition of acid mucopolysaccharides [hyaluronic acid] in the papillary and reticular dermis). Pseudohypoparathyroidism (Answer D) can be associated with subcutaneous calcifications. Familial hypercholesterolemia (Answer E) can be associated with xanthomas (biopsy would show deposition of lipid and associated inflammation in the skin).

EDUCATIONAL OBJECTIVE
Diagnose necrobiosis lipoidica and recognize its association with diabetes mellitus.

REFERENCE(S)

Murphy-Chutorian B, Han G, Cohen SR. Dermatologic manifestations of diabetes mellitus: a review. *Endocrinol Metab Clin North Am.* 2013;42(4):869-898. PMID: 24286954

Reid SD, Ladizinski B, Lee K, Baibergenova A, Alavi A. Update on necrobiosis lipoidica: a review of etiology, diagnosis, and treatment options. *J Am Acad Dermatol.* 2013;69(5):783-791. PMID: 23969033

Jabbour SA. Skin manifestations of hormone-secreting tumors. *Dermatol Ther.* 2010;23(6):643-650. PMID: 21054708

11 ANSWER: C) Tissue transglutaminase IgA antibodies

About 5% of persons with type 1 diabetes develop celiac disease. Only a minority of children and adolescents with type 1 diabetes and celiac disease present with gastrointestinal symptoms. More common initial findings include unpredictable blood glucose measurements and recurrent episodes of hypoglycemia because of erratic intestinal absorption of nutrients. Thus, elevated tissue transglutaminase IgA antibodies (Answer C) would most likely explain her hypoglycemia.

Less than 1% of children with type 1 diabetes have autoimmune adrenalitis (Addison disease) (Answer A). In one report, about 2% of children with type 1 disease had circulating antibodies to steroid 21-hydroxylase (Answer D). Although less common than celiac disease, this condition is associated with decreased insulin requirement and increased frequency of hypoglycemia, hyperpigmentation, hypotension, hyponatremia, and hyperkalemia (none of which is present in this patient). Hyperthyroidism (Answer B) is rare in patients with type 1 diabetes (1%-2%) and can lead to higher blood glucose values due to insulin resistance, not hypoglycemia. In addition, except for weight loss, this patient has no symptoms or physical findings to suggest Graves disease. Antibodies to glutamic acid decarboxylase (a 65-kD protein) (Answer E) are found in about 70% of patients with type 1 diabetes at the time of diagnosis. They could very well be high in this patient, but this would not explain or be the cause of her hypoglycemia.

EDUCATIONAL OBJECTIVE
Describe the association of celiac disease with type 1 diabetes mellitus and recognize its presentation.

REFERENCE(S)

Khoury N, Semenkovich K, Arbeláez AM. Coeliac disease presenting as severe hypoglycaemia in youth with type 1 diabetes. *Diabet Med*. 2014;31(12):e33-e36. PMID: 24805141

Abid N, McGlone O, Cardwell C, McCallion W, Carson D. Clinical and metabolic effects of gluten free diet in children with type 1 diabetes and coeliac disease. *Pediatr Diabetes*. 2011;12(4 Pt 1):322-325. PMID: 21615651

Warncke K, Fröhlich-Reiterer EE, Thon A, Hofer SE, Wiemann D, Holl RW; DPV Initiative of the German Working Group for Pediatric Diabetology; German BMBF Competence Network for Diabetes Mellitus. Polyendocrinopathy in children, adolescents, and young adults with type 1 diabetes: a multicenter analysis of 28,671 patients from the German/Austrian DPV-Wiss database. *Diabetes Care*. 2010;33(9):2010-2012. PMID: 20551013

12 ANSWER: D) Begin monitoring glucose levels with a continuous glucose sensor

This patient exhibits hypoglycemia unawareness. He also has fasting hyperglycemia, which should raise the suspicion that he is experiencing hypoglycemia overnight that is going undetected, and is followed by rebound hyperglycemia in the morning. Therefore, increasing the basal rate 1 or 2 hours before morning hyperglycemia is typically observed (Answer A) is not the correct recommendation. Changing the method of insulin delivery would not be expected to correct the fasting hyperglycemia, and including long-acting insulin as you would find in a multiple daily injection regimen (Answer C) might increase the incidence of hypoglycemia. Eliminating the bedtime snack (Answer B) would only help if the patient were hyperglycemic throughout the night, which is unknown. To determine whether this is the case, it would be necessary to check the overnight glucose level by fingerstick (not an offered option) or a continuous glucose sensor (Answer D), which would also aid with hypoglycemia detection at other times of the day.

EDUCATIONAL OBJECTIVE
Recommend continuous glucose monitoring to detect hypoglycemia and devise strategies for its reduction in patients with longstanding type 1 diabetes mellitus.

REFERENCE(S)

Vloemans AF, van Beers CAJ, de Wit M, et al. Keeping safe. Continuous glucose monitoring (CGM) in persons with type 1 diabetes and impaired awareness of hypoglycaemia: a qualitative study. *Diabet Med*. 2017;34(10):1470-1476. PMID: 28731509

Oyer DS. The science of hypoglycemia in patients with diabetes. *Curr Diabetes Rev*. 2013;9(3):195-208. PMID: 23506375

Yeh H-C, Brown TT, Maruthur N, et al. Comparative effectiveness and safety of methods of insulin delivery and glucose monitoring for diabetes mellitus: a systematic review and meta-analysis. *Ann Intern Med*. 2012;157(5):336-347. PMID: 22777524

13 ANSWER: C) Gastric emptying study

In insulin-treated diabetic patients, gastroparesis (delayed gastric emptying) may lead to unexplained hypoglycemia, particularly early in the postprandial period. Gastroparesis often occurs in patients with longstanding diabetes and concomitant microvascular complications. Most patients with gastroparesis present with upper gastrointestinal symptoms, although the correlation of symptoms with delayed gastric emptying is weak, and some patients are asymptomatic. The rate of gastric emptying regulates the delivery of carbohydrates to the small intestine, and it has a major impact on postprandial blood glucose. Variations in the rate of gastric emptying account for 35% of the variance in the initial rise of blood glucose after a 75-g glucose load in healthy persons and those with diabetes. Nuclear medicine scintigraphy, or gastric emptying study (Answer C), remains the criterion standard for assessing gastric emptying, although inconsistency in its use may affect its diagnostic accuracy.

Although adrenal insufficiency can be a cause of unexplained hypoglycemia in a patient with type 1 diabetes, it is a less likely diagnosis in a patient with normal blood pressure and electrolytes and without symptoms of orthostasis. Thus, an ACTH stimulation test (Answer B) is incorrect. This patient is frustrated and stressed about her situation, and although psychiatric counseling (Answer A) may be helpful in dealing with any chronic condition, it is unlikely to uncover the cause of her hypoglycemia. Similarly, because she has had ongoing and recent nutrition counseling, poor carbohydrate counting skills (Answer D) are unlikely to be the reason for her frequent unexplained hypoglycemia.

EDUCATIONAL OBJECTIVE
Diagnose the etiology of unexplained recurrent hypoglycemia and glycemic variability.

REFERENCE(S)

Phillips LK, Deane AM, Jones KL, Rayner CK, Horowitz M. Gastric emptying and glycaemia in health and diabetes mellitus. *Nat Rev Endocrinol.* 2015;11(2):112-128. PMID: 25421372

Chang J, Rayner CK, Jones KL, Horowitz M. Diabetic gastroparesis and its impact on glycemia. *Endocrinol Metab Clin North Am.* 2010;39(4):745-762. PMID: 21095542

Samsom M, Bharucha A, Gerich JE, Hermann K, Limmer J, Linke R, et al. Diabetes mellitus and gastric emptying: questions and issues in clinical practice. *Diabetes Metab Res Rev.* 2009;25(6):502-514. PMID: 19610128

Ma J, Rayner CK, Jones KL, Horowitz M. Diabetic gastroparesis: diagnosis and management. *Drugs.* 2009;69(8):971-986. PMID: 19496627

14 **ANSWER: A) Improve glucose control to achieve a hemoglobin A_{1c} level <7.0% (<53 mmol/mol)**

This patient's poorly controlled diabetes could be due to lack of regular monitoring and insulin adjustment. She recognizes the need to improve her control, but she has lacked the motivation (and/or education) to do so, until faced with the facts that her father has had a myocardial infarction and that she may be able to do something to reduce her future risk for the same fate. Long-term follow-up of participants in the Diabetes Control and Complications Trial and the Epidemiology of Diabetes Interventions and Complications trial (DCCT/EDIC) clearly showed that those who had early, intensive glycemic control vs more

conventional control had reduced incidence of cardiovascular events, even though later control was similar in the 2 groups (thus, Answer A is correct). Intensive treatment reduced the risk of any cardiovascular disease event by 42%. This phenomenon is referred to as "metabolic memory" or the "legacy effect"—ie, a period of excellent glycemic control during early treatment has positive effects many years later.

No real clinical trial data exist to show that starting a statin (Answer B) in a young patient (<40 years) with a 2-year history of diabetes and this lipid profile would lower cardiovascular risk. There is also no evidence to support starting an ACE inhibitor (Answer C). Lowering her basal insulin (Answer D) would not be helpful, as it is not the primary cause of her hypoglycemic events and would worsen her glycemic control.

EDUCATIONAL OBJECTIVE
Counsel patients with type 1 diabetes mellitus regarding the potential long-term benefits of early, good glycemic control on later cardiovascular risk.

REFERENCE(S)

American Diabetes Association. 9. Cardiovascular disease and risk management: standards of medical care in diabetes-2018. *Diabetes Care.* 2018;41(Suppl 1):S86-S104. PMID: 29222380

Nathan DM, Cleary PA, Backlund JY, et al; Diabetes Control and Complications Trial/Epidemiology of Diabetes Interventions and Complications (DCCT/EDIC) Study Research Group. Intensive diabetes treatment and cardiovascular disease in patients with type 1 diabetes. *N Engl J Med.* 2005;353(25):2643-2653. PMID: 16371630

15 **ANSWER: B) Start treatment with a statin**

The American College of Cardiology/American Heart Association Blood Cholesterol and the National Lipid Association Guidelines recommend statin treatment (Answer B) for patients such as the one described in this vignette (ie, individuals with diabetes aged 40 to 75 years with LDL-cholesterol levels between 70 and 189 mg/dL [1.81-4.90 mmol/L] and without clinical atherosclerotic cardiovascular disease).

After 19 years of diabetes, it is not clear whether a relatively minor reduction in hemoglobin A_{1c} from 7.2% to less than 7.0% (Answer A) would have any impact on his cardiovascular disease risk. His previous degree of glycemic control is much more important. Without clinical albuminuria, adding an ACE inhibitor (Answer C) would not be expected to result in a cardiovascular disease benefit in a normotensive, normoalbuminuric patient with type 1 diabetes. His BMI of 25.5 kg/m² is minimally elevated, thus much benefit from any weight loss (Answer D) is not expected.

EDUCATIONAL OBJECTIVE
Recommend statin use as part of cardiovascular risk reduction in patients with type 1 diabetes mellitus.

REFERENCE(S)

American Diabetes Association. 9. Cardiovascular disease and risk management: standards of medical care in diabetes-2018. *Diabetes Care.* 2018;41(Suppl 1):S86-S104. PMID: 29222380

Stone NJ, Robinson JG, Lichtenstein AH, et al; American College of Cardiology/American Heart Association Task Force on Practice Guidelines. 2013 ACC/AHA guideline on the treatment of blood cholesterol to reduce atherosclerotic cardiovascular risk in adults: a report of the American College of Cardiology/American Heart Association Task Force on Practice Guidelines [published correction appears in *Circulation.* 2014;129(25 Suppl 2):S46-S48]. *Circulation.* 2014;129(25 Suppl 2):S1-S45. PMID: 24222016

Jacobson TA, Ito MK, Maki KC, et al. National Lipid Association recommendations for patient-centered management of dyslipidemia: part 1 - executive summary. *J Clin Lipidol.* 2014;8(5):473-488. PMID: 25234560

Nathan DM, Cleary PA, Backlund JY, et al; Diabetes Control and Complications Trial/Epidemiology of Diabetes Interventions and Complications (DCCT/EDIC) Study Research Group. Intensive diabetes treatment and cardiovascular disease in patients with type 1 diabetes. *N Engl J Med.* 2005;353(25):2643-2653. PMID: 16371630

16 ANSWER: C) Myocardial infarction (decreased), stroke (decreased), cardiovascular death (decreased)

Published in 1993, the Diabetes Control and Complications Trial (DCCT) was a landmark study that compared the effects of intensive vs conventional control on the onset and progression of diabetes-related complications over 6.5 years in more than 1400 patients with type 1 diabetes. The DCCT demonstrated a substantial benefit of intensive insulin therapy in the primary prevention of diabetic retinopathy: at 9 years (mean 6.5 years), the incidence of new-onset retinopathy was 12% in the intensive therapy group vs 54% in the conventional therapy group. In addition to its efficacy in primary prevention, intensive insulin therapy also slows the rate of progression of mild to moderate retinopathy. At follow-up of up to 9 years (mean 6.5 years), intensive therapy led to a significant reduction in the incidence of new-onset microalbuminuria (16.4% vs 23.9%; adjusted risk reduction 39%). There was also a significant reduction in new-onset macroalbuminuria in the entire study population (3.2% vs 7.2%; adjusted risk reduction 51%). The incidence of confirmed clinical neuropathy (defined as findings from the history and physical examination that were confirmed by neurologic testing) was reduced with intensive insulin therapy by 64%. The DCCT documented a nonsignificant trend toward fewer cardiovascular events with intensive therapy (3.2% vs 5.4%; $P = .08$). The incidence of death was not reduced.

Following completion of the DCCT in 1993, the conventional treatment group was offered intensive treatment, and 93% of DCCT participants (n = 1394) agreed to participate in the observational Epidemiology of Diabetes Interventions and Complications (EDIC) study. Differences in glycated hemoglobin levels between the intensive and conventional treatment groups at the end of the DCCT trial (7.4% and 9.1%, respectively) narrowed at the end of the 11-year follow-up EDIC study (7.9% and 7.8%, respectively). Cardiovascular outcomes for the EDIC study were defined as the occurrence of nonfatal myocardial infarction, stroke, cardiovascular death, documented angina, or coronary revascularization. The analysis of cardiovascular events according to original DCCT treatment assignment was predetermined to conclude when 50 patients in the original conventional treatment group had experienced a cardiovascular event. During the entire follow-up period (mean 17 years), 46 events had occurred in 31 patients from the DCCT intensive therapy group, compared with 98 events in 52 patients from the conventional therapy group (0.38 vs 0.80 events per 100 patient-years). This represented a 42% decrease in any cardiovascular event (95% confidence interval, 9%-63%); there was also a 57% reduction in a serious cardiovascular event (nonfatal myocardial infarction, stroke, or death of cardiovascular disease [95% confidence interval, 12%-79%]) in the original DCCT intensive therapy group compared with the DCCT conventional treatment group (thus, Answer C is correct and Answers A, B, and D are incorrect).

EDUCATIONAL OBJECTIVE
Recall the findings of the Epidemiology of Diabetes Interventions and Complications study with regard to myocardial infarction, stroke, and death.

REFERENCE(S)
Diabetes Control and Complications Trial Research Group. The effect of intensive treatment of diabetes on the development and progression of long-term complications in insulin-dependent diabetes mellitus. *N Engl J Med.* 1993;329(14):977-986. PMID: 8366922

Diabetes Control and Complications Trial Research Group. Progression of retinopathy with intensive versus conventional treatment in the Diabetes Control and Complications Trial. *Ophthalmology.* 1995;102(4):647-661. PMID: 7724182

Nathan DM, Clearly PA, Backlund JY, et al; Diabetes Control and Complications Trial/Epidemiology of Diabetes Interventions and Complications (DCCT/EDIC) Study Research Group. Intensive diabetes treatment and cardiovascular disease in patients with type 1 diabetes. *N Engl J Med.* 2005;353(25):2643-2653. PMID: 16371630

17 ANSWER: D) Perform basal rate testing from breakfast until dinner

Changes to insulin pump settings should be based on identified patterns, such as the very frequent hypoglycemia that this patient is experiencing several days a week in the midafternoon. Either an excessive basal rate or a prelunch bolus may be the cause. To diagnose which component is responsible, one should perform basal rate testing (Answer D). In this case, with the hypoglycemia occurring midafternoon, the patient should fast and take no insulin bolus for at least 5 hours before the time in question. Fingerstick glucose values should be checked approximately hourly; if the value does not change by more than 30 mg/dL (1.7 mmol/L) over this period, then one can conclude that the basal rate is appropriate and that the bolus before the previous meal is causing the hypoglycemia. If the value drops by more than 30 mg/dL (1.7 mmol/L), the basal rate should be lowered at least 2 hours before the time that the hypoglycemia is occurring.

Increasing her carbohydrate intake at lunch (Answer A) or eating a carbohydrate snack at 2 or 3 PM (Answer B) may help some, but these options are not the best choices because they require the patient to ingest extra carbohydrate to counteract excessive insulin and they do nothing to help uncover or correct the cause of the hypoglycemia. Changing the prelunch carbohydrate ratio to 1:8 (Answer C) is incorrect because it would mean the patient would be getting *more*, not *less*, insulin before lunch, and this would most likely make the problem worse and/or cause the hypoglycemia to occur earlier.

EDUCATIONAL OBJECTIVE
Devise a strategy to identify and correct a common problem encountered with the use of continuous subcutaneous insulin infusion.

REFERENCE(S)
Bolderman KM. *Putting Your Patients on the Pump: Initiation and Maintenance Guidelines.* Alexandria, VA: American Diabetes Association; 2013.

Walsh J, Roberts R. *Pumping Insulin: Everything You Need for Success on a Smart Insulin Pump.* 5th ed. San Diego, CA: Torrey Pines Press; 2012.

Hirsch IB. Practical pearls in insulin pump therapy. *Diabetes Technol Ther*. 2010;12(Suppl 1):S23-S27. PMID: 20515302

18 ANSWER: B) Reduce all insulin doses by 10% to 20%

The "honeymoon" phase in type 1 diabetes mellitus is characterized by reduced exogenous insulin requirements in the face of well-maintained glycemic control. It may develop relatively soon after the diagnosis and is a transient phase of "remission," thought to be due either to adaptive immune tolerance or to some improvement in β-cell function. Improved residual insulin secretory function reduces the need for all exogenous insulins (thus, Answer B is correct), not only premeal or basal insulins (Answers A and C). Increasing her carbohydrate intake to at least 50 g with each meal (Answer D) is not the best choice, as it does not correct the problem of excessive insulin at mealtimes and it requires that the patient ingest extra calories.

EDUCATIONAL OBJECTIVE
Develop a strategy to manage glycemic levels during the "honeymoon" phase of type 1 diabetes mellitus.

REFERENCE(S)
Aly H, Gottlieb P. The honeymoon phase: intersection of metabolism and immunology. *Curr Opin Endocrinol Diabetes Obes*. 2009;16(4):286-292. PMID: 19506474

Akirav E, Kushner JA, Herold KC. Beta-cell mass and type 1 diabetes: going, going, gone? *Diabetes*. 2008;57(11):2883-2888. PMID: 18971435

19 ANSWER: A) Temporarily relax his tight glucose targets

Up to 30% of patients with type 1 or longstanding type 2 diabetes mellitus have impaired or absent awareness of hypoglycemia. As plasma glucose levels fall, compromised physiologic counterregulatory defenses include failure of an increase in glucagon secretion and attenuated epinephrine secretion. This, together with inability to reduce circulating insulin levels, results in the clinical syndrome of defective counterregulation, which markedly increases the risk of recurrent severe hypoglycemia. Hypoglycemia-attenuating defense

against subsequent hypoglycemia is a concept referred to as hypoglycemia-associated autonomic failure (HAAF). The mainstay therapy for HAAF is the scrupulous avoidance of hypoglycemia. Patients with hypoglycemia unawareness and/or severe hypoglycemia and tight control should be advised to relax their glucose targets for a period to allow awareness to potentially return with adrenergic symptoms (Answer A).

While clearly a patient should be advised to carry with them a source of readily absorbed glucose, if he only has neuroglycopenic symptoms, there would be nothing triggering him to use them, so it would be unlikely to prevent his hypoglycemia. Also, carrying a glucagon emergency kit (Answer B) would not help either as this is used by another person, not the patient, and a companion should be aware of the presence of the kit, as well as how to use it. Although an insulin pump (Answer C) may help reduce hypoglycemia, it would not address the underlying cause of the hypoglycemia unawareness (repetitive hypoglycemic episodes) or guarantee its avoidance. There would also be a delay in initiating pump therapy and a learning curve regarding its use. Even a pump with an automatic suspend function is only as good as its integrated continuous glucose sensor, which can be inaccurate. A patient using this type of pump must be reminded that he still must actively treat the hypoglycemia to prevent it from worsening. While a number of educational programs focusing on hypoglycemia detection and avoidance (Answer D) (Dose Adjustment for Normal Eating [DAFNE], Blood Glucose Awareness Training [BGAT], Hypoglycemia Awareness and Avoidance [HAAT]) have demonstrated effectiveness in reducing the occurrence of hypoglycemia, such an education program is not the most immediate fix for the patient, nor would it address the cause.

EDUCATIONAL OBJECTIVE
Recommend management for severe hypoglycemia and hypoglycemia unawareness in type 1 diabetes mellitus.

REFERENCE(S)

Little SA, Leelarathna L, Barendse SM, et al. Severe hypoglycaemia in type 1 diabetes mellitus: underlying drivers and potential strategies for successful prevention. *Diabetes Metab Res Rev.* 2014;30(3):175-190. PMID: 24185859

Morales J, Schneider D. Hypoglycemia. *Am J Med.* 2014;127(Suppl 10):S17-S24. PMID: 25282009

Alsahli M, Gerich JE. Hypoglycemia. *Endocrinol Metab Clin North Am.* 2013;42(4):657-676. PMID: 24286945

Awoniyi O, Rehman R, Dagogo-Jack S. Hypoglycemia in patients with type 1 diabetes: epidemiology, pathogenesis, and prevention. *Curr Diab Rep.* 2013;13(5):669-678. PMID: 23912765

Oyer DS. The science of hypoglycemia in patients with diabetes. *Curr Diabetes Rev.* 2013;9(3):195-208. PMID: 23506375

Choudhary P, Amiel SA. Hypoglycaemia: current management and controversies. *Postgrad Med.* 2011;87(1026):298-306. PMID: 21296797

Cryer PE. Mechanisms of hypoglycemia-associated autonomic failure in diabetes. *N Engl J Med.* 2013;69(4):362-372. PMID: 23883381

20 ANSWER: B) Add sitagliptin, 100 mg daily, to current metformin therapy

Unless there is intolerance or a contraindication, a combination of metformin as monotherapy plus lifestyle changes (eg, lifestyle counseling, weight-loss education, and exercise) is the preferred initial treatment of type 2 diabetes. The American Diabetes Association recommends that if the hemoglobin A_{1c} level is not 7.0% or lower (≤53 mmol/mol) after approximately 3 months of lifestyle management and metformin, therapy should be initiated with a dual combination of metformin and 1 of the following 6 treatment options: sulfonylurea, thiazolidinedione, DPP-4 inhibitor, GLP-1 agonist, SGLT-2 inhibitor, or basal insulin. Thus, because the patient has moderate to poor glycemic control on metformin monotherapy, the best course of action is to add sitagliptin (Answer B), an FDA-approved DPP-4 inhibitor, to her current regimen. The other 3 options (Answers A, C, and D) would result in monotherapy.

EDUCATIONAL OBJECTIVE
Guide therapy for type 2 diabetes mellitus when lifestyle efforts and metformin therapy fail to provide adequate glycemic control.

REFERENCE(S)

American Diabetes Association. Standards of medical care in diabetes-2018. *Diabetes Care.* 2018;41(Suppl 1):S1-S153.

Garber AJ, Abrahamson MJ, Barzilay JI, et al. Consensus statement by the American Association of Clinical Endocrinologists and American College of Endocrinology on the comprehensive type 2 diabetes management algorithm – 2018 executive summary. *Endocr Pract.* 2018;24(1):91-120. PMID: 29368965

21 ANSWER: B) Rosuvastatin, 20 mg daily

Current recommendations for statin treatment have been revised such that treatment initiation and the initial statin dosage are personalized on the basis of risk profile, rather than LDL-cholesterol levels. In patients with type 2 diabetes who are 40 years or older, moderate-intensity statin treatment, if clinically indicated, is recommended in addition to lifestyle counseling and behavioral modification. However, for patients with a high risk for cardiovascular disease such as this patient with a history of cardiovascular disease, high-intensity statin therapy is advised. Clinical trials have shown that individuals at high risk for cardiovascular disease have a significant reduction in further cardiovascular events with an aggressive regimen of high-intensity statin therapy. Currently, limited clinical trial evidence is available for statin therapy for persons older than 75 years or younger than 40 years. The only high-intensity statin therapy listed in the answer options is rosuvastatin, 20 mg daily (Answer B). Answers A, C, and D are all moderate-intensity statin therapy options.

EDUCATIONAL OBJECTIVE
Recommend appropriate statin intensity dosing in patients with type 2 diabetes mellitus.

REFERENCE(S)

Stone NJ, Robinson JG, Lichtenstein AH, Bairey Merz CN, Blum CB, et al. 2013 ACC/AHA guideline on the treatment of blood cholesterol to reduce atherosclerotic cardiovascular risk in adults: a report of the American College of Cardiology/American Heart Association Task Force on Practice Guidelines [published correction appears in *J Am Coll Cardiol.* 2014;63(25 Pt B):3024-3025]. *J Am Coll Cardiol.* 2014;63(25 Pt B):2889-2934. PMID: 24239923

American Diabetes Association. 9. Cardiovascular disease and risk management. Standards of medical care in diabetes-2018. *Diabetes Care.* 2018;41(Suppl 1):S86-S104. PMID: 29222380

22 ANSWER: C) Transferrin saturation

Whenever diabetes is diagnosed, the possibility of secondary diabetes should be considered. Secondary diabetes occurs when a separate condition leads to hyperglycemia; these are considered distinct from routine type 1 or type 2 diabetes, although clinical features are often shared. Broad categories of secondary diabetes include medication-induced (eg, corticosteroids), other endocrinopathies (eg, acromegaly), pancreatic diseases (eg, pancreatitis), infections (eg, cytomegalovirus), and genetic conditions (eg, Rabson-Mendenhall syndrome). One relatively common condition that should be considered is hemochromatosis, or iron overload. Primary hemochromatosis is the most common genetic disorder in the United States, affecting approximately 1 in every 200 to 300 Americans. It is more common in persons of Western European heritage. It results from increased absorption of iron through the gastrointestinal tract, with excess iron deposition in many tissues. Traditional teaching has been that hyperglycemia results from iron deposition in the pancreas, resulting in islet-cell dysfunction. However, recent data suggest that the pathogenesis involves primarily insulin resistance with secondary β-cell decompensation, as in routine cases of type 2 diabetes. Secondary hemochromatosis includes conditions characterized by increased red blood cell breakdown or a history of many blood transfusions (thalassemia, sideroblastic anemia, hemolytic anemia). The clues in this case include amenorrhea (due to hypogonadotropic hypogonadism from pituitary iron deposition) and hepatic dysfunction and enlargement. The initial approach to diagnosis is assessing markers of iron stores such as transferrin saturation (Answer C) and/or ferritin.

The presence of an *HNF1A* mutation (Answer A) is diagnostic of maturity-onset diabetes of the young, which does not apply to this case. Zinc transporter 8 antibodies (Answer B) would be elevated if this were type 1 diabetes or latent autoimmune diabetes of adults, but these diagnoses seem unlikely. Measuring serum ceruloplasmin (Answer D) would not be helpful since Wilson disease is unlikely in this patient (diabetes does not typically occur in Wilson disease). Mitochondrial antibodies (Answer E) are increased in primary biliary cirrhosis, but this is not associated with diabetes.

EDUCATIONAL OBJECTIVE
Diagnose hemochromatosis as a cause of secondary diabetes mellitus.

REFERENCE(S)

Barton JC, Acton RT. Diabetes in *HFE* hemochromatosis. *J Diabetes Res.* 2017;2017:9826930. PMID: 28331855

Hatunic M, Finucane FM, Brennan AM, Norris S, Pacini G, Nolan JJ. Effect of iron overload on glucose metabolism in patients with hereditary hemochromatosis. *Metabolism.* 2010;59(3):380-384. PMID: 19815242

Bacon BR, Adams PC, Kowdley KV, Powell LW, Tavill AS; American Association for Study of Liver Diseases. Diagnosis and management of hemochromatosis: 2011 practice guideline by the American Association for the Study of Liver Diseases. *Hepatology.* 2011;54(1):328-343. PMID: 21452290

23 ANSWER: A) Glucagon

The development of type 2 diabetes after age 65 to 70 years, particularly in a relatively abrupt fashion, is unusual and should prompt consideration of a secondary cause. Categories of secondary diabetes include medication-induced (eg, corticosteroids), other endocrinopathies (eg, acromegaly), pancreatic diseases (eg, pancreatitis), infections (eg, cytomegalovirus), and genetic conditions (eg, Rabson-Mendenhall syndrome). In this older patient with cachexia and rash on his feet, glucagonoma syndrome should be considered and glucagon measurement (Answer A) is most likely to reveal the cause of his diabetes.

Glucagonomas are rare neuroendocrine tumors of the pancreas (others include insulinomas, somatostatinomas, carcinoid, and nonsecreting neuroendocrine tumors). In this setting, hyperglycemia, which is typically quite severe, results predominantly through the counterregulatory effects of glucagon. In larger tumors, destruction of nearby islet cells and pancreatic insulin secretion may also have an etiologic role. Glucagonomas are often malignant and frequently present already metastatic to the liver. If localized, surgical resection is necessary. Unless large portions of the pancreas are sacrificed, hyperglycemia typically resolves relatively rapidly postoperatively. If metastatic or residual tumor is demonstrated after surgery, somatostatin receptor agonist therapy (eg, octreotide, lanreotide) should be considered. Necrolytic migratory erythema is the typical rash associated with glucagonoma syndrome, as observed in this patient. It can be itchy and painful and it often affects the genital and anal region, groin, and lower legs, but any site may be involved. The rash progresses through an initial ring-shaped red area that blisters, erodes, then crusts over and leaves behind a brown mark.

CA 19-9 (carbohydrate antigen) (Answer B) is elevated in adenocarcinoma of the pancreas, as well as in colorectal and hepatocellular carcinomas. While any tumor of the pancreas can lead to diabetes mellitus, pancreatic adenocarcinoma is not associated with necrolytic migratory erythema. Somatostatinomas are very rare and also not associated with rash, so somatostatin (Answer C) does not need to be measured in this patient. No clinical features in this vignette suggest Cushing syndrome; therefore, measurement of urinary free cortisol (Answer D) is unlikely to be helpful.

EDUCATIONAL OBJECTIVE
Diagnose glucagonoma as a secondary cause of diabetes mellitus.

REFERENCE(S)
Warner RR. Enteroendocrine tumors other than carcinoid: a review of clinically significant advances. *Gastroenterology.* 2005;128(6):1668-1684. PMID: 15887158

Jabbour SA. Skin manifestations of hormone-secreting tumors. *Dermatol Ther.* 2010;23(6):643-650. PMID: 21054708

24 ANSWER: D) Fructosamine measurement

Hemoglobin A_{1c} measurement is the criterion standard test to assess the quality of glycemic control in patients with diabetes mellitus. Unfortunately, hemoglobin A_{1c} (Answer A) cannot be used as a metric of glycemic control in all patients. Of greatest importance is its unreliability in the setting of hemoglobinopathies, such as sickle-cell disease, or other causes of increased red blood cell turnover. Because glycation of hemoglobin A increases over the life of a red cell, conditions that shorten red blood cell lifespan cause an artificially reduced hemoglobin A_{1c} level, whether measurement is point of care or done in the laboratory. In this setting, other markers of long-term glucose control should be considered. Fructosamine (Answer D), a measure of glycosylated plasma proteins, is proportional to the mean blood glucose over the previous 2 weeks and may be used in place of the hemoglobin A_{1c} in this patient because it is not dependent on red blood cell turnover.

Measuring postprandial glucose levels (Answer B) is not likely to add much in this case, as they are generally proportional to fasting values. Urinary glucose testing (Answer C) is imprecise and only estimates recent levels of circulating glucose concentrations. Continuous glucose monitoring (Answer E) is best used to fine-tune glycemic control in patients on intensive insulin regimens, especially insulin pumps.

EDUCATIONAL OBJECTIVE
Explain the relationship between hemoglobinopathy and hemoglobin A_{1c}.

REFERENCE(S)

National Glycohemoglobin Standardization Program (NGSP) Web site. Factors that interfere with HbA1c test results. Available at: http://www.ngsp.org/factors.asp. Accessed for verification April 2018.

Lorenzo-Medina M, De-La-Iglesia S, Ropero P, Nogueria-Salgueriro P, Santana-Benitez J. Effects of hemoglobin variants on hemoglobin A1c values measured using a high-performance liquid chromatography method. *J Diabetes Sci Technol.* 2014;8(6):1168–1176. PMID: 25355712

Sacks DB, Arnold M, Bakris GL, et al; National Academy of Clinical Biochemistry; Evidence-Based Laboratory Medicine Committee of the American Association for Clinical Chemistry. Guidelines and recommendations for laboratory analysis in the diagnosis and management of diabetes mellitus. *Diabetes Care.* 2011;34(6):e61-e99. PMID: 21617108

25 ANSWER: C) Familial renal glucosuria

Isolated glucosuria in the absence of diabetes or other renal dysfunction is diagnostic of familial renal glucosuria (Answer C). The incidence of this autosomal codominant condition is 3 in 1000 persons, and it is due to mutations in the sodium-glucose transporter 2 (*SLC5A2* gene) that impair glucose transport in the proximal tubule of the kidney. Familial renal glucosuria has variable penetrance, but affected patients have life-long excretion of abnormal amounts of glucose in the urine (1 to 150 g/24 h). The otherwise benign course of this condition has been used to justify the development of SGLT-2 inhibitors to treat diabetes.

IgA nephropathy (Answer A) is the most common form of glomerulonephritis and causes hematuria but not glucosuria. Renal Fanconi syndrome (Answer B) involves more general proximal tubular dysfunction with wasting of amino acids and phosphate, as well as glucose, renal tubular acidosis, and osteomalacia. Hereditary galactosemia (Answer D) is a disorder of impaired metabolism of galactose and lactose. It is typically detected by newborn screening and is fatal in the first weeks of life if not treated. It does not affect renal glucose handling.

EDUCATIONAL OBJECTIVE
Describe syndromes associated with glucosuria.

REFERENCE(S)

Lee H, Han KH, Park HW, et al. Familial renal glucosuria: a clinicogenetic study of 23 additional cases. *Pediatr Nephrol.* 2012;27(7):1091-1095. PMID: 22314875

Santer R, Calado J. Familial renal glucosuria and SGLT2: from a mendelian trait to a therapeutic target. *Clin J Am Soc Nephrol.* 2010;5(1):133-141. PMID: 19965550

26 ANSWER: D) Change to U500 insulin

This patient has severe insulin resistance and uncontrolled diabetes, probably related to long-term use of high-dosage steroids. She is taking 300 to 350 units of insulin daily (3.5 to 4.0 units/kg), reflecting severe insulin resistance. Although there is evidence that the addition of insulin sensitizers can improve glycemic control in type 2 diabetes treated with insulin, this patient is too severely affected to get much benefit from a thiazolidinedione (Answer C) or metformin. And while GLP-1 receptor agonists (Answer B) can cause modest weight loss that can improve insulin sensitivity, these too are unlikely to make much difference in such an extreme case of insulin resistance. Addition of another dose of insulin glargine (Answer A), even at a dose of 100 units, is unlikely to get her to target and would require her taking more than 5 injections per day. The most effective approach in this woman is to give her substantially more insulin, and U500 (Answer D), which is 5 times more concentrated than standard U100, is most likely to give good results.

In patients requiring more than 200 units of insulin a day, the volume of insulin given becomes a problem, both in terms of patient comfort and pharmacokinetics; large-volume insulin injections are poorly absorbed. This is true of U100 insulins given by injection or pump. There is increasing evidence of more reliable delivery of insulin and successful outcomes with the use of U500 insulin in patients such as the one presented. Although the formulation of U500 is similar to that of regular insulin, the duration of action is up to 13 to 24 hours, permitting adequate delivery with 2 or 3 injections per day.

EDUCATIONAL OBJECTIVE
Treat extreme insulin resistance.

REFERENCE(S)

Hood RC, Arakaki RF, Wysham C, Li YG, Settles JA, Jackson JA. Two treatment approaches for human regular U-500 insulin in patients with type 2 diabetes not achieving adequate glycemic control on high-dose U-100 insulin therapy with or without oral agents: a randomized, titration-to-target clinical trial. *Endocr Pract*. 2015;21(7):782-793. PMID: 25813411

Garg R, Johnston V, McNally P, Davies MJ, Lawrence IG. U-500 insulin: why, when and how to use in clinical practice. *Diabetes Metab Res Rev*. 2007;23(4):265-268. PMID: 17109474

Lane WS, Cochran EK, Jackson JA, et al. High-dose insulin therapy: is it time for U-500 insulin? *Endocr Pract*. 2009;15(1):71-79. PMID: 19211405

27 ANSWER: B) Dulaglutide

Although metformin is generally accepted as the first-line treatment for type 2 diabetes, there is no consensus about the second-line agent when additional medication is needed. All of the listed medications could be used with an expectation of improved glycemic control. However, selection of medications must also include consideration of the adverse effects of the drug with the patient's profile. This man has already discontinued one agent because of weight gain; this is likely to bother him with other drugs as well. Therefore, repaglinide (Answer A), pioglitazone (Answer D), and insulin glargine (Answer E), which all cause weight gain, are problematic. Sitagliptin (Answer C) is weight neutral and would thus probably be acceptable to this man. However, the average hemoglobin A_{1c} reduction with sitagliptin (0.7%-1.0%) is unlikely to shift his hemoglobin A_{1c} level to goal, and a third medication might be needed. GLP-1 receptor agonists are more potent than DPP-4 inhibitors, and, in clinical trials, patients with hemoglobin A_{1c} levels comparable to that of this patient have had an approximately 50% chance of reaching the hemoglobin A_{1c} target of 7.0% (53 mmol/mol). Dulaglutide (Answer B) is likely to cause weight loss and move his hemoglobin A_{1c} to goal. If the patient is willing to accept the risk of gastrointestinal adverse effects and to use an injectable agent, dulaglutide is the best choice for him.

EDUCATIONAL OBJECTIVE
Select an appropriate second-line agent to manage hyperglycemia in a patient with type 2 diabetes mellitus.

REFERENCE(S)

American Diabetes Association. Standards of medical care in diabetes-2018. *Diabetes Care*. 2018;41(Suppl 1);S1-S153.

Tasyurek HM, Altunbas HA, Balci MK, Sanlioglu S. Incretins: their physiology and application in the treatment of diabetes mellitus. *Diabetes Metab Res Rev*. 2014;30(5):354-371. PMID: 24989141

28 ANSWER: C) Weight loss and exercise to prevent type 2 diabetes

The diagnostic abnormality on the oral glucose tolerance test is impaired fasting glucose and impaired glucose tolerance, both signifying prediabetes and consistent with the patient's hemoglobin A_{1c} level. Therefore, you should recommend weight loss and exercise to prevent type 2 diabetes (Answer C). He does not have diabetes (Answer B) because the fasting glucose level is less than 126 mg/dL (<7.0 mmol/L), the hemoglobin A_{1c} level is less than 6.5% (<48 mmol/mol), and the 2-hour value from the oral glucose tolerance test is less than 200 mg/dL (<11.1 mmol/L). The 1-hour value is elevated, but this can occur in persons with prediabetes, and this is not a standard parameter for the diagnosis of diabetes. Diagnosis of diabetes on the basis of fasting glucose requires 2 separate abnormal values, but repeating this measurement (Answer D) in a patient such as this one who has a nondiagnostic level is not indicated.

The common forms of maturity-onset diabetes of the young are associated with autosomal dominant inheritance, and the presented family history (with neither parent being affected) is not consistent with this diagnosis. Thus, genetic screening (Answer E) is incorrect.

Although insulin resistance can be inferred from measurement of insulin (Answer A) during an oral glucose tolerance test, this is not likely to affect management in this patient.

The American Diabetes Association criteria for the diagnosis of diabetes are as follows:

1. Hemoglobin A_{1c} ≥6.5% (≥48 mmol/mol). The test should be performed in a laboratory using a method that is certified by the National Glycohemoglobin Standardization Program and standardized to the Diabetes Control and Complications Trial assay.*

   OR

2. Fasting plasma glucose ≥126 mg/dL (≥7.0 mmol/L). Fasting is defined as no caloric intake for at least 8 hours.*

   OR

3. Two-hour plasma glucose value ≥200 mg/dL (≥11.1 mmol/L) during an oral glucose tolerance test. The test should be performed as described by the World Health Organization, using a glucose load containing the equivalent of 75-g anhydrous glucose dissolved in water.*

   OR

4. In a patient with classic symptoms of hyperglycemia or hyperglycemic crisis, a random plasma glucose value ≥200 mg/dL (≥11.1 mmol/L).

*In the absence of unequivocal hyperglycemia, criteria 1 to 3 should be confirmed by repeated testing.

EDUCATIONAL OBJECTIVE
Diagnose prediabetes on the basis of results from oral glucose tolerance testing.

REFERENCE(S)
American Diabetes Association. Standards of medical care in diabetes-2018. *Diabetes Care.* 2018;41(1):S1-S153.

Inzucchi SE. Diagnosis of type 2 diabetes. *N Engl J Med.* 2012;367(6):542-550. PMID: 22873534

29 **ANSWER: B) Ketosis-prone diabetes**
Although diabetic ketoacidosis has long been the hallmark of type 1 diabetes, in recent years it has become clear that a subset of patients of African or Hispanic descent can present with ketoacidosis as the first manifestation of diabetes (Answer B). Often these patients have dramatic presentations (weight loss, severe polyuria/polydipsia, and diabetic ketoacidosis) and require insulin treatment, but steady improvement in control over weeks to months may permit a change to long-term oral agent therapy. The pathophysiology of this syndrome is not known, but it seems to be due to a transient and reversible loss of β-cell function.

Autoimmune diabetes (type 1 diabetes or latent autoimmune diabetes in adults, LADA) (Answer A) is possible but not as likely as ketosis-prone diabetes in this vignette. His strong family history of diabetes and elevated BMI are more consistent with type 2 diabetes. Moreover, relative to the degree of hyperglycemia, the ketoacidosis is not as severe as it is in most cases of type 1 diabetes. Diabetes due to LADA and maturity-onset diabetes of the young type 1 (Answer C) almost never present with ketoacidosis. Alcoholic ketoacidosis (Answer D) can be associated with moderately elevated blood glucose, but rarely with levels greater than 300 mg/dL (>16.7 mmol/L), and this man has no evidence of recent intoxication. Pancreatitis (Answer E) can present with severe hyperglycemia and ketoacidosis, but this is typically associated with more dramatic abdominal signs and symptoms, as well as high amylase and lipase.

EDUCATIONAL OBJECTIVE
Diagnose ketosis-prone diabetes.

REFERENCE(S)
Seok H, Jung CH, Kim SW, et al. Clinical characteristics and insulin independence of Koreans with new-onset type 2 diabetes presenting with diabetic ketoacidosis. *Diabetes Metab Res Rev.* 2013;29(6):507-513. PMID: 23653323

Gaba R, Gambhire D, Uy N, et al. Factors associated with early relapse to insulin dependence in unprovoked A-β+ ketosis-prone diabetes. *J Diabetes* Complications. 2015;29(7):918-922. PMID: 26071380

Balasubramanyam A, Yajnik CS, Tandon N. Nontraditional forms of diabetes worldwide: implications for translational investigation. *Transl Endocrinol Metab.* 2011;2(1):43-67.

30 ANSWER: A) Oral glucose tolerance test

With improved treatment, the life expectancy of patients with cystic fibrosis is increasing and non-pulmonary manifestations of the disease are becoming more prevalent. Cystic fibrosis–related diabetes affects 2% of children, 20% of adolescents, and nearly 50% of adults with cystic fibrosis. The principle etiology is islet-cell damage as a result of pancreatic fibrosis, but patients with cystic fibrosis–related diabetes also have slightly reduced insulin sensitivity compared with that of nondiabetic patients with cystic fibrosis. The hallmark of cystic fibrosis–related diabetes is postprandial hyperglycemia out of proportion with the fasting blood glucose level; that is, most patients present with results from oral glucose tolerance tests indicative of diabetes and normal fasting blood glucose levels. Thus, measurement of fasting blood glucose on 2 occasions (Answer E) is not the best diagnostic strategy. The oral glucose tolerance test (Answer A) has become the criterion standard for diagnosis, and it is the test that has been studied most frequently in patients with cystic fibrosis.

Continuous glucose monitoring (Answer B) has been evaluated recently and gives comparable diagnostic results to the oral glucose tolerance test, but it has not yet been standardized for clinical practice. Hemoglobin A_{1c} measurement (Answer C) tends to underestimate the degree of glucose intolerance in cystic fibrosis and is not used for diagnosis. The response to mixed-meal tests (Answer D) is often abnormal in the setting of cystic fibrosis–related diabetes, and it provides a more physiologic challenge to glucose regulation. However, this test has not been developed into a diagnostic standard.

EDUCATIONAL OBJECTIVE
Recommend the oral glucose tolerance test to confirm the diagnosis of cystic fibrosis–related diabetes.

REFERENCE(S)

Moran A, Pillay K, Becker DJ, Acerini CL; International Society for Pediatric and Adolescent Diabetes. ISPAD Clinical Practice Consensus Guidelines 2014. Management of cystic fibrosis-related diabetes in children and adolescents. *Pediatr Diabetes.* 2014;15(Suppl 20):65-76. PMID: 25182308

Kelly A, Moran A. Update on cystic fibrosis-related diabetes [published correction appears in *J Cyst Fibros.* 2014;13(1):119]. *J Cyst Fibros.* 2013;12(4):318-331. PMID: 23562217

Moran A, Brunzell C, Cohen RC, et al; CFRD Guidelines Committee. Clinical care guidelines for cystic fibrosis-related diabetes: a position statement of the American Diabetes Association and a clinical practice guideline of the Cystic Fibrosis Foundation, endorsed by the Pediatric Endocrine Society. *Diabetes Care.* 2010;33(12):2697-2708. PMID: 21115772

Adrenal Board Review

Richard J. Auchus, MD, PhD ● University of Michigan

ANSWER: E) Plasma ACTH measurement

The biochemical diagnosis of hypercortisolemia relies on 3 screening tests: 24-hour urinary free cortisol excretion, late-night salivary cortisol measurement, and overnight 1-mg dexamethasone suppression test. None of these studies is perfect and they all have limitations. The value of any of these tests depends greatly on the pretest probability of Cushing syndrome. This patient has a high pretest probability of Cushing syndrome on the basis of her history and physical examination findings. In addition, she has a known adrenal mass. Although the referral was to evaluate the adrenal mass, most adenomas that produce clinically significant hypercortisolemia are larger than 2.5 cm in diameter, so it is unlikely that this tumor is causing cortisol excess.

Biopsy of the mass (Answer D) would only reveal cortical cells or other tissue, and it would not address the functional state of the adrenal mass. Similarly, adrenal MRI (Answer B) might confirm that the tumor is a lipid-rich cortical adenoma, but this will not aid in the evaluation. She has 2 very abnormal salivary cortisol values and a very abnormal result following an overnight dexamethasone suppression test, so hypercortisolemia is established. Therefore, another type of screening such as urinary free cortisol measurement is not necessary. Instead, subtyping is the next step to determine whether the cortisol excess is ACTH-dependent or ACTH-independent. This is accomplished with a plasma ACTH measurement (Answer E). In this case, the plasma ACTH value was 60 pg/mL (13.2 pmol/L), and the patient had pituitary Cushing disease. The adrenal tumor was a red herring.

The purpose of the dexamethasone corticotropin-releasing hormone test (Answer C) is to distinguish physiologic hypercortisolism (pseudocushing state) from pathologic hypercortisolism when other testing and physical examination findings are equivocal. This patient has significant biochemical abnormalities and suggestive physical exam findings, so this distinction is not necessary. Plasma renin activity (Answer A) would be relevant if one were screening for primary aldosteronism but not for the evaluation of hypercortisolemia.

EDUCATIONAL OBJECTIVE

Recommend measurement of plasma ACTH as the initial differential diagnostic test in the subtyping of Cushing syndrome.

REFERENCE(S)

Findling JW, Raff H. Cushing's syndrome: important issues in diagnosis and treatment. *J Clin Endocrinol Metab.* 2006;91(10):3746-3753. PMID: 16868050

Kidambi S, Raff H, Findling JW. Limitations of nocturnal salivary cortisol and urine free cortisol in the diagnosis of mild Cushing's syndrome. *Eur J Endocrinol.* 2007;157(6):725-731. PMID: 18057379

Alexandraki KI, Grossman AB. Is urinary free cortisol of value in the diagnosis of Cushing syndrome? *Curr Opin Endocrinol Diabetes Obes.* 2011;18(4):259-263. PMID: 21681089

Pecori Giraldi F, Saccani A, Cavagnini F; Study Group on the Hypothalamo-Pituitary-Adrenal Axis of the Italian Society of Endocrinology. Assessment of ACTH assay variability: a multicenter study. *Eur J Endocrinol.* 2011;164(4):505-512. PMID: 21252174

ANSWER: A) Measure very-long-chain fatty acids

The finding of primary adrenal insufficiency in a young man with neurologic symptoms should always raise suspicion for adrenoleukodystrophy (ALD). ALD is an inherited metabolic storage disease associated with a defect in an enzyme that results in defective peroxisomal β-oxidation and accumulation of very-long-chain fatty acids (C24, C26) (Answer A) in body tissues, especially the brain and the adrenal glands. The accumulation of very-long-chain fatty acids causes demyelination associated with an intense inflammatory response in white matter. Neurologic manifestations include psychiatric symptoms (symptoms of attention deficit hyperactivity disorder), neuromuscular problems, slurred speech, and even dementia. Because it is an X-linked disorder (estimated to occur in 1:17,000 newborns), ALD affects only boys. However, female carriers can manifest some degree of disability. Approximately 70% of boys with ALD develop adrenal insufficiency. The presence of elevated plasma very-long-chain fatty acids is highly reliable, and the diagnosis can be confirmed by mutation analysis of the *ABCD1* gene. Marker studies to determine carrier status may be helpful in prenatal diagnosis. Adrenomyeloneuropathy is a milder form of this disorder that can coexist with ALD in the same family. Adrenomyeloneuropathy may actually present as primary adrenal insufficiency in young male patients and the milder neurologic deficits portend a more favorable prognosis.

When autoimmune adrenalitis is suspected, 21-hydroxylase antibodies (Answer B) are often positive. However, they are rarely positive in patients with adrenoleukodystrophy, so their measurement would not provide a specific diagnosis. Other more common autoimmune conditions (hypothyroidism, vitiligo) are absent, and the characteristic neurologic impairments of ALD are not seen with autoimmune adrenal insufficiency. Adrenal CT (Answer C) is a good option when fungal infections are suspected (histoplasmosis for example), but his absence of fever and pulmonary symptoms in the presence of neurologic findings disfavor an infectious etiology. Serum aldosterone will be low or low-normal in any form of primary adrenal insufficiency, which is already established in this case from the high ACTH and low morning cortisol, so measuring serum aldosterone (Answer D) is incorrect. An ACTH stimulation test (Answer E) does not add much information when the ACTH is already very high, and the results will not identify a specific etiology of the adrenal insufficiency.

EDUCATIONAL OBJECTIVE
Include adrenoleukodystrophy in the differential diagnosis of any young male patient with primary adrenal insufficiency of unknown cause, especially in the presence of concomitant neurologic symptoms.

REFERENCE(S)
Dubey P, Raymond GV, Moser AB, Kharkar S, Bezman L, Moser HW. Adrenal insufficiency in asymptomatic adrenoleukodystrophy patients identified by very long-chain fatty acid screening. *J Pediatr.* 2005;146(4):528-532. PMID: 15812458

Mosser J, Douar AM, Sarde CO, et al. Putative X-linked adrenoleukodystrophy gene shares unexpected homology with ABC transporters. *Nature.* 1993;361(6414):726-730. PMID: 8441467

Davis LE, Snyder RD, Orth DN, Nicholson WE, Kornfeld M, Seelinger DF. Adrenoleukodystrophy and adrenomyeloneuropathy associated with partial adrenal insufficiency in three generations of a kindred. *Am J Med.* 1979;66(2):342-347. PMID: 218453

Sadeghi-Nejad A, Senior B. Adrenomyeloneuropathy presenting as Addison's disease in childhood. *N Engl J Med.* 1990;322(1):13-16. PMID: 2294415

3 **ANSWER: E) Make no changes in his corticosteroid dosages**

The treatment of primary adrenal insufficiency with glucocorticoid and mineralocorticoid replacement has evolved over the past 30 years. Hydrocortisone dosages as high as 30 to 40 mg daily (Answer C) were routinely administered years ago. These dosages were often associated with signs and symptoms of excessive glucocorticoid exposure, such as decreased bone mineral density. In healthy individuals, the daily secretion of cortisol is only 6 to 7 mg/m^2 (or approximately 8 to 12 mg daily). Most patients with primary adrenal insufficiency need only 15 to 20 mg of hydrocortisone in divided daily doses (even less in many patients with secondary adrenal insufficiency). Almost all patients with primary adrenal insufficiency require mineralocorticoid replacement. Fludrocortisone is the treatment of choice. The fludrocortisone dosage is usually titrated on the basis of electrolyte composition, blood pressure, and plasma renin activity. A plasma renin activity less than 5 mg/mL per h is a reasonable treatment target.

This patient has evidence of adequate mineralocorticoid replacement and a dosage increase in fludrocortisone (Answer D) is not indicated. However, monitoring the adequacy of glucocorticoid replacement is more difficult. It is currently impossible to mimic the diurnal rhythm of cortisol. It is well known that the early-morning increase in cortisol begins at approximately 3:00 AM in patients with normal sleep–wake cycles. Glucocorticoid negative feedback on ACTH is complex, and ACTH levels usually remain elevated in patients with primary adrenal insufficiency despite adequate glucocorticoid replacement. Measurement of plasma ACTH in patients with adrenal insufficiency may be helpful if low-normal or subnormal levels are found. This suggests excessive glucocorticoid exposure and the need for a dosage reduction.

Because this patient is doing very well on his current replacement therapy, the modest increase in ACTH is of no concern and no change in treatment is warranted (Answer E). Some clinicians prescribe prednisone therapy (Answer A). However, there is no acceptable physiologic replacement dosage of prednisone. Because its active metabolite, prednisolone, has a very high affinity for the glucocorticoid receptor and a long plasma half-life, it is often associated with clinical features of excessive glucocorticoid exposure. The addition of 0.75 mg of dexamethasone at bedtime (Answer B) may suppress ACTH to near the reference range, but it would most likely cause iatrogenic Cushing syndrome. Reviewing the stress dosing of glucocorticoid replacement in patients with adrenal insufficiency is always indicated and should be done at nearly every visit.

EDUCATIONAL OBJECTIVE
Assess the adequacy of glucocorticoid and mineralocorticoid support in patients with primary adrenal insufficiency and recognize that plasma ACTH is usually elevated in this setting.

REFERENCE(S)
Bleicken B, Hahner S, Loeffler M, Ventz M, Allolio B, Quinkler M. Impaired subjective health status in chronic adrenal insufficiency: impact of different glucocorticoid replacement regimens. *Eur J Endocrinol.* 2008;159(6):811-817.

Hahner S, Loeffler M, Bleicken B, et al. Epidemiology of adrenal crisis in chronic adrenal insufficiency: the need for new prevention strategies. *Eur J Endocrinol.* 2010;162(3):597-602.

Bornstein SR, Allolio B, Arlt W, et al. Diagnosis and treatment of primary adrenal insufficiency: an Endocrine Society Clinical Practice Guideline. *J Clin Endocrinol Metab.* 2016;101(2):364-389.

4 **ANSWER: B) Perform a 1-mg overnight dexamethasone suppression test**

Because of hypertension and hypokalemia, this patient was evaluated for primary aldosteronism, and the screening aldosterone-to-renin ratio is marginally positive. Ordinarily, one would proceed to confirmatory testing, followed by CT, and then adrenal venous sampling to localize the source(s) of aldosterone. The CT showed a fairly large adrenal tumor—significantly larger than those that usually cause primary aldosteronism. On careful inspection, one can discern that the contralateral adrenal gland is somewhat atrophic, suggesting hypercortisolism from the adrenal tumor. When the diameter of adrenal cortical tumors is larger than 2.4 cm, the risk of hypercortisolism rises, and additional dynamic testing of cortisol production should be undertaken (Answer B) before proceeding along the pathway of the normal evaluation for primary aldosteronism.

In this case, the results of the adrenal venous sampling are confusing and appear to lateralize cortisol production to the atrophic left adrenal and away from the large adenoma on the right side. Closer inspection shows aldosterone values in the thousands for both the left and right adrenal veins, more 50 times higher than the mixed venous aldosterone values and confirming adequate access to the adrenal veins. The odd feature is the unusually low cortisol values in the left adrenal vein, yet still 2 to 3 times higher than in the mixed venous blood. The reason is suppression of cortisol from the left adrenal due to cortisol excess from the right adrenal.

Additional testing revealed the following laboratory values:

- ACTH = <5 pg/mL (SI: <1.1 pmol/L)
- DHEA-S = 18 µg/dL (SI: 0.49 µmol/L)
- Urinary free cortisol = 260 µg/24 h (SI: 718 nmol/d)
- 8 AM cortisol after 1 mg dexamethasone = 22.5 µg/dL (SI: 620.7 nmol/L)

Testing revealed ACTH-independent hypercortisolism from the right adrenal tumor. She had moderate features of hypercortisolism on careful physical examination. Following right adrenalectomy, she had resolution of her hypertension, a period of adrenal insufficiency, and subsequently carried pregnancies to term.

Spironolactone (Answer A) would treat the mineralocorticoid excess, but not glucocorticoid manifestations, and this patient needs further evaluation. While the screening aldosterone-to-renin ratio might have been equivocal and ordinarily followed up with confirmatory testing for primary aldosteronism (Answer C), the size of the adrenal tumor indicates a greater need for cortisol testing. Left adrenalectomy (Answer D) is incorrect, despite ostensible lateralization of aldosterone production to the left, due to the greater importance of cortisol excess. Adrenal MRI (Answer E) would only confirm that the tumor is a lipid-rich mass, but it would not determine function.

EDUCATIONAL OBJECTIVE
Correlate the size of adrenal cortical adenomas with hormone production or coproduction and pursue appropriate evaluation and management.

REFERENCE(S)
Spath M, Korovkin S, Antke C, Anlauf M, Willenberg HS. Aldosterone- and cortisol-cosecreting adrenal tumors: the lost subtype of primary aldosteronism. *Eur J Endocrinol.* 2011;164(4):447-455. PMID: 21270113

Morelli V, Reimondo G, Giordano R, et al. Long-term follow-up in adrenal incidentalomas: an Italian multicenter study. *J Clin Endocrinol Metab.* 2014;99(3):827-834. PMID: 24423350

Fallo F, Bertello C, Tizzani D, et al. Concurrent primary aldosteronism and subclinical cortisol

hypersecretion: a prospective study. *J Hypertens.* 2011;29(9):1773-1777. PMID: 21720261

5 ANSWER: C) Urine synthetic glucocorticoid testing

Corticosteroid injections for back pain are commonly administered in pain clinics, and patients are often unaware that the pain medicine is a mixture of anaesthetics and potent synthetic corticosteroids. A typical history includes the abrupt onset of cushingoid features and metabolic consequences. Because these drugs do not activate the mineralocorticoid receptor as do high concentrations of cortisol, hypertension and hypokalemia are usually absent. When soluble preparations such as methylprednisolone are injected into the synovial fluid of a joint space, the drug is absorbed and cleared within several days, limiting the cumulative consequences. When a suspension preparation is injected into a relatively avascular space, the drug is absorbed very slowly, and the endocrinologic action can be profound and sustained. The most common agent causing long-term problems is triamcinolone acetonide, 0.1% suspensions, when given as facet joint or myofascial injections. The cumulative effect of 40 mg of triamcinolone acetonide is equivalent to roughly 1.2 g of hydrocortisone, more than the average person produces in 100 days. The particulate formulation prolongs the absorption of the triamcinolone acetonide over weeks to months, which creates a sustained toxic exposure. Patients with HIV infection taking the potent CYP3A4 inhibitor ritonavir are particularly susceptible due to delayed metabolism of the triamcinolone.

Although late-night salivary cortisol measurement (Answer A) might generally be the most sensitive test for ACTH-dependent hypercortisolism, this patient has low serum cortisol and plasma ACTH values, suggesting exogenous hypercortisolism. Imaging studies (Answers B, D, and E) would only be indicated if the screening laboratory tests suggested endogenous hypercortisolism. In this case, the urine synthetic glucocorticoid screen (Answer C) was positive for triamcinolone acetonide, despite the last injection being 4 months ago.

EDUCATIONAL OBJECTIVE

Confirm the diagnosis of iatrogenic Cushing syndrome and describe the magnitude and duration of glucocorticoid excess caused by injectable corticosteroids.

REFERENCE(S)

Danaher PJ, Salsbury TL, Delmar JA. Metabolic derangement after injection of triamcinolone into the hip of an HIV-infected patient receiving ritonavir. *Orthopedics*. 2009;32(6):450. PMID: 19634808

Iglesias P, González J, Díez JJ. Acute and persistent iatrogenic Cushing's syndrome after a single dose of triamcinolone acetonide. *J Endocrinol Invest*. 2005;28(11):1019-1023. PMID: 16483182

Taylor RL, Grebe SK, Singh RJ. Quantitative, highly sensitive liquid chromatography-tandem mass spectrometry method for detection of synthetic corticosteroids. *Clin Chem*. 2004;50(12):2345-2352. PMID: 15486026

6 ANSWER: C) Adrenocortical carcinoma

Functional benign adrenal adenomas generally produce a single major active hormone. Large cortisol-producing adenomas sometimes cosecrete aldosterone, but usually one hormone excess is dominant, while the second is mild. In contrast, overt, clinically manifested excess of more than one active steroid, such as androgen and mineralocorticoid excess, is characteristic of adrenocortical carcinomas (Answer C). Furthermore, the rapid progression of androgen excess alone, with very high testosterone and virilization (voice deepening), is worrisome for an adrenal or ovarian tumor. Coexistence of mineralocorticoid excess, disproportionate to the cortisol and aldosterone concentrations, suggests elevation of cortisol precursors, primarily corticosterone and 11-deoxycorticosterone. Adrenal carcinomas tend to be relatively deficient in 11β-hydroxylase activity, leading to elevation of 11-deoxycortisol and further upstream intermediates, which can account for the robust androgen and mineralocorticoid excess with normal or modestly elevated cortisol.

Macronodular adrenocortical hyperplasia (Answer A) typically manifests with pure cortisol excess, and the mineralocorticoid excess is due to high cortisol and thus rises in parallel with cortisol production. DHEA-S is usually normal in hypercortisolemic patients with macronodular hyperplasia rather than suppressed as is often the case in hypercortisolemic patients with unilateral adrenal cortical adenomas, but this preservation of DHEA-S does not account for the profound androgen excess in this patient. While mild or nonclassic 11β-hydroxylase deficiency (Answer B) has been described, these patients have mild androgen excess and rarely have hypertension; the abrupt onset in adulthood as in this vignette is also inconsistent with a genetic etiology. Licorice ingestion (Answer D) can cause hypertension despite normal amounts of cortisol, but it does not lead to androgen excess. Glycyrrhetinic acid, derived from the glycyrrhizic acid found in licorice, inhibits 11β-hydroxysteroid dehydrogenase type 2, not 11β-hydroxylase. Anabolic steroid abuse (Answer E) could account for the androgen excess but not the mineralocorticoid excess.

EDUCATIONAL OBJECTIVE

Suspect adrenal cortical carcinoma on the basis of clinical features.

REFERENCE(S)

Arlt W, Biehl M, Taylor AE, et al. Urine steroid metabolomics as a biomarker tool for detecting malignancy in adrenal tumors. *J Clin Endocrinol Metab*. 2011;96(12):3775-3784. PMID: 21917861

Messer CK, Kirschenbaum A, New MI, Unger P, Gabrilove JL, Levine AC. Concomitant secretion of glucocorticoid, androgens, and mineralocorticoid by an adrenocortical carcinoma: case report and review of literature. *Endocr Pract*. 2007;13(4):408-412. PMID: 17669719

7 ANSWER: A) Unable to localize

For adrenal venous sampling, the cortisol concentrations in the adrenal vein samples are used to determine whether the adrenal veins were accessed and to correct for the fractional dilution of the adrenal vein blood with mixed venous blood. This ratio of cortisol in the adrenal vein blood to the cortisol in the mixed venous blood is often called the selectivity index. The selectivity index on both sides should be greater than 2 if adrenal venous sampling is performed without cosyntropin and greater than 3 if performed with cosyntropin infusion. Otherwise, the sample does not contain sufficient adrenal vein blood to interpret the results, and the study should not be interpreted unless both selectivity indices are greater than these minimum values. Usually, the right side, which is more difficult to access, fails the selectivity index test. If the aldosterone-to-cortisol ratio in the left adrenal vein is much lower than in the mixed venous blood, also called "contralateral suppression," aldosterone production can sometimes be confidently localized to the right adrenal, but conclusive cut-off values are not known. Note that contralateral suppression is not always observed in studies with convincing lateralization, so lack of contralateral suppression does not equate to bilateral aldosterone production.

Because the selectivity index on the right side is only 1.1 times higher than that of the mixed venous blood, the study was not successful (thus, Answer A is correct and Answer D is incorrect). Although it is possible that both adrenal glands are the source (Answer C), this interpretation cannot be drawn because of the low selectivity index on the right side. For the reasons stated above, the adrenal venous sampling study did not yield enough information to localize the aldosterone production (thus, Answer B is incorrect), even though all the information required for interpretation (aldosterone and cortisol from the adrenal veins and mixed venous blood) was available. Plasma metanephrines can also be used to confirm successful access of the adrenal veins, but the values cannot be used mathematically to correct for dilution with mixed venous blood.

EDUCATIONAL OBJECTIVE
Interpret results of adrenal venous sampling.

REFERENCE(S)

Rossi GP, Auchus RJ, Brown M, et al. An expert consensus statement on the use of adrenal vein sampling for the subtyping of primary aldosteronism. *Hypertension.* 2014;63(1):151-160. PMID: 24218436

Dekkers T, Deinum J, Schultzekool LJ, et al. Plasma metanephrine for assessing the selectivity of adrenal venous sampling. *Hypertension.* 2013;62(6):1152-1157. PMID: 24082051

Funder JW, Carey RM, Mantero F, et al. The management of primary aldosteronism: case detection, diagnosis, and treatment: an Endocrine Society Clinical Practice Guideline. *J Clin Endocrinol Metab.* 2016;101(5):1889-1916. PMID: 26934393

8 ANSWER: A) No changes

The treatment of 21-hydroxylase deficiency requires glucocorticoid to replace the cortisol deficiency and to limit the rise in ACTH, thus controlling the adrenal-derived androgen excess. Relatively tight control of androgen (and thus estrogen) excess is necessary in childhood to prevent premature development of secondary sexual characteristics and bone maturation. Serum 17-hydroxyprogesterone, which accumulates immediately before the enzymatic block, is used for diagnosis and is also measured to titrate therapy in children. 17-Hydroxyprogesterone is a very sensitive measure of disease control when small amounts of androgens and estrogens are detrimental. In adults, disease control is relaxed somewhat as tolerated, because small amounts of adrenal-derived sex steroid compared to gonadal synthesis are not damaging. Overtreatment can cause iatrogenic Cushing syndrome with long-term complications. Periods requiring intensified therapy in adults include when women are attempting pregnancy and when men have testicular adrenal rest tumors.

This woman, who has no androgen excess symptoms, regular menses, and absence of cushingoid features, has disease control that is clinically at goal. Not surprisingly, her androstenedione and testosterone are in the normal female reference range, and her plasma renin activity is normal. 17-Hydroxyprogesterone tends to rise before the next dose of hydrocortisone, but a high 17-hydroxyprogesterone level alone—especially just before a hydrocortisone dose—is not an indication for intensified therapy. Hence, no change in therapy is indicated (Answer A).

Increasing the hydrocortisone dosage (Answer B) or further dividing her dose (Answer D) is not necessary. In fact, her hydrocortisone dosage could be reduced slightly, but that is not a listed option. Note that DHEA-S is typically low and rarely elevated in the setting of classic 21-hydroxylase deficiency. Dexamethasone given at bedtime is the most effective way to prevent the early-morning ACTH rise and thus control the androgen excess. However, dexamethasone is difficult to titrate and easily causes iatrogenic Cushing syndrome, particularly when given at bedtime (Answer C), and a dosage of 1 mg is far too high for a small adult such as this patient. Stopping fludrocortisone (Answer E) will cause volume depletion and it should not be discontinued.

EDUCATIONAL OBJECTIVE
Guide the treatment of congenital adrenal hyperplasia on the basis of clinical and laboratory information.

REFERENCE(S)

Auchus RJ, Arlt W. Approach to the patient: the adult with congenital adrenal hyperplasia. *J Clin Endocrinol Metab*. 2013;98(7):2645-2655. PMID: 23837188

Arlt W, Willis DS, Wild SH, et al; United Kingdom Congenital Adrenal Hyperplasia Adult Study Executive (CaHASE). Health status of adults with congenital adrenal hyperplasia: a cohort study of 203 patients. *J Clin Endocrinol Metab*. 2010;95(11):5110-5121. PMID: 20719839

Casteràs A, De Silva P, Rumsby G, Conway GS. Reassessing fecundity in women with classical congenital adrenal hyperplasia (CAH): normal pregnancy rate but reduced fertility rate. *Clin Endocrinol (Oxf)*. 2009;70(6):833-837. PMID: 19250265

9 **ANSWER: D) ⁶⁸Ga-DOTATATE PET/CT scan**

Multiple modalities can be used to detect paragangliomas. Standard cross-sectional imaging (CT or MRI) (Answers A and C) is a standard approach to the initial evaluation, but CT and MRI techniques are insensitive for detecting small primary tumors or metastases, especially to bone, with detection rates of 50% to 60%. In contrast, for *SDHB*-related tumors, the somatostatin-receptor imaging agent DOTATATE, when labeled with the PET nuclide ⁶⁸Ga (Answer D), detects more than 98% of lesions, whereas ¹⁸F-fluorodeoxyglucose PET detects more than 85%. *SDHB*-related tumors—even primary tumors—are routinely negative with ¹²³I-metaiodobenzguanine (MIBG) scans (Answer

B). The ⁹⁹Tc-sestamibi scan (Answer E) is used for detecting parathyroid tumors, not paragangliomas.

EDUCATIONAL OBJECTIVE
Compare imaging modalities for detecting metastatic *SDHB*-related paragangliomas.

REFERENCE(S)

Fonte JS, Robles JF, Chen CC, et al. False-negative ¹²³I-MIBG SPECT is most commonly found in SDHB-related pheochromocytoma or paraganglioma with high frequency to develop metastatic disease. *Endocr Relat Cancer*. 2012;19(1):83-93. PMID: 22167067

Janssen I, Blanchet EM, Adams K, et al. Superiority of [68Ga]-DOTATATE PET/CT to Other Functional Imaging Modalities in the Localization of SDHB-Associated Metastatic Pheochromocytoma and Paraganglioma. *Clin Cancer Res*. 2015;21(17):3888-3895. PMID: 25873086

Jha A, Ling A, Millo C, et al. Superiority of ⁶⁸Ga-DOTATATE over ¹⁸F-FDG and anatomic imaging in the detection of succinate dehydrogenase mutation (SDHx)-related pheochromocytoma and paraganglioma in the pediatric population. *Eur J Nucl Med Mol Imaging*. 2017;45(5):787-797. PMID: 29204718

Timmers HJ, Chen CC, Carrasquillo JA, et al. Comparison of 18F-fluoro-L-DOPA, 18F-fluorodeoxyglucose, and 18F-fluorodopamine PET and 123I-MIBG scintigraphy in the localization of pheochromocytoma and paraganglioma. *J Clin Endocrinol Metab*. 2009;94(12):4757-4767. PMID: 19864450

10 **ANSWER: A) Add eplerenone, 50 mg twice daily**

Unlike 21-hydroxylase deficiency, 11β-hydroxylase deficiency is a hypertensive form of congenital adrenal hyperplasia. As in 21-hydroxylase deficiency, these patients require glucocorticoid therapy to replace the cortisol deficiency and to limit the rise in ACTH, thus controling the adrenal-derived androgen excess. In addition, glucocorticoid reduces the production of 11-deoxycorticosterone, an upstream precursor with mineralocorticoid activity.

Treatment is a difficult balance between steroid excess and adverse effects of glucocorticoids.

In this example, the minimum tolerable dosage of prednisolone affords normal testicular function and androgen production but persistent mineralocorticoid-dependent hypertension, as evidenced from the suppressed renin and hypokalemia. Although not measured, the 11-deoxycorticosterone is high by inference, because aldosterone is suppressed and 11-deoxycortisol is high. We are told that he does not tolerate higher glucocorticoid dosages (Answers B and C), and potassium supplementation alone (Answer D) will not improve his blood pressure. Similar to the glucocorticoid-sparing effect of fludrocortisone for 21-hydroxylase deficiency, one can use mineralocorticoid receptor antagonist in 11β-hydroxylase deficiency to minimize the prednisolone dosage. Since the patient is male and is likely to experience antiandrogen adverse effects of spironolactone at the stated dosage (Answer E), the drug of choice is eplerenone (Answer A). If the patient were female, then spironolactone, used with contraception, might mitigate both mineralocorticoid and androgen excess consequences. Although not given as an answer option, amiloride is also an alternative choice.

EDUCATIONAL OBJECTIVE
Guide therapy of congenital adrenal hyperplasia due to 11β-hydroxylase deficiency on the basis of clinical and laboratory information.

REFERENCE(S)
Auchus RJ. The classic and nonclassic concenital adrenal hyperplasias. *Endocr Pract.* 2015;21(4):383-389. PMID: 25536973

Mantero F, Opocher G, Rocco S, Carpenè G, Armanini D. Long-term treatment of mineralocorticoid excess syndromes. *Steroids.* 1995;60(1):81-86. PMID: 7792822

11 ANSWER: B) Serum glucose
Pasireotide is a pan-somatostatin agonist, which has high affinity for receptor subtypes 1, 2, 3, and 5. Its effectiveness in treating Cushing disease is largely due to the expression of receptor subtype 5 on corticotrope adenomas. In the pivotal trial, pasireotide improved urinary free cortisol in 93% of patients and normalized urinary free cortisol in 26% of patients. The most common adverse effect was onset or worsening of hyperglycemia in 73% of patients. Thus, serum glucose should be monitored frequently (Answer B).

Serum potassium (Answer A) should be normal before starting mifepristone, which can also cause vaginal bleeding (Answer C) in 20% of reproductive-aged women. These concerns do not apply to pasireotide therapy, which lowers rather than increases cortisol and does not have progesterone receptor antagonist properties. Liver enzyme elevation (Answer D) is uncommon with pasireotide, although it occurs in 20% to 30% of patients treated with ketoconazole. Blood pressure (Answer E) generally improves with all medical therapies for Cushing disease, including pasireotide.

EDUCATIONAL OBJECTIVE
Monitor for adverse effects of pasireotide therapy in patients with Cushing disease.

REFERENCE(S)
Colao A, Petersenn S, Newell-Price J,; Pasireotide B2305 Study Group. A 12-month phase 3 study of pasireotide in Cushing's disease [*N Engl J Med.* 2012;367(8):780]. *N Engl J Med.* 2012;366(10):914-924. PMID: 22397653

Schopohl J, Gu F, Rubens R, et al; Pasireotide B2305 Study Group. Pasireotide can induce sustained decreases in urinary cortisol and provide clinical benefit in patients with Cushing's disease: results from an open-ended, open-label extension trial. *Pituitary.* 2015;18(5):604-612. PMID: 25537481

Pivonello R, Petersenn S, Newell-Price J, et al; Pasireotide B2305 Study Group. Pasireotide treatment significantly improves clinical signs and symptoms in patients with Cushing's disease: results from a phase III study. *Clin Endocrinol (Oxf).* 2014;81(3):408-417. PMID: 24533697

12 ANSWER: E) Measure serum aldosterone and plasma renin activity
The recommended evaluation of an incidentally discovered adrenal mass includes:

- Measurement of plasma or urinary metanephrines to exclude pheochromocytoma
- Overnight dexamethasone suppression test to exclude hypercortisolemia

- Measurement of plasma renin and serum aldosterone (Answer E) to exclude primary aldosteronism (only in hypertensive patients)

This patient had normal results for the first 2 tests. While plasma metanephrine measurement has many false-positive results, the test has high negative predictive value, and further testing for pheochromocytoma (Answer A) is not necessary. If the dexamethasone suppression test were equivocal, plasma ACTH and serum DHEA-S (Answer C) could be used to further assess for autonomous cortisol excess, but these tests are not necessary if the dexamethasone suppression test is normal. Furthermore, clinically significant hypercortisolemia is uncommon if an adrenal adenoma is smaller than 2.4 cm in diameter. Because this patient has hypertension, he should be screened for primary aldosteronism, even with a normal serum potassium level. Of normokalemic hypertensive patients with an incidental adrenal tumor, 5% to 10% have primary aldosteronism. In fact, this patient did have primary aldosteronism, and after evaluation, he underwent left adrenalectomy with marked improvement in his blood pressure.

Although it is customary to repeat CT scans in a year (Answer D) when the adrenal tumor is determined not to have any significant autonomous hormone production, the evaluation for primary aldosteronism should be conducted first. MRI (Answer B) might confirm a lipid-rich adenoma, but it would not determine the hormonal activity of an adrenal tumor.

EDUCATIONAL OBJECTIVE
Evaluate an incidentally discovered adrenal tumor for hormone production.

REFERENCE(S)
Zeiger MA, Siegelman SS, Hamrahian AH. Medical and surgical evaluation and treatment of adrenal incidentalomas. *J Clin Endocrinol Metab.* 2011;96(7):2004-2015. PMID: 21632813

Bernini G, Moretti A, Argenio G, Salvetti A. Primary aldosteronism in normokalemic patients with adrenal incidentalomas. *Eur J Endocrinol.* 2002;146(4):523-529. PMID: 11916621

13 **ANSWER: C) Etomidate**
Drugs that inhibit cortisol synthesis include aminoglutethimide, ketoconazole, metyrapone, and etomidate (Answer C), as well as new drugs under development such as the 11β-hydroxylase inhibitor osilodrostat. Etomidate is frequently administered intravenously in preparation for rapid intubation in the emergency department. Etomidate inhibits 11β-hydroxylase, the last step in cortisol synthesis and an enzyme unique to the cortisol pathway. Etomidate is very effective for control of hypercortisolemia in acutely ill patients with Cushing syndrome. Sedation is the limiting adverse effect, which is why it is usually used in intubated patients as in the stem. It has the advantages of intravenous administration and rapid onset.

Mitotane (Answer A) is adrenolytic, but it takes weeks to have an effect. Pasireotide (Answer B) is only effective in treating Cushing disease. Ketoconazole (Answer D) is relatively contraindicated due to elevated transaminases and must be administered orally. Mifepristone (Answer E) can be used to treat any form of hypercortisolemia and it might be effective in this patient, but it is orally administered, and hypokalemia should be corrected before dosing.

EDUCATIONAL OBJECTIVE
Differentiate among drugs that lower cortisol production.

REFERENCE(S)
Alexandraki KI, Grossman AB. Therapeutic strategies for the treatment of severe Cushing's syndrome. *Drugs.* 2016;76(4):447-458. PMID: 26833215

Preda VA, Sen J, Karavitaki N, Grossman AB. Etomidate in the management of hypercortisolaemia in Cushing's syndrome: a review. *Eur J Endocrinol.* 2012;167(2):137-143. PMID: 22577107

Fleseriu M, Petersenn S. Medical therapy for Cushing's disease: adrenal steroidogenesis inhibitors and glucocorticoid receptor blockers. *Pituitary.* 2015;18(2):245-252. PMID: 25560275

14
ANSWER: D) Increase the hydrocortisone dosage to 40 mg on arising and 20 mg in the early afternoon

This woman had quite severe Cushing disease for a prolonged period. Her pituitary surgery was successful with histologic confirmation of adenoma resection plus undetectable cortisol and ACTH, as well as DHEA-S. Her hypothalamic-pituitary-adrenal axis will remain suppressed for many months, and she requires cortisol replacement therapy. Not surprisingly, she is suffering from cortisol withdrawal syndrome. Laboratory testing confirms central adrenal insufficiency, so no further testing for recurrent disease (Answers A and C) is required. Instead, she needs to have her hydrocortisone dosage increased (Answer D). While the current dosage might seem supraphysiologic, it is still very low relative to her cortisol exposure when she had Cushing disease. Patients even experience cortisol withdrawal syndrome when their Cushing disease is not cured but ACTH and cortisol production is significantly lowered.

Because her cortisol deficiency is central, her renin-angiotensin-aldosterone axis is functional, and both standing blood pressure and serum potassium are normal. Fludrocortisone (Answer B) is therefore unnecessary. DHEA-S decreases following cure of Cushing disease and can remain low for years despite recovery of cortisol production. Some literature suggests that DHEA replacement (Answer E) is beneficial for women with permanent adrenal insufficiency in the chronic setting, but the benefits are mostly for sexuality and do not address cortisol withdrawal. In several months, it might be appropriate to consider DHEA supplementation.

Ancillary medications to aid symptoms include selective serotonin reuptake inhibitors for mood problems and nonsteroidal anti-inflammatory drugs for myalgias. The hydrocortisone dosage is gradually tapered as symptoms abate to allow axis recovery. For those with severe glucocorticoid-induced myopathy, physical therapy is very important from the midpoint of the recovery phase.

EDUCATIONAL OBJECTIVE
Manage the cortisol withdrawal syndrome following cure of Cushing disease.

REFERENCE(S)
Bhattacharyya A, Kaushal K, Tymms DJ, Davis JR. Steroid withdrawal syndrome after successful treatment of Cushing's syndrome: a reminder. *Eur J Endocrinol.* 2005;153(2):207-210. PMID: 16061825

Kleiber H, Rey F, Temler E, Gomez F. Dissociated recovery of cortisol and dehydroepiandrosterone sulphate after treatment for Cushing's syndrome. *J Endocrinol Invest.* 1991;14(6):489-492. PMID: 1663528

El Asmar N, Rajpal A, Selman WR, Arafah BM. The value of perioperative levels of ACTH, DHEA, and DHEA-S and tumor size in predicting recurrence of Cushing disease. *J Clin Endocrinol Metab.* 2018;103(2):477-445. PMID: 29244084

Nieman LK, Biller BM, Findling JW, et al; Endocrine Society. Treatment of Cushing's syndrome: an Endocrine Society Clinical Practice Guideline. *J Clin Endocrinol Metab.* 2015;100(8):2807-2831. PMID: 26222757

15
ANSWER: E) Serum glucose level

Mifepristone is a competitive antagonist for both the glucocorticoid receptor and the progesterone receptor. It is used for the treatment of Cushing syndrome in patients with glucose intolerance or diabetes mellitus. Because mifepristone also antagonizes the feedback inhibition of cortisol on the adenoma, ACTH and cortisol production often rise in Cushing disease when patients are on treatment but not enough to offset the beneficial effects of glucocorticoid receptor blockade in peripheral tissues. Consequently, serum cortisol, urinary free cortisol (Answer A), or plasma ACTH (Answer C) cannot be used to titrate therapy.

Because of potent progesterone receptor antagonism, menses cease during mifepristone therapy. Furthermore, endometrial hypertrophy and vaginal bleeding can occur weeks to months after starting therapy. Thus, return of regular monthly menses (Answer B) cannot be used as a guide.

Blood pressure (Answer D) can decrease after several weeks of treatment, but blood pressure can also rise if the cortisol increases sufficiently. A rise in cortisol increases mineralocorticoid receptor activation, yet mifepristone does not antagonize the mineralocorticoid receptor. Thus, hypertension and hypokalemia can also occur or worsen on treatment. Hence, blood pressure is not a reliable measure of therapeutic adequacy.

If elevated, serum glucose (Answer E) decreases rapidly with mifepristone treatment, and the improved glycemic control is a reliable indicator of therapeutic effect. Additional parameters include weight loss and regression of cushingoid features, but these changes take much longer than the immediate reduction in glucose.

EDUCATIONAL OBJECTIVE
Titrate mifepristone therapy for Cushing disease on the basis of clinical and biochemical data.

REFERENCE(S)

Castinetti F, Fassnacht M, Johanssen S, et al. Merits and pitfalls of mifepristone in Cushing's syndrome. *Eur J Endocrinol.* 2009;160(6):1003-1010. PMID: 19289534

Fleseriu M, Biller BM, Findling JW, Molitch ME, Schteingart DE, Gross C; SEISMIC Study Investigators. Mifepristone, a glucocorticoid receptor antagonist, produces clinical and metabolic benefits in patients with Cushing's syndrome. *J Clin Endocrinol Metab.* 2012;97(6):2039-2049. PMID: 22466348

16 ANSWER: E) No further testing

During critical illness, cortisol rises and remains elevated without circadian rhythm for days to weeks until recovery occurs. Furthermore, cortisol production is resistant to suppression from exogenous glucocorticoids such as dexamethasone. The more gravely ill the patient, the greater the stimulus for cortisol production and the less the cortisol rises with cosyntropin. Viewed this way, cortisol and its attenuated rise with cosyntropin are prognostic factors in critical illness. In addition, many critically ill patients are hypoproteinemic, with low albumin and low plasma cortisol-binding capacity as in this patient, such that the total serum cortisol underestimates the concentration of free and biologically active cortisol. For patients with serum albumin concentrations less than 2.5 g/dL (<25 g/L), the serum free cortisol is uniformly normal even when the serum total cortisol concentration is 12 to 18 µg/dL (331.1 to 496.6 nmol/L), which is below the conventional cut-off for a normal response. In addition, newer cortisol immunoassays and mass spectrometry assays yield values about 30% lower than older immunoassays. For these reasons, this patient does not have adrenal insufficiency and requires no further testing (Answer E).

Serum DHEA-S (Answer B) is a useful measure of adrenal function in combination with cortisol, as DHEA-S production is also ACTH-dependent. However, in critical illness, DHEA-S falls and DHEA rises. Thus, serum DHEA-S cannot be used to adjudicate adrenal function in critical illness. Plasma ACTH (Answer C) will not influence the interpretation of the ACTH-stimulation test and can be low or low-normal after several days of crucial illness. Critical illness is a contraindication to an insulin tolerance test (Answer A), and cortisol values from a low-dose ACTH-stimulation test (Answer D) would have to be corrected for hypoproteinemia as well.

EDUCATIONAL OBJECTIVE
Interpret cortisol dynamics in critical illness.

REFERENCE(S)

Sprung CL, Annane D, Keh D, et al; CORTICUS Study Group. Hydrocortisone therapy for patients with septic shock. *N Engl J Med.* 2008;358(2):111-124. PMID: 18184957

Arafah BM. Hypothalamic pituitary adrenal function during critical illness: limitations of current assessment methods. *J Clin Endocrinol Metab.* 2006;91(10):3725-3745. PMID: 16882746

Sam S, Corbridge TC, Mokhlesi B, Comellas AP, Molitch ME. Cortisol levels and mortality in severe sepsis. *Clin Endocrinol (Oxf).* 2004;60(1):29-35. PMID: 14678284

Hamrahian AH, Oseni TS, Arafah BM. Measurements of serum free cortisol in critically ill patients. *N Engl J Med.* 2004;350(16):1629-1638. PMID: 15084695

Annane D, Sebille V, Troche G, Raphael JC, Gajdos P, Bellissant E. A 3-level prognostic classification in septic shock based on cortisol levels and cortisol response to corticotropin. *JAMA.* 2000;283(8):1038-1045. PMID: 10697064

Al-Aridi R, Abdelmannan D, Arafah BM. Biochemical diagnosis of adrenal insufficiency: the added value of dehydroepiandrosterone sulfate measurements. *Endocr Pract.* 2011;17(2):261-270. PMID: 21134877

Arlt W, Hammer F, Sanning P, et al. Dissociation of serum dehydroepiandrosterone and dehydroepiandrosterone sulfate in septic shock. *J Clin Endocrinol Metab*. 2006;91(7):2548-2554. PMID: 16608898

Raverot V, Richet C, Morel Y, Raverot G, Borson-Chazot F. Establishment of revised diagnostic cut-offs for adrenal laboratory investigation using the new Roche Diagnostics Elecsys® Cortisol II assay. *Ann Endocrinol (Paris)*. 2016;77(5):620-622. PMID: 27449530

17 ANSWER: D) Hydrocortisone, 10 mg twice daily

Two large studies have shown that in women with untreated nonclassic 21-hydroxylase deficiency, more than 80% become pregnant in 1 year with or without medical therapy. However, the risk of miscarriage is up to 26%. In these cohorts, patients with nonclassic 21-hydroxylase deficiency who are treated with hydrocortisone have a 6% risk of miscarriage. If treatment is prescribed, glucocorticoid alone (Answer D) is sufficient.

Anastrozole (Answer A), clomiphene (Answer C), and metformin (Answer E) are treatments to improve fertility in women with polycystic ovary syndrome, which is a diagnosis of exclusion after ruling out Cushing syndrome, hyperprolactinemia, and nonclassic 21-hydroxylase deficiency. For nonclassic 21-hydroxylase deficiency, the dosage of 1 mg of dexamethasone daily (Answer B) is much too high and is contraindicated for pregnancy. Furthermore, fludrocortisone is not necessary.

EDUCATIONAL OBJECTIVE
Manage a patient with nonclassic 21-hydroxylase deficiency and infertility.

REFERENCE(S)
Finkielstain GP, Chen W, Mehta SP, et al. Comprehensive genetic analysis of 182 unrelated families with congenital adrenal hyperplasia due to 21-hydroxylase deficiency. *J Clin Endocrinol Metab*. 2011;96(1):E161-E172. PMID: 20926536

Nandagopal R, Sinaii N, Avila NA, et al. Phenotypic profiling of parents with cryptic nonclassic congenital adrenal hyperplasia: findings in 145 unrelated families. *Eur J Endocrinol*. 2011;164(6):977-984. PMID: 21444649

Moran C, Azziz R, Weintrob N, et al. Reproductive outcome of women with 21-hydroxylase-deficient nonclassic adrenal hyperplasia. *J Clin Endocrinol Metab*. 2006;91(9):3451-3456. PMID: 16822826

Bidet M, Bellanné-Chantelot C, Galand-Portier MB, et al. Fertility in women with nonclassical congenital adrenal hyperplasia due to 21-hydroxylase deficiency. *J Clin Endocrinol Metab*. 2010;95(3):1182-1190. PMID: 20080854

18 ANSWER: A) Serum corticosterone and 11-deoxycorticosterone measurement

In a patient with a 46,XY karyotype and sex reversal, the elevated LH and low testosterone indicate gonadal dysgenesis or a testosterone biosynthetic defect. The elevated ACTH and low cortisol indicate a simultaneous adrenal problem, yet the patient also has hypertension and hypokalemia. The diagnosis rests at the intersection of 3 differentials. First, the differential diagnosis for ACTH-dependent mineralocorticoid excess is best approached considering the pathologic mineralocorticoid in each case:

Aldosterone
- Glucocorticoid-remediable aldosteronism (familial hyperaldosteronism)

Cortisol
- Cushing syndrome; apparent mineralocorticoid excess (genetic or licorice)

11-Deoxycorticosterone
- 17α-hydroxylase/17,20-lyase deficiency, 11β-hydroxylase deficiency

Second, consider the enzymes common to the adrenal and gonad (*see image*): the cholesterol side-chain cleavage enzyme (CYP11A1), 17α-hydroxylase/17,20-lyase (CYP17A1), and 3β-hydroxysteroid dehydrogenase/isomerase type 2 (3βHSD2).

Third, for completeness, the main considerations for primary amenorrhea with a 46,XY karyotype in a phenotypic female include testosterone biosynthesis defects, steroid 5α-reductase type 2 deficiency, and androgen insensitivity syndrome.

Thus, enzymatic defects that do not include the adrenal gland cannot explain the low cortisol hypertension (eg, 17β-hydroxysteroid dehydrogenase type

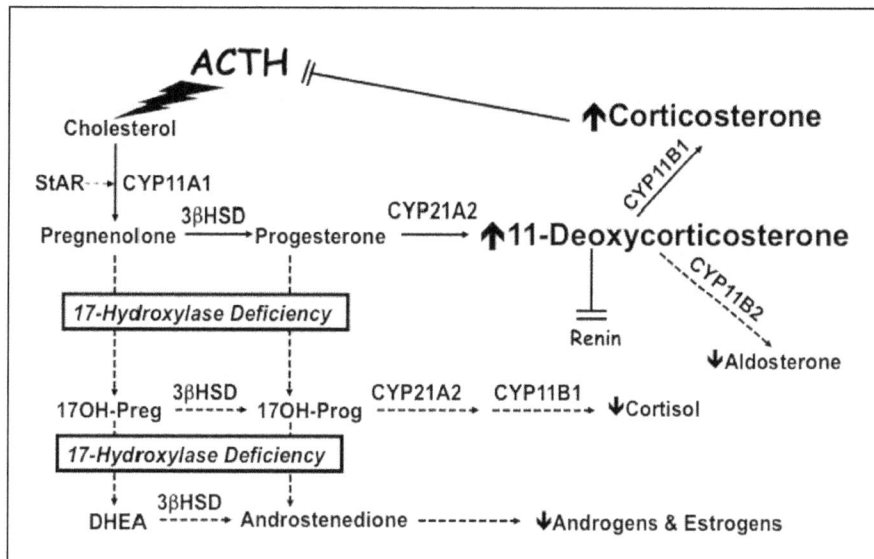

Disordered steroidogenesis in 17-hydroxylase deficiency. Abbreviations: CYP21A2, 21-hydroxylase; CYP11B1, 11β-hydroxylase; CYP11B2, aldosterone synthase.

3 and 5α-reductase type 2 deficiencies [Answer B] or aromatase deficiency [Answer D]). Androgen insensitivity (Answer C) is excluded with the low testosterone and absent breast development. Although 3β-hydroxysteroid dehydrogenase/isomerase type 2 (Answer E) is common to the adrenal and gonad, testosterone is produced in moderate amounts via the type 1 isoenzyme in the liver and skin.

The remaining etiology is 17α-hydroxylase deficiency, and the diagnosis relies on demonstration of elevated steroids proximal to the enzymatic blockade: corticosterone, 11-deoxycorticosterone, and progesterone (Answer A). In patients with 17α-hydroxylase deficiency, corticosterone in high amounts substitutes for cortisol as their glucocorticoid, so they rarely develop adrenal crises. The diagnosis is often delayed until adolescence or early adulthood, when primary amenorrhea with absent secondary sexual characteristics and hypertension are present. Serum 11-deoxycorticosterone is also elevated in 11β-hydroxylase deficiency, but testosterone is high and corticosterone is not elevated.

The management of 17-hydroxylase deficiency aims to replace the deficient gonadal steroids and to mitigate the mineralocorticoid-mediated hypertension and hypokalemia. Because patients are phenotypically female, estrogen replacement is prescribed as it is for other forms of gonadal dysfunction such as Turner syndrome. Glucocorticoid replacement is not strictly necessary since corticosterone substitutes for cortisol, and mineralocorticoid excess can be managed with spironolactone titrated to achieve normal blood pressure and serum potassium. Nevertheless, it is standard practice to treat with glucocorticoid to reduce ACTH and 11-deoxycorticosterone, thus accomplishing the same goal. In patients with a 46,XY karyotype and intra-abdominal testes, gonadectomy should be strongly considered because of the increased risk of malignancy and absence of spermatogenesis. In patients with a 46,XX karyotype, large ovarian cysts commonly develop due to chronically elevated gonadotropins, and cyclic withdrawal bleeding is necessary. Recently, the first pregnancy was achieved in a patient with some residual enzyme activity.

EDUCATIONAL OBJECTIVE
Perform the differential diagnosis of ACTH-dependent mineralocorticoid excess.

REFERENCE(S)

Auchus RJ. Steroid 17-hydroxylase and 17,20-lyase deficiencies, genetic and pharmacologic. *J Steroid Biochem Mol Biol.* 2017;165(Pt A):71-78. PMID: 26862015

Costa-Santos M, Kater CE, Auchus RJ; Brazilian Congenital Adrenal Hyperplasia Multicenter Study Group. Two prevalent CYP17 mutations and genotype-phenotype correlations in 24 Brazilian patients with 17-hydroxylase deficiency. *J Clin Endocrinol Metab.* 2004;89(1):49-60. PMID: 2004;89(1):49-60.

Zhang M, Sun S, Liu Y, et al. New, recurrent, and prevalent mutations: clinical and molecular characterization of 26 Chinese patients with 17alpha-hydroxylase/17,20-lyase deficiency. *J Steroid Biochem Mol Biol.* 2015;150:11-16. PMID: 25697092

Miller WL, Auchus RJ. The molecular biology, biochemistry, and physiology of human steroidogenesis and its disorders [published correction appears in *Endocr Rev.* 2011;32(4):579]. *Endocr Rev.* 2011;32(1):81-151. PMID: 21051590

Bianchi PH, Gouveia GR, Costa EM, et al. Successful live birth in a woman with 17α-hydroxylase deficiency through IVF frozen-thawed embryo transfer. *J Clin Endocrinol Metab.* 2016;101(2):345-348. PMID: 26647153

19 ANSWER: C) Increase the fludrocortisone acetate dosage to 0.2 mg at bedtime

Adrenal replacement therapy is guided primarily on clinical grounds with limited laboratory testing. In particular, the plasma ACTH does not normalize with physiologic replacement doses and should not be used to titrate glucocorticoid as the TSH is used for thyroxine replacement. Weight regain is a good sign that glucocorticoid dosing is adequate, and lack of cushingoid stigmata suggests that she is not overtreated. Fatigue persists in some patients, and if it is due to glucocorticoid deficiency, this will transiently improve following each hydrocortisone dose, which is not the case in this woman. Consequently, a more distributed dose (Answer A) of hydrocortisone, a higher dose (Answer D) of hydrocortisone, or a switch to a longer-acting drug such as prednisone (Answer B) is unlikely to help.

Chronic volume depletion is another cause of fatigue in patients with adrenal insufficiency. This patient has constant fatigue, a mild increase in heart rate, and borderline-low blood pressure. More importantly, the plasma renin activity is quite elevated and the serum potassium value is high-normal. The patient was asked to stand for 2 minutes, and her blood pressure fell to 92/66 mm Hg and her pulse rate rose to 105 beats/min. Thus, her mineralocortoid replacement is inadequate, and the dosage of fludrocortisone acetate should be increased (Answer C). The laboratory data alone are sufficient to justify this change. Therefore, a change is indeed indicated in her treatment regimen (thus, Answer E is incorrect). For many patients with primary adrenal insufficiency, the "standard" dosage of 0.1 mg daily of fludrocortisone acetate is inadequate. For her, the dosage might need to be increased further to 0.3 to 0.6 mg daily in gradual increments.

EDUCATIONAL OBJECTIVE
Guide therapy of adrenal insufficiency on the basis of clinical and laboratory information.

REFERENCE(S)
Bornstein SR, Allolio B, Arlt W, et al. Diagnosis and treatment of primary adrenal insufficiency: an Endocrine Society Clinical Practice Guideline. *J Clin Endocrinol Metab.* 2016;101(2):364-389. PMID: 26760044

Bancos I, Hahner S, Tomlinson J, Arlt W. Diagnosis and management of adrenal insufficiency. *Lancet Diabetes Endocrinol.* 2015;3(3):216-226. PMID: 25098712

Esposito D, Pasquali D, Johannsson G. Primary adrenal insufficiency: managing mineralocorticoid replacement therapy. *J Clin Endocrinol Metab.* 2018;103(2):376-387. PMID: 29156052

20 ANSWER: E) Increase sodium intake

The chronic vasoconstriction in patients with pheochromocytoma induces a state of volume depletion. Often the hematocrit is slightly increased, and patients can be hypertensive but show orthostatic hypotension, especially with α-adrenergic blockade. After just a few doses of phenoxybenzamine, the patient was still hypertensive but now has an orthostatic rise in heart rate. Preoperative volume expansion via sodium loading (Answer E) is critical to mitigate postoperative hypotension. Often a β-adrenergic blocker is added once adequate α-blockade is established and volume expansion is completed, but the rise in heart rate with standing is maintaining the blood pressure with standing. Adding metoprolol now (Answer A) could dangerously drop the patient's blood pressure. The phenoxybenzamine dosage will need to be increased later but not until his orthostasis improves (thus, Answer B is incorrect). Nicardipine (Answer C) is sometimes used as an alternative to α-blockade, but phenoxybenzamine is effective in this patient; he simply needs time to allow volume expansion at the lower dose using either drug. Water intake alone (Answer D) will not suffice—only sodium-containing food and drinks.

EDUCATIONAL OBJECTIVE
Manage volume depletion in pheochromocytoma.

REFERENCE(S)

Lenders JW, Duh QY, Eisenhofer G, et al; Endocrine Society. Pheochromocytoma and paraganglioma: an Endocrine Society Clinical Practice Guideline. *J Clin Endocrinol Metab*. 2014;99(6):1915-1942. PMID: 24893135

Young WF Jr. Adrenal causes of hypertension: pheochromocytoma and primary aldosteronism. *Rev Endocr Metab Disord*. 2007;8(4):309-320. PMID: 17914676

21 ANSWER: C) Normal testosterone, high androstenedione, low LH

This patient has a history of adrenal insufficiency with bilateral testicular masses and medication nonadherence. This is an unfortunately common situation for young men with classic 21-hydroxylase deficiency who develop testicular adrenal rest tumors (TARTs). These are ACTH-responsive masses that are either ectopic adrenal tissue or reprogrammed steroidogenic stem cells in the testes that grow and produce a pattern of steroids similar to that of the adrenal cortex of these patients. The major clue is the bilateral nature of the tumors and their firm, irregular texture. In 21-hydroxylase deficiency, the adrenal produces abundant androstenedione and inefficiently converts this precursor to testosterone, so the major laboratory feature is the elevated androstenedione, disproportionate to the testosterone, which is typically "normal" but not derived from the normal testicular Leydig cells. The high adrenal androgen production suppresses LH. Initially, FSH is also low, but with time the masses compromise blood flow to the normal testis and cause irreversible damage to the Sertoli and germ cells, and FSH rises. Both the testicular mass and the suppressed gonadotropins cause infertility. The presence of TART and high FSH are poor prognostic factors for fertility in men with classic 21-hydroxylase deficiency. Intensification of glucocorticoid therapy can allow regression of the rests and restoration of fertility, but this can take many months. Surgical removal of TARTs often provides long-term control of the tumors, but it does not restore testicular function. The pattern of laboratory results expected in this patient is normal testosterone, high androstenedione, and low LH (Answer C).

The pattern depicted in Answer A implies LH-dependent androstenedione and testosterone production, which is incorrect. The pattern depicted in Answer B is typical of a Leydig-cell tumor producing estradiol but presents as a solitary, often small and round mass in one testis. The pattern in Answer D is typical of primary testicular failure and ignores the adrenal-derived androgens. The pattern in Answer E is typical of a nonfunctional testicular tumor such as a seminoma early in the disease course, and these cancers are also unilateral.

EDUCATIONAL OBJECTIVE
Diagnose testicular adrenal rest tumors in a man with 21-hydroxylase deficiency and predict patterns of laboratory test results.

REFERENCE(S)

Finkielstain GP, Chen W, Mehta SP, et al. Comprehensive genetic analysis of 182 unrelated families with congenital adrenal hyperplasia due to 21-hydroxylase deficiency. *J Clin Endocrinol Metab*. 2011;96(1):E161-E172. PMID: 20926536

Arlt W, Willis DS, Wild SH, et al; United Kingdom Congenital Adrenal Hyperplasia Adult Study Executive (CaHASE). Health status of adults with congenital adrenal hyperplasia: a cohort study of 203 patients. *J Clin Endocrinol Metab*. 2010;95(10):5110-5121. PMID: 20719839

Auchus RJ, Arlt W. Approach to the patient: the adult with congenital adrenal hyperplasia. *J Clin Endocrinol Metab*. 2013;98(7):2645-2655. PMID: 23837188

Reisch N, Rottenkolber M, Greifenstein A, et al. Testicular adrenal rest tumors develop independently of long-term disease control: a longitudinal analysis of 50 adult men with congenital adrenal hyperplasia due to classic 21-hydroxylase deficiency. *J Clin Endocrinol Metab*. 2013;98(11):E1820-E1826. PMID: 23969190

Claahsen-van der Grinten HL, Otten BJ, Takahashi S, et al. Testicular adrenal rest tumors in adult males with congenital adrenal hyperplasia:

evaluation of pituitary-gonadal function before and after successful testis-sparing surgery in eight patients. *J Clin Endocrinol Metab.* 2007;92(2):612-615. PMID: 17090637

King TF, Lee MC, Williamson EE, Conway GS. Experience in optimizing fertility outcomes in men with congenital adrenal hyperplasia due to 21 hydroxylase deficiency. *Clin Endocrinol (Oxf).* 2016;84(6):830-836. PMID: 26666213

22 ANSWER: C) Micronodular adrenocortical hyperplasia

This young man has strong clinical evidence of Cushing syndrome, and biochemical testing confirms hypercortisolemia. The surprising finding is that, despite low ACTH, an adrenal tumor (Answer A) is not identified. ACTH measurement was documented to be low on 2 occasions, ruling out ACTH-dependent Cushing disease (Answer B) or ectopic ACTH syndrome (Answer D). Because cortisol is high in the serum and urine, he is not receiving exogenous synthetic glucocorticoids (Answer E). His Cushing syndrome is due to micronodular adrenocortical hyperplasia (Answer C). When the nodules are pigmented, the pathology is called primary pigmented nodular adrenal disease (PPNAD). Often the adrenal glands appear normal or just slightly irregular on CT because multiple small adenomas (<1 cm) form in both glands.

Many patients with micronodular adrenocortical hyperplasia have Carney complex, which is caused by mutations in the tumor suppressor gene *PRKAR1A*, encoding the regulatory subunit of protein kinase A. Carney complex is inherited in an autosomal dominant manner, and its manifestations are caused by loss or mutation of the wild-type *PRKAR1A* allele in a cell of a susceptible tissue, leading to constant and unregulated elevation of cyclic AMP. In the adrenal cortex, cyclic AMP drives the growth of clonal adrenal cell clusters, which exhibit autonomous cortisol production. Carney complex includes many other clinical features, such as mucosal lentigines, blue nevi, cardiac myxomas, and several additional tumors. These Carney complex-associated tumors include pituitary adenomas, which most often produce growth hormone, thyroid adenomas, Sertoli-cell tumors of the testes in men, and uterine tumors in women.

EDUCATIONAL OBJECTIVE
Identify the clinical and radiographic features of micronodular adrenocortical hyperplasia.

REFERENCE(S)

Bertherat J, Horvath A, Groussin L, et al. Mutations in regulatory subunit type 1A of cyclic adenosine 5′-monophosphate-dependent protein kinase (PRKAR1A): phenotype analysis in 353 patients and 80 different genotypes. *J Clin Endocrinol Metab.* 2009;94(6):2085-2091. PMID: 19293268

Kirschner LS. PRKAR1A and the evolution of pituitary tumors. *Mol Cell Endocrinol.* 2010;326(1-2):3-7. PMID: 20451576

23 ANSWER: B) Perform bilateral adrenalectomy

This woman has an indolent but metastatic medullary thyroid cancer, which is one type of foregut neuroendocrine tumor. She had been managed expectantly with imaging, biochemical monitoring, and levothyroxine replacement. At some point, clones from her tumor acquired the capacity to produce other hormones, and the rapidly progressive hypercortisolism suggests ectopic ACTH syndrome. Medullary thyroid cancer and other neuroendocrine tumors can cause ectopic ACTH syndrome, which is consistent with the history, physical examination findings, and laboratory findings. The most important point in this patient's management is that the tumor burden is not her most pressing immediate problem; rather, it is her hypercortisolism. She is at high risk for psychosis, opportunistic infections, and venous thrombosis. Prompt control of her Cushing syndrome is indicated with medical and/or surgical management. Bilateral adrenalectomy (Answer B) is the best immediate step in her management. An important consideration is that the patient's malignancy is incurable, and any tumor-directed therapies are palliative and unlikely to correct the hypercortisolism.

Biopsy of the liver mass (Answer A) will only reveal medullary thyroid cancer/neuroendocrine tumor. Given the delayed onset of Cushing syndrome with the preexisting tumor, it is likely that not all of the cells will stain for ACTH, and the biopsy findings would not add to the management plan.

Although octreotide (Answer C) can be helpful in managing any hormonal secretion from a neuroendocrine tumor, the drug is not formally indicated for medullary thyroid cancer, and biochemical responses in this situation are uncommon. Cytotoxic chemotherapy (Answer D) for neuroendocrine tumors is reserved for high-grade tumors such as small cell lung cancer. It is not indicated for a low-grade malignancy and will not correct the hypercortisolism. While vandetanib (Answer E) is active in medullary thyroid cancer, it is not curative but generally helps to delay progression. Although vandetanib might be considered in this patient, it should be initiated after correction of the hypercortisolism with bilateral adrenalectomy.

EDUCATIONAL OBJECTIVE
Manage ectopic ACTH syndrome resulting from a metastatic neuroendocrine tumor.

REFERENCE(S)

Kamp K, Alwani RA, Korpershoek E, Franssen GJ, de Herder WW, Feelders RA. Prevalence and clinical features of the ectopic ACTH syndrome in patients with gastroenteropancreatic and thoracic neuroendocrine tumors. *Eur J Endocrinol.* 2016;174(3):271-280. PMID: 26643855

Ejaz S, Vassilopoulou-Sellin R, Busaidy NL, et al. Cushing syndrome secondary to ectopic adrenocorticotropic hormone secretion: the University of Texas MD Anderson Cancer Center Experience. *Cancer.* 2011;117(19):4381-4389. PMID: 21412758

Isidori AM, Kaltsas GA, Pozza C, et al. The ectopic adrenocorticotropin syndrome: clinical features, diagnosis, management, and long-term follow-up. *J Clin Endocrinol Metab.* 2006;91(2):371-377. PMID: 16303835

Ilias I, Torpy DJ, Pacak K, Mullen N, Wesley RA, Nieman LK. Cushing's syndrome due to ectopic corticotropin secretion: twenty years' experience at the National Institutes of Health. *J Clin Endocrinol Metab.* 2005;90(8):4955-4962. PMID: 15914534

24 ANSWER: B) Rescreen after correcting hypokalemia

Although many medications interact with the renin-angiotensin-aldosterone axis, most antihypertensive agents act by vasodilation or volume depletion, which tends to raise plasma renin activity. Thus, when the plasma renin activity is low (<1), the aldosterone-to-renin ratio (ARR) screen is generally valid. β-Adrenergic blockers can lower renin, but aldosterone falls as well. The ARR in this case is greater than 13, which is intermediate between a clearly positive screen (>20) (Answer E) and a normal screen (<4) (Answer A). During proper preparation for screening, however, it is important to first correct hypokalemia (Answer B), as low potassium impairs aldosterone production. Thus, in a setting of high clinical suspicion and an unusual result with a very low potassium, the screen cannot be dismissed as normal and should be repeated after correcting the hypokalemia.

Candesartan and nifedipine are not significantly interfering with the screening since the plasma renin activity is less than 1 (thus, Answers C and D are incorrect). However, these drugs can cause false-negative screens if the renin is elevated.

EDUCATIONAL OBJECTIVE
Identify causes of false-negative screening for primary aldosteronism.

REFERENCE(S)

Raizman JE, Diamandis EP, Holmes D, Stowasser M, Auchus R, Cavalier E. A renin-ssance in primary aldosteronism testing: obstacles and opportunities for screening, diagnosis, and management. *Clin Chem.* 2015;61(8):1022-1027. PMID: 26106077

Funder JW, Carey RM, Mantero F, et al. The management of primary aldosteronism: case detection, diagnosis, and treatment: an Endocrine Society Clinical Practice Guideline. *J Clin Endocrinol Metab.* 2016;101(5):1889-1916. PMID: 26934393

25 ANSWER: C) Prolonged hyperkalemia

With sustained autonomous aldosterone excess, the normal zona glomerulosa can become suppressed. In this case, hyperkalemia can develop after adrenalectomy. Risk factors that have been identified include older age, longer duration of hypertension, proteinuria, and most importantly, reduced renal function. This older man with long-standing hypertension, microalbuminuria, and elevated serum creatinine is therefore at significant risk for postoperative hyperkalemia (Answer C), which can be prolonged. Hyperkalemia can be treated with dietary potassium restriction, a thiazide diuretic, or fludrocortisone acetate, depending on the patient's blood pressure.

Patients with primary aldosteronism often have a slight rise in creatinine after adrenalectomy or upon addition of mineralocorticoid receptor antagonist therapy, but they rarely experience renal failure (Answer A). Unlike patients with pheochromocytoma who are receiving potent $\alpha 1$ receptor blockade, refractory hypotension (Answer B) does not develop postoperatively. Because the tumor was localized with adrenal venous sampling, recurrence of hyperaldosteronism (Answer D) is unlikely. Adrenal insufficiency (Answer E) can occur after removal of an aldosterone-secreting adenoma that is cosecreting cortisol, but these tumors tend to be larger than 3 cm, and cortisol withdrawal is very unlikely given the small size of the adenoma.

EDUCATIONAL OBJECTIVE
Identify risk factors for postadrenalectomy hyperkalemia in patients with primary aldosteronism.

REFERENCE(S)

Chiang WF, Cheng CJ, Wu ST, et al. Incidence and factors of post-adrenalectomy hyperkalemia in patients with aldosterone producing adenoma. *Clin Chim Acta.* 2013;424:114-118. PMID: 23727469

Fischer E, Hanslik G, Pallauf A, et al. Prolonged zona glomerulosa insufficiency causing hyperkalemia in primary aldosteronism after adrenalectomy. *J Clin Endocrinol Metab.* 2012;97(11):3965-3973. PMID: 22893716

Park KS, Kim JH, Ku EJ, et al. Clinical risk factors of postoperative hyperkalemia after adrenalectomy in patients with aldosterone-producing adenoma. *Eur J Endocrinol.* 2015;172(6):725-731. PMID: 25766046

Calcium and Bone Board Review

Carolyn B. Becker, MD ● Brigham & Women's Hospital

ANSWER: A) Genetic testing for a calcium-sensing receptor (*CASR*) gene mutation

Does this patient have familial hypocalciuric hypercalcemia (FHH) or primary hyperparathyroidism? Answering this question might be easier if she had documentation of previous serum calcium measurements (normal serum calcium values in the past would make FHH unlikely) or relatives in whom serum calcium measurements could be obtained. She is young (<50 years), so surgery would be recommended if she has primary hyperparathyroidism. In pregnancy, the optimal time for surgery is the second trimester (thus, Answer B is incorrect). However, surgery (Answer C) should not be performed until her diagnosis is confirmed, particularly given her very mild presentation. The key to this question is to recognize the impact of pregnancy on urinary calcium excretion in a patient with FHH.

The 24-hour urine calcium-to-creatinine clearance ratio (CCCR) in FHH is generally less than 0.01 and is calculated using the following formula:

$$[\text{urine calcium (mg/24 h)} \times \text{serum creatinine (mg/dL)}] / [\text{urine creatinine (mg/24 h)} \times \text{serum calcium (mg/dL)}]$$

In this patient, the CCCR is 0.016, more consistent with primary hyperparathyroidism than with FHH. However, due to increased calcium flux and glomerular filtration rate in pregnancy, the CCCR can approach that usually seen in women with primary hyperparathyroidism.

The most common form of FHH, known as FHH type 1, is caused by inactivating mutations in the gene encoding the calcium-sensing receptor (*CASR*), and genetic testing for a *CASR* mutation is the best next step now (Answer A). Recently, mutations in the *GNA11* gene were shown to cause FHH type 2. Additionally, mutations affecting codon 15 in the *AP2S1* gene have been described as causing FHH type 3.

Persons with FHH continue to secrete PTH because the inactivated calcium-sensing receptor is reading a low serum calcium level. This also occurs in the renal tubular calcium-sensing receptor where it leads to renal calcium conservation (decreased renal calcium excretion). The end result is hypercalcemia and hypocalciuria. A low CCCR (<0.01) is consistent with FHH and should be followed by confirmatory genetic testing.

If the patient has FHH, one of her parents most likely had the same mutation, as transmission is autosomal dominant (although this cannot be confirmed because her parents are deceased). Several different mutations have been described, and a negative result for any of the known mutations would not conclusively exclude FHH. Because primary hyperparathyroidism is much more common than FHH, should the diagnosis still be unclear after genetic testing for a *CASR* mutation, parathyroid surgery could be considered. In the older literature, primary hyperparathyroidism during pregnancy was associated with high fetal loss and adverse pregnancy outcomes. More recent experience suggests that mild, asymptomatic primary hyperparathyroidism with serum calcium levels less than 11.4 mg/dL (<2.9 mmol/L) can be watched conservatively and closely monitored without surgical intervention.

MRI of the neck and mediastinum (Answer D) would be an option if the diagnosis of primary hyperparathyroidism were definite and surgery was to be done before delivery. Otherwise, sestamibi scanning and/or 4D CT scanning to localize an adenoma are generally contraindicated during pregnancy, although in rare cases, they have been done. Testing for an *MEN1* gene mutation (Answer E) would be strongly recommended if the diagnosis of primary hyperparathyroidism were confirmed in this young person.

EDUCATIONAL OBJECTIVE
Distinguish familial hypocalciuric hypercalcemia from primary hyperparathyroidism during pregnancy.

REFERENCE(S)
Ghaznavi SA, Saad NM, Donovan LE. The biochemical profile of familial hypocalciuric hypercalcemia and primary hyperparathyroidism during pregnancy and lactation: two case reports and review of the literature. *Case Rep Endocrinol*. 2016;2725486. PMID: 27957351

Maltese G, Izatt L, McGowan BM, Hafeez K, Hubbard JG, Carroll PV. Making (mis) sense of asymptomatic marked hypercalcemia in pregnancy. *Clin Case Rep*. 2017;5(10):1587-1590. PMID: 29026550

Rubin MR, Silverberg SJ. Use of cinacalcet and 99mTc-sestamibi imaging during pregnancy. *J Endocr Soc*. 2017;1(9):1156-1159. PMID: 29264570

Hovden S, Rejnmark L, Ladefoged SA, Nissen PH. AP2S1 and NA11 mutations – not a common cause of familial hypocalciuric hypercalcemia. *Eur J Endocrinol*. 2017;176(2):177-185. PMID: 27913609

Christensen SE, Nissen PH, Vestergaard P, Mosekilde L. Familial hypocalciuric hypercalcaemia: a review. *Curr Opin Endocrinol Diabetes Obes*. 2011;18(5):359-370. PMID: 21986511

Shinall MC Jr, Dahir KM, Broome JT. Differentiating familial hypocalciuric hypercalcemia from primary hyperparathyroidism. *Endocr Pract*. 2013;19(4):697-702. PMID: 23425644

2   ANSWER: E) Measure serum pyridoxal 5′ phosphate

This man has hypophosphatasia, a rare metabolic bone disorder in which tissue nonspecific alkaline phosphatase (TNSALP) deficiency in osteoblasts and chondrocytes impairs mineralization, leading to a rickets-like syndrome in children and osteomalacia in adults. The pathognomonic finding is subnormal serum activity of the TNSALP enzyme, which may result from any one of hundreds of genetic mutations in the gene encoding TNSALP (*ALPL*). Genetic inheritance is autosomal recessive for the infantile forms but either autosomal recessive or autosomal dominant in the milder, adult forms with variable penetrance. The prevalence of severe hypophosphatasia is approximately 1 in 100,000 among Anglo-Saxon populations and is particularly prevalent among the Mennonites in Manitoba, Canada, where 1 in every 25 persons is a carrier.

The clinical presentation depends on the age at presentation. Adult hypophosphatasia can be associated with premature loss of deciduous teeth or early loss of adult teeth. Osteomalacia results in painful feet with poor healing of metatarsal stress fractures, as well as thigh or hip pain from femoral pseudofractures located in the lateral cortices of the femora. Some patients experience attacks of arthritis (pseudogout from calcium pyrophosphate crystal deposition), cartilage degeneration, and pyrophosphate arthropathy.

TNSALP is tethered to osteoblasts and chondrocytes and hydrolyzes inorganic pyrophosphate and 5′-phosphate, a major form of vitamin B_6. When TNSALP is low, inorganic pyrophosphate inhibits formation of hydroxyapatite, causing rickets or osteomalacia.

Characteristic laboratory findings include low serum activity of alkaline phosphatase. In general, the lower the alkaline phosphatase, the more severe the symptoms. The decrease in alkaline phosphatase activity leads to an increase in pyridoxal 5′-phosphate; thus, once the condition is suspected, serum 5′-phosphate (Answer E) should be measured. Genetic testing for a mutation in the TNSALP gene (*ALPL*) is confirmatory.

Screening for *COL1A1/COL1A2* gene mutations (Answer A) would be appropriate if osteogenesis imperfecta were being considered, but in that condition, the alkaline phosphatase level should be normal. Treating with an antiresorptive agent such as alendronate (Answer B) or denosumab would not be indicated in hypophosphatasia, although the anabolic agent teriparatide has been used in rare cases. Measuring fasting serum C-telopeptide (Answer C) is not going to be useful. In general, bone turnover is low in hypophosphatasia, but a low marker of bone resorption such as C-telopeptide will not be diagnostic. Tetracycline-labeled iliac crest bone biopsy (Answer D) can diagnose osteomalacia, but it would not indicate the specific cause of the metabolic bone disorder. Since 2015, enzyme replacement with asfotase alfa for hypophosphatasia has been available. Indications for enzyme treatment and duration of treatment are not well established.

EDUCATIONAL OBJECTIVE
Diagnose hypophosphatasia.

REFERENCE(S)
Whyte MP. Hypophosphatasia: an overview for 2017. *Bone*. 2017;102:15-25. PMID: 28238808

Whyte MP, Mumm S, Deal C. Adult hypophosphatasia treated with teriparatide. *J Clin Endocrinol Metab*. 2007;92(4):1203-1208. PMID: 17213282

3 **ANSWER: C) Adynamic bone disease**

The PTH level in this patient is lower than the goal in patients undergoing dialysis and that, coupled with the very low alkaline phosphatase level and multiple fragility fractures, is most consistent with adynamic bone disease (Answer C). Adynamic bone disease, a type of renal osteodystrophy (now called chronic kidney disease–mineral bone disorder [CKD-MBD]), is present in at least one-third of patients receiving dialysis. Adynamic bone disease is characterized by markedly low bone turnover, reduction of both osteoclast and osteoblast activity, no accumulation of osteoid, and high fracture risk. Serum PTH levels in adynamic bone disease are relatively low (usually <150 pg/mL [<150 ng/L]) compared with levels in patients undergoing dialysis who have other forms of CKD-MBD. This patient's very low alkaline phosphatase level is also consistent with a low bone turnover state.

In patients with end-stage kidney disease, there is resistance to PTH due at least in part to increased N-terminal truncated PTH (7-84), which counteracts the effect of the 1-84 whole molecule on bone. This can be exacerbated by the use of cinacalcet, as well as overly aggressive treatment with calcitriol, both of which reduce PTH secretion. Excessive use of calcium-containing phosphate binders may also contribute.

Osteitis fibrosa cystica (Answer A) would be associated with very high levels of PTH, often with hypercalcemia and elevated alkaline phosphatase. Osteomalacia (Answer B) in patients on long-term hemodialysis is very unusual now that aluminum-based phosphate binders have been abandoned and given the strict limits on aluminum content in dialysate fluids. Mixed uremic osteodystrophy (Answer D) is characterized by osteitis fibrosa cystica coupled with a mineralization defect (osteomalacia) and would not be the most likely finding here.

Diabetes-related osteoporosis (Answer E) in patients with type 2 diabetes is characterized by low bone turnover, inferior bone quality, and increased fracture risk, often despite relatively normal or high bone mineral density. The risk of diabetes-related osteoporosis is correlated with longer duration of diabetes, use of insulin, and presence of diabetes-related complications such as retinopathy and neuropathy. Given that this patient has had a relatively short duration of diabetes without complications and very low bone density, diabetes-related osteoporosis is unlikely.

EDUCATIONAL OBJECTIVE
Diagnose adynamic bone disease in a patient undergoing dialysis.

REFERENCE(S)
Cannata-Andía JB, Rodriguez García M, Gómez Alonso C. Osteoporosis and adynamic bone in chronic kidney disease. *J Nephrol*. 2013;26(1):73-80. PMID: 23023723

Hruska KA, Mathew S. Chronic kidney disease mineral bone disorder (CKD-MBD). In: Rosen CJ, Compston JE, Lian JB, eds. *Primer on the Metabolic Bone Diseases and Disorders of Mineral Metabolism*. Washington, DC: The American Society for Bone and Mineral Research; 2008:343-349.

Brandenburg VM, Floege J. Adynamic bone disease: bone and beyond. *Clin Kidney J*. 2008;1(3):135-147. PMID: 25983860

Kidney Disease: Improving Global Outcomes (KDIGO) CKD-MBD Work Group. KDIGO clinical practice guideline for the diagnosis, evaluation, prevention, and treatment of chronic kidney disease-mineral and bone disorder (CKD-MBD). *Kidney Int*. 2009;(Suppl 113):S1-S130. PMID: 19644521

Paschou SA, Dede AD, Anagnostis PG, Vryonidou A, Morganstein D, Goulis DG. Type 2 diabetes and osteoporosis: a guide to optimal management. *J Clin Endocrinol Metab.* 2017;102(10):3621-3634. PMID: 28938433

Rubin MR. Skeletal fragility in diabetes. *Ann N Y Acad Sci.* 2017;1402(1):18-30. PMID: 28926113

4. ANSWER: D) Vitamin D intoxication

This patient has non-PTH–mediated severe hypercalcemia. Although both *Mycobacterium avium intracellulare* and *Mycobacterium tuberculosis* can be associated with hypercalcemia, *Mycobacterium bovis* infection (Answer A) is not. Nonmycobacterial infections (eg, cytomegalovirus and fungal), as well as lymphomas (eg, Burkitt, T-cell, and others) (Answer C), can present with calcitriol-induced hypercalcemia in patients with HIV/AIDS, but the data in this vignette are not consistent with this etiology. HIV-associated immune reconstitution syndrome (Answer E) occurs during therapy for HIV when there is a massive, acute inflammatory reaction to an infectious agent causing hypercalcemia, but this man has not yet started any therapy for HIV/AIDS. Finally, HIV-associated increase in vitamin D–binding protein (Answer B), which could lead to elevated 25-hydroxyvitamin D and 1,25-dihydroxyvitamin D levels as seen in this case, has never been reported.

The most likely etiology of this patient's hypercalcemia is vitamin D intoxication (Answer D). This is clear by the elevation in both 25-hydroxyvitamin D and 1,25-dihydroxyvitamin D. The culprit in this case was an over-the-counter "vitamin" supplement found in the Dominican Republic and Upper Manhattan containing massive doses of vitamin D (864,000 IU) and vitamin A (123,000 IU) in a 5-mL bottle. In a series of 9 patients with vitamin D intoxication, there were often other reasons for hypercalcemia (such as lymphoma, granulomatous disease, etc), so that the homeostatic and detoxifying mechanisms were overwhelmed. Treatment of vitamin D intoxication includes vigorous intravenous hydration, bisphosphonates, and glucocorticoids, but the resolution of the high 25-hydroxyvitamin D levels may take weeks or months.

EDUCATIONAL OBJECTIVE
Diagnose vitamin D intoxication as the cause of severe hypercalcemia.

REFERENCE(S)
Lowe H, Cusano NE, Binkley N, Blaner WS, Bilezikian JP. Vitamin D toxicity due to a commonly available "over the counter" remedy from the Dominican Republic. *J Clin Endocrinol Metab.* 2011;96(2):291-295. PMID: 21123442

Araki T, Holick MF, Alfonso BD, et al. Vitamin D intoxication with severe hypercalcemia due to manufacturing and labeling errors of two dietary supplements made in the United States. *J Clin Endocrinol Metab.* 2011;96(12):3603-3608. PMID: 21917864

5. ANSWER: A) PTHrP measurement

This case illustrates the point that patients with primary hyperparathyroidism have a higher incidence of cancer and that the 2 conditions may coexist. Initially, this patient presented with elevated calcium and PTH, consistent with primary hyperparathyroidism, and underwent successful resection of a parathyroid adenoma. However, her hypercalcemia did not resolve and in fact worsened, a pattern that is common with coexisting primary hyperparathyroidism and malignant hypercalcemia. The key to diagnosis is to measure PTHrP (Answer A), which is the most common mechanism of hypercalcemia in so-called humoral hypercalcemia associated with many solid cancers.

Without bone pain or elevated alkaline phosphatase, extensive bony metastases are less likely to be the etiology of the hypercalcemia and therefore a total body bone scan (Answer E) would not be the best next test. The mildly detectable PTH level is most likely due to renal insufficiency and there would be no role for measuring PTH antibodies (Answer C). Similarly, a 4D CT scan (Answer B) would only be warranted if there were evidence of recurrent or persistent primary hyperparathyroidism. A 24-hour urinary calcium measurement (Answer D) would not offer any additional diagnostic information in this case.

EDUCATIONAL OBJECTIVE
Diagnose the coexistence of primary hyperparathyroidism and humoral hypercalcemia of malignancy.

REFERENCE(S)

Casez J, Pfammatter R, Nguyen Q, Lippuner K, Jaeger P. Diagnostic approach to hypercalcemia: relevance of parathyroid hormone and parathyroid hormone-related protein measurements. *Eur J Intern Med.* 2001;12(4):344-349. PMID: 11395297

Gomes Lda S, Kulak CA, Costa TM, Vasconcelos EC, Carvalho MD, Borba VZ. Association of primary hyperparathyroidism and humoral hypercalcemia of malignancy in a patient with clear cell renal carcinoma. *Arch Endocrinol Metab.* 2015;59(1):84-88. PMID: 25926120

Richey DS, Welch BJ. Concurrent primary hyperparathyroidism and humoral hypercalcemia of malignancy in a patient with clear cell endometrial cancer. *South Med J.* 2008;101(12):1266-1268. PMID: 19005452

6   ANSWER: D) Pseudohypoparathyroidism type 1A

This young woman has classic signs of pseudohypoparathyroidism type 1A. Pseudohypoparathyroidism is a group of disorders defined by end-organ resistance to PTH that results in hypocalcemia, hyperphosphatemia, and elevated PTH levels. The syndrome is caused by mutations in the *GNAS1* gene that encodes the α subunit of the G protein, which is linked to the PTH receptor. The mutations prevent generation of adenyl cyclase when PTH binds to its receptor and therefore, failure of signal transduction by PTH. Interestingly, *GNAS1* is imprinted in humans, so that expression of the allele for a specific tissue is dependent on whether the allele is inherited from the mother or father. Thus, pseudohypoparathyroidism type 1A (Answer D) is an autosomal dominant disease with a loss-of-function mutation in *GNAS1* that only manifests when the mutation is inherited from the mother. Affected patients have the biochemical abnormalities listed above, as well as a classic phenotypic appearance known as Albright hereditary osteodystrophy. Such patients have round facies, short stature, obesity, developmental delay, and short fourth metacarpal bones as shown in the x-ray in the vignette. Additionally, patients with pseudohypoparathyroidism type 1A have resistance to various other G-protein–coupled hormones, including TSH, LH, FSH, and GnRH.

In contrast, those with paternally transmitted mutations in the *GNAS1* gene have the physical phenotype of Albright hereditary osteodystrophy but normal serum calcium, phosphate, and PTH concentrations. This is referred to as pseudopseudohypoparathyroidism (Answer E).

DiGeorge syndrome (22q11.2 deletion syndrome) (Answer A) results from abnormal development of the third and fourth branchial pouches and is associated with parathyroid aplasia or hypoplasia, thymic aplasia or hypoplasia, cardiac abnormalities, developmental delay, and characteristic facial appearance. In this setting, PTH would be low, not high. An activating mutation in the gene encoding the calcium-sensing receptor (*CASR*) (Answer B) is the usual cause of autosomal dominant hypocalcemia and manifests with hypocalcemia and inappropriately "normal" PTH concentrations. The high PTH seen in this case would not be consistent with autosomal dominant hypocalcemia. Autoimmune polyglandular syndrome type 1 (Answer C) results in immunologic destruction of the parathyroid glands and presents with hypoparathyroidism, primary adrenal insufficiency, and mucocutaneous candidiasis, none of which is present in this patient.

EDUCATIONAL OBJECTIVE
Diagnose pseudohypoparathyroidism type 1A.

REFERENCE(S)

Virágh K, Toke J, Sallai A, Jakab Z, Racz K, Toth M. Gradual development of brachydactyly in pseudohypoparathyroidism. *J Clin Endocrinol Metab.* 2014;99(6):1945-1946. PMID: 24684469

Mantovani G. Clinical review: pseudohypoparathyroidism: diagnosis and treatment. *J Clin Endocrinol Metab.* 2011;96(10):3020-3030. PMID: 21816789

7   ANSWER: B) Recommend that her antidepressant be changed to a different class

This patient has hyponatremia from syndrome of inappropriate antidiuretic hormone secretion (SIADH), most likely from the selective serotonin reuptake inhibitor fluoxetine. As a class, the selective serotonin reuptake inhibitors have been associated with significantly increased risks of syndrome of inappropriate antidiuretic hormone secretion and hyponatremia, particularly in the elderly population. Other antidepressants such as mirtazapine, bupropion, trazodone, and the tricyclic antidepressants are associated with lower rates of hyponatremia. It would be important to offer a combined approach of calcium, vitamin D, fall reduction, and reversal of hyponatremia to this patient at very high risk.

A number of studies have shown that hyponatremia (serum sodium <135 mEq/L) is associated with increased risk for osteoporosis and falls. Although there are no clinical trials showing that reversal of hyponatremia leads to reductions in falls and fractures, it makes sense to try this in such a high-risk patient who refuses other interventions. The mechanisms by which hyponatremia may predispose to falls and fractures are complex and not completely understood, but there is evidence for both bone loss and gait instability in association with hyponatremia.

Treating this elderly woman with salt tablets (Answer C) may actually worsen her hyponatremia, and a chronic 1000 cc per day fluid restriction (Answer D) is unrealistic and may result in volume depletion and increased fall risk. An intensive weightlifting program (Answer A) could lead to injury in an elderly woman with very low spinal bone mineral density, but other forms of exercise, such as mild to moderate muscle strengthening and balance and gait training would be beneficial. Prescribing a high-calorie diet to promote weight gain (Answer E) is unrealistic in this patient.

EDUCATIONAL OBJECTIVE
Explain the link between hyponatremia and osteoporosis.

REFERENCE(S)
Upala S, Sanguankeo A. Association between hyponatremia, osteoporosis, and fracture: a systematic review and meta-analysis. *J Clin Endocrinol Metab*. 2016;101(4):1880-1886. PMID: 26913635

Usala RL, Fernandez SJ, Mete M, Cowen L, Shara NM, Barsony J, Verbalis JG. Hyponatremia is associated with increased osteoporosis and bone fractures in a large US health system population. *J Clin Endocrinol Metab*. 2015;100(8):3021-3031. PMID: 26083821

Sejling A-S, Thorsteinsson A-L, Pedersen-Bjergaard U, Eiken P. Recovery from SIADH-associated osteoporosis: a case report. *J Clin Endocrinol Metab*. 2014;99(10):3527-3530. PMID: 24971663

8 ANSWER: C) Cinacalcet, 30 mg orally twice daily

This patient has primary hyperparathyroidism and is acutely ill with multiple comorbidities that make her a poor surgical candidate. Therefore, urgent surgery (Answer A) is inappropriate. In 2011, the US FDA approved cinacalcet (Answer C) for treatment of severe primary hyperparathyroidism in patients who are poor surgical candidates. The peak action of cinacalcet in lowering serum calcium is observed at 1 week, but significant calcium reduction can be seen in a few days and long-term treatment is effective in maintaining eucalcemia. Cinacalcet may be a useful "bridge" to surgery for patients requiring medical stabilization.

Zoledronic acid, 5 mg intravenously (Answer B), would lower serum calcium within 4 to 5 days, but it is contraindicated in patients with an estimated glomerular filtration rate less than 35 mL/min. Moreover, intravenous bisphosphonates may be associated with atrial fibrillation. Intravenous normal saline, 500 cc/h (Answer D), is contraindicated in a patient with congestive heart failure. Nasal calcitonin (Answer E) is not an effective treatment for hypercalcemia. Subcutaneous calcitonin can provide a temporary decrease in calcium levels but is limited by tachyphylaxis within 24 to 48 hours. Denosumab, a very potent antiresorptive agent approved for osteoporosis and hypercalcemia of malignancy, would effectively lower serum calcium but does not specifically target PTH excess. Additionally, denosumab could precipitate symptomatic hypocalcemia and may not be desirable in a patient with pneumonia due to some immunosuppressive activity.

EDUCATIONAL OBJECTIVE
Recommend cinacalcet as an appropriate treatment for primary hyperparathyroidism in patients with hypercalcemia who are poor surgical candidates.

REFERENCE(S)

Khan A, Bilezikian J, Bone H, et al. Cinacalcet normalizes serum calcium in a double-blind randomized, placebo-controlled study in patients with primary hyperparathyroidism with contraindications to surgery. *Eur J Endocrinol*. 2015;172(5):527-535. PMID: 25637076

Marcocci C, Bollerslev J, Khan AA, Shoback DM. Medical management of primary hyperparathyroidism: proceedings of the fourth International Workshop on the Management of Asymptomatic Primary Hyperparathyroidism. *J Clin Endocrinol Metab*. 2014;99(10):3607-3618. PMID: 25162668

ANSWER: B) 21-Hydroxylase antibodies

This patient has autoimmune polyendocrine syndrome type 1 (APS type 1) due to a mutation in the autoimmune regulator gene (*AIRE*). APS type 1 is also known by the acronym APECED (autoimmune polyendocrinopathy-candidiasis-ectodermal dystrophy). The classic presentation includes at least 2 of the following 3 major clinical components: chronic mucocutaneous candidiasis, primary hypoparathyroidism, and autoimmune adrenal insufficiency. Studies have shown that primary adrenal insufficiency may be diagnosed before clinical symptoms by checking for antibodies against the 21-hydroxylase enzyme (Answer B). A normal 8-AM serum cortisol level does not detect preclinical disease. Inclusion of an ACTH measurement with the morning cortisol might show early adrenal insufficiency with a high ACTH, but that was not one of the choices.

Serum ceruloplasmin (Answer A) is used to diagnose Wilson disease, a genetic syndrome in which copper accumulates in tissues, including the parathyroid glands. Classic findings are Kayser-Fleischer rings, liver damage, and neuropsychiatric symptoms. PTH antibody assessment (Answer D) is not necessary to diagnose hypoparathyroidism in APS type 1. Glutamic acid decarboxylase (GAD_{65}) antibodies (Answer C) are often present in patients with APS type 1, but they have not been shown to predict the development of type 1 diabetes mellitus, which occurs in about 18% of those with the syndrome. Anti-islet cell antibodies are a better predictor. TPO antibodies (Answer E) are positive in patients with autoimmune thyroid disease, but this is not a feature of autoimmune polyendocrine syndrome type 1.

EDUCATIONAL OBJECTIVE
Diagnose autoimmune polyendocrine syndrome type 1 as a cause of hypoparathyroidism and recommend appropriate screening.

REFERENCE(S)

Weiler FG, Dias-da-Silva MR, Lazaretti-Castro M. Autoimmune polyendocrine syndrome type 1: case report and review of literature. *Arq Bras Endocrinol Metabol*. 2012;56(1):54-66. PMID: 22460196

Akirav EM, Ruddle NH, Herold KC. The role of AIRE in human autoimmune disease. *Nat Rev Endocrinol*. 2011;7(1):25-33. PMID: 21102544

Eisenbarth GS, Gottlieb PA. Autoimmune polyendocrine syndromes. *N Engl J Med*. 2004;350(20):2068-2079. PMID: 15141045

ANSWER: E) Hypercalcemia

Hypercalcemia (Answer E) and hypercalciuria are the 2 most common adverse effects from teriparatide. Serum calcium is often slightly (and transiently) elevated in the hours immediately following the day's dose of teriparatide, but it will usually be back within normal limits on samples drawn 16 or more hours after the last dose. Patients who take teriparatide in the morning who need blood work done should be told to delay their teriparatide dose until after samples for lab tests have been drawn. In the comparator trial against abaloparatide, 6.4% of patients on teriparatide developed hypercalcemia. For persistent hypercalcemia on teriparatide, the first step is to reduce calcium intake by 50% or to stop it completely. If this doesn't resolve the hypercalcemia, some clinicians recommend reducing the injections to every other day for a period.

Despite hypercalciuria while on teriparatide, nephrocalcinosis (Answer D) has not been reported and new-onset nephrolithiasis during treatment (Answer C) is very rare. Osteosarcoma (Answer B) was reported in Fischer rats receiving high doses of teriparatide, resulting in a "black box" warning by the US FDA. However, in more than 1 million humans treated with the drug, there have been only 3 reported cases of osteosarcoma.

Finally, although uric acid increases with both teriparatide and abaloparatide, attacks of gout (Answer A) are not common.

EDUCATIONAL OBJECTIVE
Identify mild hypercalcemia as one of the most common adverse effects during teriparatide therapy for osteoporosis.

REFERENCE(S)
Satterwhite J, Heathman M, Miller PD, Marin F, Glass EV, Dobnig H. Pharmacokinetics of teriparatide (rhPTH[1-34]) and calcium pharmacodynamics in postmenopausal women with osteoporosis. *Calcif Tiss Int*. 2010;87(6):485-492. PMID: 20953593

Miller PD, Hattersley G, Riis BJ, et al; ACTIVE Study Investigators. Effect of abaloparatide vs placebo on new vertebral fractures in postmenopausal women with osteoporosis: a randomized clinical trial. *JAMA*. 2016;316(7):722-733. PMID: 27533157

Neer RM, Arnaud CD, Zanchetta JR, et al. Effect of parathyroid hormone (1-34) on fractures and bone mineral density in postmenopausal women with osteoporosis. *N Engl J Med*. 2001;344(19):1434-1441. PMID: 11346808

11 ANSWER: A) Calcitriol plus oral phosphate

This patient has X-linked hypophosphatemic rickets, an X-linked dominant form of rickets that is relatively unresponsive to vitamin D. The hypophosphatemia arises as a consequence of a defective *PHEX* gene product (phosphate-regulating gene with homology to endopeptidases on the X chromosome), which ultimately results in elevated fibroblast growth factor 23 (FGF-23) levels and impaired renal proximal tubule phosphate reabsorption. In addition, despite severe hypophosphatemia, 1,25-dihydroxyvitamin D_3 production is not appropriately enhanced due to FGF-23–mediated suppression of 1α-hydroxylase activity. Thus, the "normal" level of 1,25-dihydroxyvitamin D_3 is inappropriate in the setting of elevated PTH and low serum phosphate.

Although children with X-linked hypophosphatemic rickets receive treatment with calcitriol and oral phosphate, it is controversial whether adults with fused epiphyses should continue to be treated. The goal of therapy in adults is to minimize bone pain and to enhance mobility. Because this patient has diffuse, severe bone pain, some treatment should be offered (thus, Answer E is incorrect). The lowest effective dosages of calcitriol and oral phosphate (Answer A) should be given to control symptoms and then stopped if and when symptoms resolve. Calcitriol and oral phosphate reduce bone pain and dental abscesses in X-linked hypophosphatemic rickets, but they do not improve radiographically proven enthesopathy (calcification of tendons, ligaments, and joint capsules). Oral calcitriol alone (Answer B) would enhance calcium and phosphate absorption from the gut and inhibit PTH secretion, but would not be effective for the bone pain without added oral phosphate. Phosphate alone (Answer C) would worsen hyperparathyroidism and therefore is not recommended. Cinacalcet (Answer D) can be useful in patients with elevated PTH levels to reduce the phosphaturic effects of PTH at the renal tubule and prevent the secondary hyperparathyroidism resulting from phosphate administration. However, cinacalcet alone has not been shown to reduce bone pain or improve the osteomalacia in X-linked hypophosphatemic rickets.

On April 17, 2018, the human monoclonal antibody burosumab received US FDA approval for treatment of patients age 1 year and older with X-linked hypophosphatemic rickets. This drug targets FGF-23. The role of burosumab in the management of adults with symptomatic X-linked hypophosphatemic rickets awaits further recommendations.

Two important complications from treatment of X-linked hypophosphatemic rickets include nephrocalcinosis and hyperparathyroidism. Up to 80% of patients with X-linked hypophosphatemic rickets have radiographic evidence of nephrocalcinosis, secondary to renal tubular acidosis and deposition of calcium phosphate in the renal tubules. Intermittent hypercalcemia and hypercalciuria are believed to contribute to the development of nephrocalcinosis. Thiazide diuretics and amiloride may be useful in the prevention of nephrocalcinosis in these patients. Hyperparathyroidism usually occurs after years of treatment, but may be present early in the disease course. When calcium forms a complex with oral phosphate supplements, this can result in intermittent hypocalcemia and stimulation of PTH release despite the suppressive effects of calcitriol. When this secondary hyperparathyroidism is not adequately controlled, autonomous (tertiary) hyperparathyroidism can occur, necessitating surgical intervention.

EDUCATIONAL OBJECTIVE
Manage X-linked hypophosphatemic rickets in adults.

REFERENCE(S)

Alizadeh Naderi AS, Reilly RF. Hereditary disorders of renal phosphate wasting. *Nat Rev Nephrol.* 2010;2(11):657-665. PMID: 20924400

Beck-Nielsen SS, Brusgaard K, Rasmussen LM, et al. Phenotype presentation of hypophosphatemic rickets in adults. *Calcif Tissue Int.* 2010;87(2):108-119. PMID: 20524110

Connor J, Olear EA, Insogna KL, et al. Conventional therapy in adults with X-linked hypophosphatemia: effects on enthesopathy and dental disease. *J Clin Endocrinol Metab.* 2015;100(10):3625-3632. PMID: 26176801

Yavropoulou MP, Kotsa K, Gotzamani Psarrakou A, et al. Cinacalcet in hyperparathyroidism secondary to X-linked hypophosphatemic rickets: case report and brief literature review. *Hormones (Athens).* 2010;9(3):274-278. PMID: 20688626

12 ANSWER: C) Adjust the FRAX scores upward by 15% at the spine and 20% at the hip

Patients taking any dosage of glucocorticoid with an anticipated duration of 3 months or longer require a metabolic bone evaluation. The goal is to identify patients at high risk for fracture who would benefit from possible pharmacologic intervention. Within 6 months of initiating glucocorticoids, clinical risk factors for fracture should be assessed and, in selected patients, DXA of the hip and spine should be performed. For this patient who does not have osteoporosis on DXA or a personal history of fracture, use of the FRAX calculator can help determine whether she is likely to benefit from pharmacologic treatment.

It is important to realize, however, that FRAX assumes that the glucocorticoid dosage is between 2.5 and 7.5 mg daily. For patients on higher dosages (>7.5 mg daily), the recommendation is to adjust the FRAX scores upward at both the spine and the hip (Answer C). In this patient, a 20% increase in her FRAX hip score will place her above the treatment threshold of 3% (ie, 2.6% + 0.52 = 3.12%). Some experts also recommend imaging the spine (via lateral spine radiographs or vertebral fracture assessments on DXA) to further identify higher-risk patients who would warrant intervention if, for example, silent spinal fractures were identified.

Close monitoring with a repeated DXA in 6 months (Answer A) is not unreasonable, but this strategy may miss vulnerable patients who could fracture within the first 6 months. Measuring fasting serum C-telopeptide (Answer B) has not been shown to help predict fractures in glucocorticoid-induced osteoporosis. Initially, bone resorption increases in glucocorticoid-induced osteoporosis, but with long-term exposure, the major defect is suppression of osteoblast function and reduced bone formation. The decrease in bone formation is due to direct inhibition of osteoblast proliferation and differentiation and to increased apoptosis of mature osteoblasts and osteocytes.

Denosumab (Answer D) is not US FDA-approved for management of glucocorticoid-induced osteoporosis and thus would not be the best therapeutic choice. Alendronate, risedronate, zoledronate, and teriparatide (Answer E) are approved by the US FDA for management of glucocorticoid-induced osteoporosis. However, teriparatide would not be indicated as first-line treatment due to cost and other considerations. Alendronate or risedronate are usually considered first-line therapies for glucocorticoid-induced osteoporosis unless there are contraindications or previous intolerance. Alendronate has recently been shown to be associated with decreased hip fractures in patients on long-term glucocorticoid therapy.

EDUCATIONAL OBJECTIVE
Adjust FRAX scores in patients on glucocorticoid dosages greater than 7.5 mg daily.

REFERENCE(S)

Kanis JA, Johansson H, Oden A, McCloskey EV. Guidance for the adjustment of FRAX according to the dose of glucocorticoids. *Osteoporos Int.* 2011;22(3):809-816. PMID: 21229233

Buckley L, Guyatt G, Fink HA, et al. 2017 American College of Rheumatology guideline for the prevention and treatment of glucocorticoid-induced osteoporosis. *Arthritis Rheumatol.* 2017;69(8):1521-1537. PMID: 28585373

Axelsson KF, Nilsson AG, Wedel H, Lundh D, Lorentzon M. Association between alendronate use and hip fracture risk in older patients using oral prednisolone. *JAMA.* 2017;318(2):146-155. PMID: 28697254

13 ANSWER: E) Switch to zoledronic acid

This patient has multiple issues that place her at highest risk for future fractures: she is elderly, frail, and female with 3 prevalent vertebral fractures, gait instability, frequent falls, and probable mild cognitive dysfunction. In addition, she has persistent osteoporosis at the hip on DXA after 5 years of alendronate. The relatively high fasting serum C-telopeptide suggests that she is not absorbing or not taking the alendronate properly. Postmenopausal women on oral bisphosphonates should have fasting serum C-telopeptide levels in the lower half of the premenopausal range. Clearly, she is too high risk for a drug holiday but is not doing well on oral alendronate. In patients with poor response to alendronate and persistent high bone turnover, switching to zoledronic acid (Answer E) can result in improvements in bone mineral density and offer protection against both spine and nonvertebral fractures. It would also be logistically easier for her to come in once per year, given her transportation issues.

A frequent clinical question is when or if to recommend a "bisphosphonate holiday" to patients with osteoporosis who have been on either oral or intravenous bisphosphonates for several years. Because bisphosphonates have a long retention in the skeleton, they may continue to exhibit antifracture effectiveness even after therapy is stopped. The decision to stop bisphosphonate therapy must be individualized. Studies have shown that after 3 years of annual intravenous zoledronic acid or 5 years of oral bisphosphonate therapy, it is reasonable to reassess each patient and determine whether a bisphosphonate holiday should be considered. Patients and physicians worry about the risk of rare but devastating adverse effects (such as osteonecrosis of the jaw and atypical femur fractures) that seem to be correlated with duration of bisphosphonate therapy.

Data from the FLEX and HORIZON extension trials show that many patients can stop bisphosphonate therapy temporarily after 3 to 5 years without loss of bone mineral density or increased fracture risk. However, some subgroups of patients appear to be at higher risk for bone loss or fractures after stopping therapy. For these patients, the options include either continuing the bisphosphonate for up to 10 years with periodic reassessment or stopping the bisphosphonate and switching to a different agent. Patients at highest risk include those with a history of hip or vertebral fractures, multiple fractures, T-score of –2.5 or lower at the hip, or other factors placing them "at high risk" for fractures.

Stopping alendronate and reassessing in 1 to 2 years (Answer A) is not acceptable given her very high risk for falls and fractures. Continuing alendronate for another 5 years (Answer B) does not make sense as she has evidence of treatment failure with multiple vertebral fractures and a nonsuppressed C-telopeptide.

It might make sense to switch from an antiresorptive agent to the anabolic agent teriparatide (Answer C), particularly with the presence of vertebral fractures. However, in an elderly patient with mild cognitive dysfunction who lives alone and has most likely been nonadherent to alendronate therapy, giving daily injections with teriparatide (or the other anabolic agent, abaloparatide) would not be a good choice.

Until recently, the best answer to this question would have been denosumab (Answer D), as this has shown excellent efficacy and safety over 10 years of continuous use, increases bone mineral density at both spine and hip without reaching a plateau, and significantly reduces fracture risk at the spine, hip, and nonvertebral areas. However, recent reports have documented that missing even 1 dose of denosumab may result in a very rapid rebound in bone resorption and loss of bone mineral density, and, in some cases, multiple vertebral fractures. Therefore, in an elderly patient with severe vertebral osteoporosis who may not be able to reliably get her denosumab injections every 6 months, intravenous zoledronate would be a safer choice.

EDUCATIONAL OBJECTIVE
Manage patients on long-term bisphosphonate therapy with high fracture risk.

REFERENCE(S)

Black DM, Schwartz AV, Ensrud KE, et al; FLEX Research Group. Effects of continuing or stopping alendronate after 5 years of treatment: the Fracture Intervention Trial Long-term Extension (FLEX): a randomized trial. *JAMA*. 2006;296(24):2927-2938. PMID: 17190893

Black DM, Reid IR, Boonen S, et al. The effect of 3 versus 6 years of zoledronic acid treatment of osteoporosis: a randomized extension to the HORIZON-Pivotal Fracture Trial (PFT) [published correction appears in *J Bone Miner Res*. 2012;27(12):2612]. *J Bone Miner Res*. 2012;27(2):243-254. PMID: 22161728

Adler RA, Fuleihan GE, Bauer DC, et al. Managing osteoporosis in patients on long-term bisphosphonate treatment: report of a Task force of the American Society for Bone and Mineral Research. *J Bone Miner Res*. 2016;31(1):16-35. PMID: 26350171

Eiken P, Vestergaard P. Treatment of osteoporosis after alendronate or risedronate. *Osteoporos Int*. 2016;27(1):1-12. PMID: 26438307

Cummings SR, Ferrari S, Eastell R, et al. Vertebral fractures after discontinuation of denosumab: a post-hoc analysis of the randomized placebo-controlled FREEDOM trial and its extension. *J Bone Miner Res*. 2018;33(2):190-198. PMID: 29105841

14 ANSWER: B) Intravenous isotonic saline, 300-500 cc/h

This is a classic case of milk-alkali syndrome leading to a hypercalcemic crisis. The triad of hypercalcemia, renal failure, and metabolic alkalosis results from ingestion of excessive amounts of calcium and absorbable alkali over a short period. In this case, the patient was taking very large doses (bottles) of calcium carbonate and aspirin, sodium bicarbonate, and anhydrous citric acid for gastrointestinal distress following an alcohol binge. Taking a careful history and recognizing the triad are keys to making the diagnosis.

In the setting of excess calcium/alkali ingestion, hypercalcemia causes renal vasoconstriction, decreases the glomerular filtration rate, and increases bicarbonate reabsorption. Metabolic alkalosis further increases renal tubular reabsorption of calcium, and hypovolemia from nausea/vomiting further reduces the glomerular filtration rate. A vicious cycle can occur with rapid clinical deterioration and death. Hyperphosphatemia may also be seen with excessive ingestion of milk as the calcium source.

Acute management of a hypercalcemic crisis generally involves saline hydration, subcutaneous calcitonin for 24 to 48 hours, intravenous bisphosphonate (or subcutaneous denosumab in selected cases), and treatment of the underlying disease. Furosemide should be added only when there is clinical evidence of volume overload or congestive heart failure. In cases of vitamin D–mediated hypercalcemia, prednisone, 40 to 60 mg daily, or another glucocorticoid equivalent may be useful, but it should not be given without biochemical evidence of inappropriate vitamin D levels. Finally, in patients with hypercalcemic crisis due to primary hyperparathyroidism, cinacalcet can be a "bridge" to parathyroidectomy.

In milk-alkali syndrome, simply stopping the exogenous calcium and alkali and providing vigorous saline hydration (Answer B) to increase the glomerular filtration rate and help clear the calcium and bicarbonate can rapidly reverse the metabolic disarray. In those with acute milk-alkali syndrome, treatment can lead to an acute drop in serum calcium to hypocalcemic levels (with rebound increase in PTH). More chronic cases with nephrocalcinosis take much longer to resolve.

Neither zoledronic acid (Answer A) nor denosumab (Answer C) would be effective because the hypercalcemia is not due to increased bone resorption. Similarly, hydrocortisone (Answer D) would not address the primary mechanism.

EDUCATIONAL OBJECTIVE
Diagnose and manage milk-alkali syndrome.

REFERENCE(S)

Beall DP, Scofield RH. Milk-alkali syndrome associated with calcium carbonate consumption. Report of 7 patients with parathyroid hormone levels and an estimate of prevalence among patients hospitalized with hypercalcemia. *Medicine (Baltimore)*. 1995;74(2):89-96. PMID: 7891547

Fiorino AS. Hypercalcemia and alkalosis due to the milk-alkali syndrome: a case report and review. *Yale J Biol Med*. 1996;69(6):517-523. PMID: 9436295

Picolos MK, Lavis VR, Orlander PR. Milk-alkali syndrome is a major cause of hypercalcaemia among non-end-stage renal disease (non-ESRD) inpatients. *Clin Endocrinol (Oxf)*. 2005;63(5):566-576. PMID: 16268810

Bazari H, Palmer WE, Baron JM, Armstrong K. Case records of the Massachusetts General Hospital. Case 24-2016. A 66-year-old man with malaise, weakness, and hypercalcemia. *N Engl J Med*. 2016;375(6):567-574. PMID: 27509105

15 ANSWER: E) Albumin

Fifty percent of circulating calcium is bound to serum proteins, primarily to albumin. In this patient with advanced cirrhosis, serum albumin (Answer E) is almost certainly low. The correction factor is to adjust the serum calcium up or down by 0.8 mg/dL (0.2 mmol/L) for each 1.0 g/dL (10 g/L) deviation of serum albumin below 4 mg/dL (<40 g/L). If his albumin level were 2.0 g/dL (20 g/L) (lower range of normal 3.5 g/dL [35 g/L]), then his adjusted serum calcium level would be 8.6 mg/dL (2.2 mmol/L). Ionized calcium measurement would be another excellent choice. He could also have low magnesium (Answer D) in addition to low albumin, but the first step in his evaluation is to determine whether there is any calcium problem at all and this requires correcting the measured serum calcium for the hypoalbuminemia. If he is truly hypocalcemic with a low corrected calcium, then measuring 25-hydroxyvitamin D (Answer B) and PTH (Answer A) would be appropriate. Measuring 1,25-dihydroxyvitamin D (Answer C) would not be helpful in this situation.

EDUCATIONAL OBJECTIVE

Investigate the etiology of hypocalcemia and correct for low albumin in this setting.

REFERENCE(S)

Ariyan CE, Sosa JA. Assessment and management of patients with abnormal calcium. *Crit Care Med*. 2004;32(Suppl 4):S146-S154. PMID: 15064673

Shoback D. Hypocalcemia: definition, etiology, pathogenesis, diagnosis, and management. In: Rosen CJ, Compston JE, Lian JB, eds. *Primer on the Metabolic Bone Diseases and Disorders of Mineral Metabolism*. Washington, DC: The American Society for Bone and Mineral Research; 2008:313-317.

16 ANSWER: E) Monitor over time without any immediate changes

According to the National Osteoporosis Foundation, osteoporosis can be diagnosed by a T-score in the hip, spine, or distal radius of less than –2.5 or by a fragility fracture. Fractures of fingers, toes, metatarsals, facial bones, and the skull are not included within the definition of osteoporotic fractures. These fractures can occur in otherwise healthy individuals with normal bone density and bone quality. Since this patient's DXA shows osteopenia and the fractures are not diagnostic of osteoporosis, the FRAX tool can be used to determine whether he should be treated pharmacologically. Pharmacologic treatment should be considered for patients with an absolute 10-year fracture risk of 20% or higher for any major fracture or 3% or higher for hip fracture. This patient's fracture risk is well below the treatment threshold, and he should therefore not be treated with a medication. The best answer is to monitor him over time (Answer E). There is no indication to start alendronate (Answers A and C).

Finasteride is approved to treat men with androgenic hair loss or benign prostatic hypertrophy. It works by inhibiting 5α-reductase, thereby reducing dihydrotestosterone levels. In a small percentage of cases, men on finasteride may experience decreased libido, sexual dysfunction, decreased sperm count, and gynecomastia. However, testosterone levels do not decrease and, in general, there has been no consistent association between finasteride use and osteoporosis or fractures. A case-control study from Taiwan did show a 1.52-fold increased risk of osteoporosis in men using finasteride for benign prostatic hypertrophy, particularly at higher dosages, but other studies have shown no association. In this man with osteopenia, there is no need to stop finasteride (Answer B or C). Given the normal level of testosterone, there is no need to treat with transdermal testosterone (Answer D).

EDUCATIONAL OBJECTIVE
Manage men with low bone density who are taking finasteride and use the FRAX tool for risk assessment.

REFERENCE(S)

Lin WL, Hsieh YW, Lin CL, Sung FC, Wu CH, Kao CH. A population-based nested case-control study: the use of 5-alpha-reductase inhibitors and the increased risk of osteoporosis diagnosis in patients with benign prostate hyperplasia. *Clin Endocrinol (Oxford)*. 2015;82(4):503-508. PMID: 25158777

Jacobsen SJ, Cheetham TC, Haque R, Shi JM, Loo RK. Association between 5-alpha reductase inhibition and risk of hip fracture. *JAMA*. 2008;300(14):1660-1664. PMID: 18840839

National Osteoporosis Foundation. *Clinician's Guide to Prevention and Treatment of Osteoporosis*. Washington, DC: National Osteoporosis Foundation; 2014.

17 **ANSWER: D) 25-Hydroxyvitamin D measurement**

This patient has classic clinical signs and symptoms of osteomalacia from profound vitamin D deficiency, most likely due to nutritional deficiencies and clothing blocking the sunlight. When screening for vitamin D deficiency, the appropriate test is 25-hydroxyvitamin D measurement (Answer D). The activated form of vitamin D, calcitriol (or 1,25-dihydroxyvitamin D) may be normal, high, or low in the setting of severe vitamin D deficiency and it is therefore not a good marker for deficiency.

Although this patient's serum phosphate was slightly low, due to vitamin D deficiency and secondary hyperparathyroidism, it is not at the level where tumor-induced osteomalacia should be considered before ruling out vitamin D deficiency.

Therefore, checking FGF-23 (Answer A) is incorrect.

A total body bone scan (Answer B) is appropriate for patients with metastatic cancer to the bone, marked by bone pain, pathologic fractures, hypercalcemia, and elevated alkaline phosphatase. In this patient, the bone scan could be "positive" with multiple "hot spots" and could lead the clinician toward a workup for malignancy. However, the low, rather than high, serum calcium points more to a metabolic bone disorder than to malignancy.

Urinary fractional excretion of phosphate (Answer E) will correctly demonstrate renal phosphate wasting in X-linked hypophosphatemic rickets, tumor-induced osteomalacia, and other causes of low phosphate, but it would not be useful here. The mild hypophosphatemia is due to profound vitamin D deficiency and hyperparathyroidism and is not the primary underlying disorder.

EDUCATIONAL OBJECTIVE
Diagnose osteomalacia due to severe vitamin D deficiency.

REFERENCE(S)

Gifre L, Peris P, Monegal A, Martinez de Osaba MJ, Alvarez L, Guañabens. Osteomalacia revisited: a report on 28 cases. *N Clin Rheumatol*. 2011;30(5):639-645. PMID: 20949298

Bhan A, Rao AD, Rao DS. Osteomalacia as a result of vitamin D deficiency. *Endocrinol Metab Clin North Am*. 2010;39(2):321-331. PMID: 20511054

18 **ANSWER: A) Monitoring only**

This young premenopausal woman has a spinal bone mineral density measurement that is well below the mean for her age group, as indicated by the low Z-score. However, this does not define "osteoporosis" since her risk for a fracture is much less than for an older postmenopausal woman with the same bone mineral density. The diagnosis of osteoporosis in premenopausal women is best defined by 1 or more low-trauma (fragility) fractures and requires exclusion of secondary causes such as connective tissue disorders, malabsorption, inflammatory/autoimmune disorders, and many others. Measurement of bone mineral density by DXA should not be used as the sole guide for the diagnosis or treatment of osteoporosis in premenopausal women. This patient presented with a stress fracture of her proximal femur, which is almost certainly due to excessive repetitive mechanical stress from running rather than true bone fragility. Therefore, simple monitoring (Answer A) is appropriate.

None of the medications used for postmenopausal osteoporosis or for men with osteoporosis 50 years or older are approved for use in premenopausal women, and they generally should not be used outside of clinical trials. All of the medications listed for osteoporosis (Answers B, C, and D) are incorrect in this clinical setting. In terms of bone health, there is no advantage to prescribing an oral contraceptive pill (Answer E) for a premenopausal woman with regular menses.

In rare cases, pharmacologic intervention may be considered in premenopausal women. These exceptions include young women with multiple or severe fragility fractures or those with prolonged exposure to illnesses or medications that can cause bone loss and skeletal fragility (eg, high-dosage glucocorticoids or ongoing anorexia nervosa). Special caution is needed before prescribing bisphosphonates to premenopausal women because of their long retention in bone and the ability to cross the placenta during pregnancy. Anecdotally, both bisphosphonates and teriparatide have been used in patients with stress fractures, including in young athletes, but this use is off-label and not substantiated by large studies.

EDUCATIONAL OBJECTIVE
Manage low bone mineral density in premenopausal women.

REFERENCE(S)

Cohen A. Premenopausal osteoporosis. *Endocrinol Metab Clin N Am.* 2017;46(1)L117-L133. PMID: 28131128

Ferrari S, Bianchi ML, Eisman JA, et al ; IOF Committee of Scientific Advisors Working Group on Osteoporosis Pathophysiology. Osteoporosis in young adults: pathophysiology, diagnosis, and management. *Osteoporos Int.* 2012;23(12):2735-2748. PMID: 22684497

Moreira CA, Bilezikian JP. Stress fractures: concepts and therapeutics. *J Clin Endocrinol Metab.* 2017;102(2):525-534. PMID: 27732325

19 ANSWER: D) Severe aromatase enzyme deficiency

This is a prototypical case of a 46,XY male with severe aromatase enzyme deficiency (Answer D) due to a mutation in the *CYP19A1 gene.* The aromatase enzyme converts androgens to estrogens in both males and females. Males with this syndrome have normal pubertal development but very low or undetectable serum estradiol levels. This results in failure to fuse the epiphyses, continued linear growth, tall stature, and osteoporosis, all due to the lack of estrogen. Since conversion of testosterone to estradiol in the pituitary is important for feedback control of gonadotropins, LH (and FSH) levels are elevated despite the high testosterone levels. The syndrome of aromatase deficiency is very rare but has provided critical insights into the importance of estrogen in male skeletal physiology.

The 5α-reductase gene is responsible for converting testosterone to dihydrotestosterone and masculinizing the external genitalia. A deficiency in 5α-reductase (Answer A) results in males born with ambiguous genitalia who are usually raised as girls until puberty when virilization and enlargement of the phallus occur. An inactivating mutation in the estrogen receptor (Answer B) could cause a presentation in a 46,XY male similar to this patient, but there would be no response to administration of exogenous estrogen. Complete androgen insensitivity syndrome (Answer C) due to mutations in the androgen receptor gene leads to impaired masculinization in 46,XY individuals and a female phenotype with marked breast development (gynecomastia). Estradiol levels would be elevated, not undetectable. Antiestrogen antibodies (Answer E) have rarely been described with women with systemic lupus erythematosus, but they do not result in the syndrome described here.

Patients with aromatase deficiency and osteoporosis respond well to estrogen therapy with fusion of epiphyses and marked accrual in bone mass.

EDUCATIONAL OBJECTIVE
Recognize the importance of estrogen in male skeletal physiology and the hallmarks of aromatase deficiency in male patients.

REFERENCE(S)

Bilezikian JP, Morishima A, Bell J, Grumbach MM. Increased bone mass as a result of estrogen therapy in a man with aromatase deficiency. *N Engl J Med*. 1998;339(9):599-603. PMID: 9718379

Morishima A, Grumbach MM, Simpson ER, Fisher C, Qin K. Aromatase deficiency in male and female siblings caused by a novel mutation and the physiological role of estrogens. *J Clin Endocrinol Metab*. 1995;80(12):3689-3698. PMID: 8530621

Carani C, Qin K, Simoni M, et al. Effect of testosterone and estradiol in a man with aromatase deficiency. *N Engl J Med*. 1997;337(2):91-95. PMID: 9211678

20 ANSWER: B) Type 1 collagen α 1 and 2 genes (*COL1A1/COL1A2*)

This patient has the mildest form of osteogenesis imperfecta, known as type 1. Inheritance is autosomal dominant, but many mutations can occur de novo so that the family history may be negative. Patients with osteogenesis imperfecta type 1 have normal stature and little or no skeletal deformity. Fractures occur in childhood or adolescence and decrease markedly after puberty. As is the case in this vignette, affected patients may then present in middle age with "osteoporosis." In 50% of patients, there is early-onset hearing loss before age 40 years. On physical examination, there may be blue sclerae and easy bruising. Joint laxity may be present, but dentinogenesis imperfecta is usually absent. Diagnosis is made by sequencing the genes that encode type 1 collagen (α1 and α2) (*COL1A1/COL1A2*) (Answer B). The main therapy for osteogenesis imperfecta remains bisphosphonates (intravenous pamidronate and zoledronic acid and oral bisphosphonates). Denosumab has been used in rare case reports. Teriparatide does not dramatically change clinical outcomes. It is hoped that the sclerostin inhibitor romosozumab may have some effectiveness in decreasing fractures in osteogenesis imperfecta, but this awaits clinical trials and drug approval.

Osteoprotegerin (Answer A) is a cytokine and decoy receptor for the receptor activator of nuclear factor kappa B ligand (RANKL). By binding to RANKL, it reduces differentiation of precursors to osteoclasts and blocks osteoclast production and proliferation, thus reducing bone resorption. Mutations in this gene have been associated with osteoarthritis but not with the phenotype illustrated in this question. Mutations in the gene encoding the LDL receptor-related protein 5 are involved with the canonical Wnt pathway. Loss-of-function mutations can cause osteoporosis-pseudoglioma syndrome, while gain-of-function mutations result in a high bone mass phenotype. Mutations in the vitamin D receptor gene (Answer D) can be found in vitamin D–resistant rickets, but this would be accompanied by a high 1,25-dihydroxyvitamin D level, as well as hypophosphatemia, hypocalcemia, and osteomalacia. Sclerostin, produced by the *SOST* gene (Answer E) is produced by osteocytes and has antianabolic effects on bone formation by suppressing Wnt signaling. Inactivating mutations in the *SOST* gene cause syndromes of high bone mass (sclerosteosis and van Buchem disease).

EDUCATIONAL OBJECTIVE

Diagnose osteogenesis imperfecta type 1 (the mildest form).

REFERENCE(S)

Van Dijk FS, Sillence DO. Osteogenesis imperfecta: clinical diagnosis, nomenclature and severity assessment [published correction appears in *Am J Med Genet A*. 2015;167A(5):1178]. *Am J Med Genet A*. 2014;164A(6):1470-1481. PMID: 24715559

Thomas IH, DiMeglio LA. Advances in the classification and treatment of osteogenesis imperfecta. *Curr Osteoporos Rep*. 2016;14(1):1-9. PMID: 26861807

Shapiro JR, Thompson CB, Wu Y, Nunes M, Gillen C. Bone mineral density and fracture rate in response to intravenous and oral bisphosphonates in adult osteogenesis imperfecta. *Calcif Tissue Int*. 2010;87(2):120-129. PMID: 20544187

21 ANSWER: B) Symptomatic hypocalcemia

Denosumab, a human monoclonal antibody against RANK ligand, is approved for treatment of osteoporosis, as well as metastatic solid tumors such as breast cancer. It is a very potent inhibitor of osteoclastic bone resorption. Unlike bisphosphonates, denosumab is not cleared via the kidneys and has no effect on renal function. Thus, worsening renal function (Answer A) is incorrect. Severe flulike syndromes (also known as acute-phase reactions [Answer C]) are much more common with intravenous bisphosphonates than with denosumab. Rarely, denosumab may have mild glucose-lowering effects, but symptomatic hypoglycemia is unusual (Answer D). Denosumab and other potent antiresorptives do not generally cause delays in fracture healing (Answer E).

The major adverse effect to be expected in this setting is profound, symptomatic hypocalcemia (Answer B) within 7 to 10 days following denosumab administration. Patients at greatest risk for this complication are those with significantly impaired renal function. At highest risk are those with impaired renal function coupled with high bone turnover and elevated alkaline phosphatase. The potent inhibition of osteoclastic bone resorption by denosumab stops the efflux of calcium from bone and can lower serum calcium dramatically. The usual physiologic responses to hypocalcemia, such as a rise in PTH and calcitriol production, that would normally lead to increased renal tubular reabsorption of calcium and increased gut absorption of calcium, will not work in the setting of renal failure. Due to this high risk for hypocalcemia, it is important to bring the patient back to recheck serum calcium levels within 7 to 10 days of the injection, which is when the serum calcium level reaches its nadir. Some experts advocate prescribing calcitriol and increased calcium intake for several weeks after the denosumab to prevent the hypocalcemia. The patient should also be warned to watch for and report immediately any symptoms of hypocalcemia such as paresthesias, numbness, and muscle twitching.

EDUCATIONAL OBJECTIVE
Anticipate the risk of symptomatic hypocalcemia following denosumab in the setting of renal failure.

REFERENCE(S)
Dave V, Chiang CY, Booth J, Mount PF. Hypocalcemia post denosumab in patients with chronic kidney disease stage 4-5. *Am J Nephrol.* 2015;41(2):129-137. PMID: 25790847

Body JJ, Bone HG, de Boer RH, et al. Hypocalcaemia in patients with metastatic bone disease treated with denosumab. *Eur J Cancer.* 2015;51(13):1812-1821. PMID: 26093811

Kinoshita Y, Arai M, Ito N, et al. High serum ALP level is associated with increased risk of denosumab-related hypocalcemia in patients with bone metastases from solid tumors. *Endocr J.* 2016;63(5):479-484. PMID: 26860123

Stopeck AT, Lipton A, Body JJ, et al. Denosumab compared with zoledronic acid for the treatment of bone metastases in patients with advanced breast cancer: a randomized, double-blind study. *J Clin Oncol.* 2010;28(35):5132-5139. PMID: 21060033

22 ANSWER: C) Cholecalciferol, 4000 IU daily

The average serum 25-hydroxyvitamin D response to 1000 IU of vitamin D daily for 8 to 12 weeks is an increase of about 12 ng/mL (30.0 nmol/L). In this vignette, the patient's level would be expected to increase from 8 to 20 ng/mL (20.0 to 49.9 nmol/L) over a period of 2 to 3 months. Instead, due to class 3 obesity, her 25-hydroxyvitamin D level may only increase by a few nanograms per deciliter, a very blunted response. Therefore, recommending cholecalciferol, 400 or 1000 IU daily (Answers A and B), will not normalize her 25-hydroxyvitamin D level.

A number of studies have shown that patients who are overweight or obese require much higher dosages of vitamin D than normal-weight participants to achieve adequate levels. Obese patients are estimated to require 2 to 3 times the usual daily dose of cholecalciferol to achieve adequate levels. The mechanism is not well understood. The closest dose to what would be needed to correct the vitamin D deficiency in this patient is cholecalciferol, 4000 IU daily (Answer C). The dose could be adjusted in 8 to 12 weeks after rechecking the 25-hydroxyvitamin D level. Giving 10,000 IU cholecalciferol weekly (Answer D) would only provide about 1700 IU daily and thus would not be adequate. Finally, there is no role for treating with activated vitamin D or calcitriol (Answer E) in this setting.

EDUCATIONAL OBJECTIVE
Recommend appropriate vitamin D supplementation for obese patients.

REFERENCE(S)

Heaney RP, Davies KM, Chen TC, Holick MF, Barger-Lux MJ. Human serum 25-hydroxychole-calciferol response to extended oral dosing with cholecalciferol [published correction appears in *Am J Clin Nutr*. 2003;78(5):1047]. *Am J Clin Nutr*. 2003;77(1):204-210. PMID: 12499343

Ekwaru JP, Zwicker JD, Holick MF, Giovannucci E, Veugelers PJ. The importance of body weight for the dose response relationship of oral vitamin D supplementation and 25-hydroxyvitamin D in healthy volunteers. *PLoS One*. 2014;9(11):e111265. PMID: 25372709

Holick MF, Binkley NC, Bischoff-Ferrari HA, et al; Endocrine Society. Evaluation, treatment, and prevention of vitamin D deficiency: an Endocrine Society clinical practice guideline. *J Clin Endocrinol Metab*. 2011;96(7):1911-1930. PMID: 21646368

23 ANSWER: D) Stop the zoledronic acid infusions and refer to orthopedics

Atypical femur fractures after long-term bisphosphonate treatment for osteoporosis occur in up to 1 in 500 patients and have a number of common features. In approximately 50% of cases, they are bilateral, as in this patient. The nuclear bone scan is the most sensitive way to evaluate both femurs and show early stress reactions or stress fractures. These can progress to complete transverse fractures and sometimes need urgent placement of rods within the femur(s) to stabilize. Thus, the zolendronic acid infusions should be stopped and she should be referred to orthopedics (Answer D). Proceeding with the zoledronic acid infusion (Answers A and B) or switching to denosumab (Answer E) are incorrect because continuing potent antiresorptive therapy is inappriopriate in the setting of pending atypical femur fractures. Treating with the anabolic agent abaloparatide (Answer C) has not yet been studied and is not advised. Teriparatide has been used anecdotally in a few cases of atypical femur fractures and may be useful, but this awaits more rigorous study and is not US FDA approved for this purpose.

A task force of the American Society for Bone and Mineral Research released new case definitions for atypical femur fractures that are located on the femoral diaphysis and include 4 of 5 major features:

- Fracture is associated with minimal or no trauma (eg, fall from standing height)
- Fracture line originates at the lateral cortex and is substantially transverse in orientation although it may become oblique as it traverses medially across the femur
- Complete fractures extend through both cortices and may be associated with a medial spike; incomplete fractures include only the lateral cortex
- Fractures are noncomminuted or only minimally comminuted
- Localized periosteal or endosteal thickening of the lateral cortex is present at the fracture site ("beaking" or "flaring")

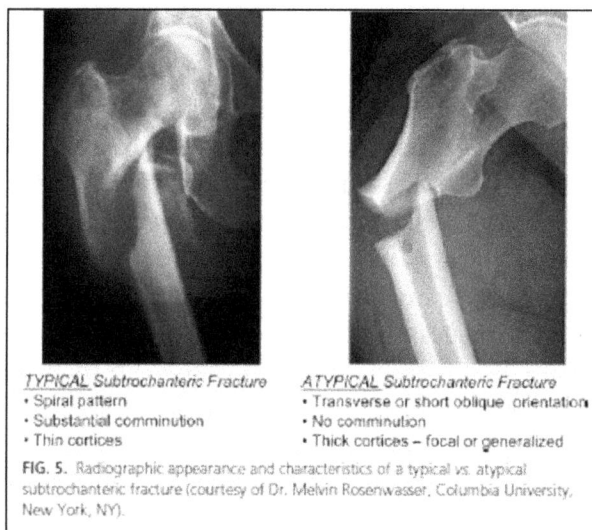

TYPICAL Subtrochanteric Fracture
• Spiral pattern
• Substantial comminution
• Thin cortices

ATYPICAL Subtrochanteric Fracture
• Transverse or short oblique orientation
• No comminution
• Thick cortices – focal or generalized

FIG. 5. Radiographic appearance and characteristics of a typical vs. atypical subtrochanteric fracture (courtesy of Dr. Melvin Rosenwasser, Columbia University, New York, NY).

The 2 images above illustrate the differences between "typical" and "atypical" femur fractures very well (reference: Khosla S, Bilezikian JP, Dempster DW, et al. Benefits and risks of bisphosphonate therapy for osteoporosis. *J Clin Endocrinol Metab*. 2012;97:2272-2282).

EDUCATIONAL OBJECTIVE
Evaluate an impending atypical femur fracture and assess for bilaterality.

REFERENCE(S)

Shane E, Burr D, Ebeling PR, et al; American Society for Bone and Mineral Research. Atypical subtrochanteric and diaphyseal femoral fractures: report of a task force of the American Society for Bone and Mineral Research [published correction appears in *J Bone Miner Res*;26(8):1987]. *J Bone Miner Res*. 2010;25(11):2267-2294. PMID: 20842676

Shaikh W 3rd, Morris D, Morris S 4th. Signs of insufficiency fractures overlooked in a patient receiving chronic bisphosphonate therapy. *J Am Board Fam Med*. 2016;29(3):404-407. PMID: 27170798

Selga J, Nuñez JH, Minguell J, Lalanza M, Garrido M. Simultaneous bilateral atypical femoral fracture in a patient receiving denosumab: case report and literature review. *Osteoporos Int*. 2016;27(2):827-832. PMID: 26501556

24 ANSWER: D) Ask the technician to reanalyze the spine region of interest

It is always important to look at the images and numbers of a DXA study, particularly when the results do not make sense. Although gains in bone mineral density at one site and loss at another are possible, this situation is very uncommon. In this patient's images, the placement of the spine analysis bars is incorrect, one level higher up than the previous study (ie, L4 on the current study is actually L3). After correct reanalysis (Answer D), the difference in her spine bone mineral density was not significant.

She appears to be responding to alendronate at the hip, so there is no need at this time to switch to denosumab (Answer A), zoledronic acid (Answer B), or teriparatide (Answer E). She also does not need another evaluation for secondary causes (Answer C).

EDUCATIONAL OBJECTIVE
Carefully review DXA images and identify common technical errors.

REFERENCE(S)

Watts NB. Fundamentals and pitfalls of bone densitometry using dual-energy X-ray absorptiometry (DXA). *Osteoporos Int*. 2004;15(11):847-854. PMID: 15322740

Schousboe JT, Shepherd JA, Bilezikian JP, Baim S. Executive summary of the 2013 international society for clinical densitometry position development conference on bone densitometry. *J Clin Densitom*. 2013;16(4):455-466. PMID: 24183638

25 ANSWER: A) Increased fluid intake

According to a comprehensive meta-analysis in patients who had a single kidney stone, increased fluid intake (Answer A) was the one intervention that was clearly shown to reduce recurrent stone disease. Of interest, reducing phosphate-containing soft drink consumption (not an answer option above) was moderately helpful. In patients with multiple stone episodes—most of whom had already increased their fluid intake—thiazide diuretics (Answer E) and citrate supplements (Answer D) were similarly effective in patients with hypercalciuria, as well as in unselected patients. Hydrochlorothiazide acts to enhance renal calcium reabsorption to reduce urinary calcium excretion and might be an additional measure to consider if he has more stones. Hypercalciuria may be caused by increased sodium intake, which leads to increased sodium excretion and an obligatory loss of calcium in the urine; however, this patient's normal urinary sodium excretion indicates that is not the case here (thus, Answer B is incorrect). His urinary oxalate level is not elevated, so there would be no benefit in reducing his dietary intake of oxalate (Answer C).

EDUCATIONAL OBJECTIVE
Recommend increased fluid intake as a means to reduce the risk of a second kidney stone.

REFERENCE(S)

Fink HA, Wilt TJ, Eldman KE, et al. Medical management to prevent recurrent nephrolithiasis in adults: a systematic review for an American College of Physicians Clinical Guideline [published correction appears in *Ann Intern Med.* 2013;159(3):230-232]. *Ann Intern Med.* 2013;158(7):535-543. PMID: 23546565

Vigen R, Weideman RA, Reilly RF. Thiazides diuretics in the treatment of nephrolithiasis: are we using them in an evidence-based fashion? *Int Urol Nephrol.* 2011;43(3):813-819. PMID: 20737209

Borghi L, Schianchi T, Meschi T, et al. Comparison of two diets for the prevention of recurrent stones in idiopathic hypercalciuria. *N Engl J Med.* 2002;346(2):77-84. PMID: 11784873

26 ANSWER: B) Parathyroidectomy with identification of all parathyroid glands

This patient has mild, asymptomatic primary hyperparathyroidism. Reduced renal function, which this patient has, is one of the major criteria for recommending parathyroid surgery in asymptomatic patients. Some studies suggest that parathyroidectomy can halt the deterioration of renal function in primary hyperparathyroidism. Parathyroidectomy with identification of all parathyroid glands (Answer B) is the correct next step.

Minimally invasive parathyroidectomy (Answer A) is not an option because of the nonlocalizing sestamibi scan. Since up to 20% of patients with biochemically proven primary hyperparathyroidism may have a nonlocalizing sestamibi scan, there is no indication to repeat this in 6 months (Answer D). Her 1,25-dihydroxyvitamin D level (Answer C) may be low, normal, or high, but knowing this will not help in the management decision. Rechecking calcium and creatinine in 6 months (Answer E) is not appropriate because she meets criteria for surgery now. One might consider other localization studies (eg, 4-dimensional CT if available), but that option was not offered.

Criteria for parathyroid surgery in patients with asymptomatic primary hyperparathyroidism include the following:

- Age <50 years
- Serum calcium >1 mg/dL above upper normal limit
- T-score less than –2.5 at any skeletal site on DXA or vertebral compression fracture identified on imaging
- Creatinine clearance <60 mL/min per 1.73 m^2
- Kidney stones on imaging or nephrocalcinosis
- Urinary calcium excretion >400 mg/24 h and increased stone risk by biochemical stone risk analysis

EDUCATIONAL OBJECTIVE

Identify decreased glomerular filtration rate as a criterion for parathyroid surgery in primary hyperparathyroidism.

REFERENCE(S)

Eastell R, Brandi ML, Costa AG, D'Amour P, Shoback DM, Thakker RV. Diagnosis of asymptomatic primary hyperparathyroidism: proceedings of the Fourth International Workshop. *J Clin Endocrinol Metab.* 2014;99(10):3570-3579. PMID: 25162666

Tassone F, Guarnieri A, Castellano E, Baffoni C, Attanasio R, Borretta G. Parathyroidectomy halts the deterioration of renal function in primary hyperparathyroidism. *J Clin Endocrinol Metab.* 2015;100(8):3069-3073. PMID: 26079781

Tassone F, Gianotti L, Baffoni C, Pellegrino M, Castellano E, Borretta G. KDIGO categories of glomerular filtration rate and parathyroid hormone secretion in primary hyperparathyroidism. *Endocr Pract.* 2015;21(6):629-633. PMID: 25716636

27 ANSWER: A) Order DXA of the one-third distal radius

This patient most likely has normocalcemic primary hyperparathyroidism. This is defined as persistently normal total and ionized serum calcium levels in the setting of persistently elevated serum intact PTH, along with normal 25-hydroxyvitamin D, serum creatinine, and 24-hour urinary calcium excretion levels. Such patients are often discovered during a workup for low bone mineral density. It is important to obtain a DXA of the one-third distal radius (Answer A) because this site, rich in cortical bone, is most susceptible to the bone-resorbing effects of sustained hyperparathyroidism. If she has osteoporosis at this site, she would meet criteria for parathyroid imaging and surgery. Longitudinal studies indicate that parathyroidectomy improves bone mineral density in patients with both hypercalcemic and normocalcemic primary hyperparathyroidism. For patients who decline surgery or are not surgical candidates, alendronate has been shown to significantly improve bone mineral density. Cinacalcet, which is US FDA approved for treatment of primary hyperparathyroidism in nonsurgical patients, has not been shown to improve bone mineral density.

Sestamibi parathyroid scans (Answer B) detect only approximately 80% of abnormal parathyroid tissue, and there can be false-negative results. Sestamibi would not be indicated unless parathyroid surgery was planned. Without a personal or family history of kidney stones or an abnormally high urinary calcium excretion, imaging for renal stones (Answer C) would not be the most appropriate next step in a woman of this age. She is already getting enough calcium, so doubling calcium supplementation (Answer D) is unlikely to affect her serum PTH level. Many patients with normocalcemic hyperparathyroidism eventually demonstrate elevated serum calcium levels but measuring calcium and PTH every 3 months is excessive. Most clinicians recommend retesting serum calcium and albumin every 6 to 12 months.

The recommendations for the evaluation of patients with asymptomatic primary hyperparathyroidism are outlined (see table).

Table 3. Recommendations for the Evaluation of Patients With Asymptomatic PHPT

Recommended
  Biochemistry panel (calcium, phosphate, alkaline
    phosphatase activity, BUN, creatinine), 25(OH)D
  PTH by second- or third-generation immunoassay
  BMD by DXA
    Lumbar spine, hip, and distal 1/3 radius
  Vertebral spine assessment
    X-ray or VFA by DXA
  24-h urine for:
    Calcium, creatinine, creatinine clearance
    Stone risk profile
  Abdominal imaging by x-ray, ultrasound, or CT scan
Optional
  HRpQCT
  TBS by DXA
  Bone turnover markers (bone-specific alkaline phosphatase
    activity, osteocalcin, P1NP [select one]; serum CTX,
    urinary NTX [select one])
  Fractional excretion of calcium on timed urine sample
  DNA testing if genetic basis for PHPT is suspected

Abbreviations: BUN, blood urea nitrogen; P1NP, procollagen type 1 N-propeptide; CTX, C-telopeptide cross-linked collagen type I; NTX, N-telopeptide of type I collagen. This evaluation is for PHPT, not to distinguish between PHPT and other causes of hypercalcemia.

Table reprinted from Bilezikian JP, Brandi ML, Eastell R, et al. Guidelines for the management of asymptomatic primary hyperparathyroidism: summary statement from the Fourth International Workshop. *J Clin Endocrinol Metab.* 2014;99(10):3561-3569.

EDUCATIONAL OBJECTIVE
Evaluate normocalcemic hyperparathyroidism.

REFERENCE(S)
Cusano NE, Maalouf NM, Wang PY, et al. Normocalcemic hyperparathyroidism and hypoparathyroidism in two community-based nonreferral populations. *J Clin Endocrinol Metab.* 2013;98(7):2734-2741. PMID: 23690312

Rejnmark L, Amstrup AK, Mollerup CL, Heickendorff L, Mosekilde L. Further insights into the pathogenesis of primary hyperparathyroidism: a nested case-control study. *J Clin Endocrinol Metab.* 2013;98(1):87-96. PMID: 23150677

Lowe H, McMahon DJ, Rubin MR, Bilezikian JP, Silverberg SJ. Normocalcemic primary hyperparathyroidism: further characterization of a new clinical phenotype. *J Clin Endocrinol Metab.* 2007;92(8):3001-3005. PMID: 17536001

Bilezikian JP, Brandi ML, Eastell R, et al. Guidelines for the management of asymptomatic primary hyperparathyroidism: summary statement from the Fourth International Workshop. *J Clin Endocrinol Metab.* 2014;99(10):3561-3569. PMID: 25162665

28 ANSWER: C) Estradiol patch
Estrogen therapy remains the most potent therapy for postmenopausal vasomotor symptoms and has also been shown to stop bone loss and reduce osteoporotic fractures in large clinical trials. For a healthy woman relatively early in menopause with both menopausal symptoms and osteoporosis, estrogen therapy (Answer C) is an excellent option. Given that she had a hysterectomy, no progestin is needed but even if she had an intact uterus, the choice of combination estrogen and progesterone would be a good therapy for her. Paroxetine (Answer A) is US FDA approved for this indication and may help with her menopausal symptoms, but it would not improve bone health. Raloxifene (Answer B) would be useful for osteoporosis, but it would actually worsen her hot flashes. Risedronate (Answer D) is a potent antiosteoporosis agent, but it would not improve her vasomotor symptoms. Calcitonin (Answer E) is an ineffective therapy for both osteoporosis and menopausal symptoms.

EDUCATIONAL OBJECTIVE
Recommend estrogen therapy as an approved option for treating menopausal symptoms and osteoporosis.

REFERENCE(S)

Manson JE, Kaunitz AM. Menopause management-- getting clinical care back on track. *N Engl J Med.* 2016;374(9):803-806. PMID: 26962899

Steunkel CA, Davis SR, Gompel A, et al. Treatment of symptoms of the menopause: an Endocrine Society clinical practice guideline. *J Clin Endocrinol Metab.* 2015;100(11):3975-4011. PMID: 26444994

29 **ANSWER: E) No treatment**

Most patients with Paget disease are asymptomatic and do not require treatment (thus, Answer E is correct). When treatment is necessary, the best pharmacologic agent for Paget disease appears to be zoledronic acid (Answer C). Head-to-head clinical trials have shown that risedronate is better than alendronate (Answer A) and zoledronic acid is better than risedronate. Calcitonin (Answer D) is considered the weakest agent and is rarely used for Paget disease. Denosumab (Answer B) is not approved for treatment of Paget disease.

Indications for treatment in an asymptomatic patient include the following:

- Involvement of a weight-bearing bone (eg, spine or leg)
- Involvement near a joint
- Involvement of the skull
- Serum alkaline phosphatase level greater than 3 times the upper normal limit

EDUCATIONAL OBJECTIVE
Determine when it is necessary to treat Paget disease.

REFERENCE(S)

Brandi ML. Current treatment approaches for Paget disease of bone. *Discov Med.* 2010;10(52):209-212. PMID: 20875342

Singer FR. Paget disease: when to treat and when not to treat. *Nat Rev Rheumatol.* 2009;5(9):483-489. PMID: 19652650

Siris ES, Lyles KW, Singer FR, Meunier PJ. Medical management of Paget's disease of bone: indications for treatment and review of current therapies. *J Bone Miner Res.* 2006;21(Suppl 2):P94-P98. PMID: 17229018

Ralston SH. Clinical practice. Paget's disease of bone. *N Engl J Med.* 2013;368(7):644-650. PMID: 23406029

30 **ANSWER: C) Intravenous bolus of 150 mg calcium gluconate followed by a continuous calcium gluconate infusion of 1 mg/kg per h**

This patient needs rapid correction of hypocalcemia. Calcium gluconate is preferred over calcium chloride because the latter is more likely to cause vein sclerosis and tissue necrosis if extravasated (thus, Answers A and B are incorrect). The dose of intravenous calcium is dangerously high in Answer D. Dosing at 1 mg/kg per h would be a total dose of 1680 mg daily for a 70-kg patient; a higher rate might be required for patients with a profound calcium deficiency, but this patient has only been without her usual calcium intake for 72 hours (thus, Answer C is correct).

Ordering intravenous calcium can be potentially confusing. For intravenous use, a 10-mL ampule of calcium gluconate contains 93 mg of calcium; a 10-mL ampule of 10% calcium chloride contains 272 mg of calcium. In some situations, adding a calcium salt to an intravenous liter bag of 0.9% saline or 5% dextrose requires removing some of the fluid to allow space for the added calcium salt.

EDUCATIONAL OBJECTIVE
Manage acute, severe hypocalcemia.

REFERENCE(S)

Zalonga GP, Chernow B. Hypocalcemia in critical illness. *JAMA.* 1986;256(14):1924-1929. PMID: 3531557

Vetter T, Lohse MJ. Magnesium and the parathyroid. *Curr Opin Nephrol Hypertens.* 2002;11(4):403-410. PMID: 12105390

al-Ghamdi SM, Cameron EC, Sutton RA. Magnesium deficiency: pathophysiologic and clinical overview.

Obesity/Lipids Board Review

Andrea D. Coviello, MD • Duke University

1 **ANSWER: C) Lorcaserin, 10 mg twice daily**
Over the last few years, the US FDA has approved 4 new weight-loss medications. These include the combinations of phentermine-topiramate ER and bupropion ER-naltrexone ER and the single agents lorcaserin, 10 mg twice daily, and liraglutide, 3 mg daily. These medications differ in their mechanisms of action, adverse effect profiles, and effectiveness. The Endocrine Society recently published a clinical practice guideline on the pharmacologic management of obesity. This guideline concurs with previous guidelines that the consideration of a weight-loss medication is appropriate for individuals with a BMI greater than 30 kg/m^2 or those with a BMI greater than 27 kg/m^2 who also have a weight-related comorbidity. The group writing the Endocrine Society guideline conducted a systematic review of the literature and reports on the risk of adverse effects from these medications. The guideline lists the following for the medications mentioned in this vignette:

- Liraglutide, 3 mg daily (Answer A): nausea occurs in 40% of treated patients compared with 15% of control patients.
- Phentermine-topiramate ER (Answer B): paresthesia occurs in 19.9% of patients treated at a dosage of 15 mg/92 mg daily compared with 1.9% of control patients.
- Lorcaserin (Answer C): nasopharyngitis occurs in 11.3% of treated patients compared with 9.9% of control patients and nausea occurs in 9.4% of treated patients compared with 7.9% of control patients.
- Bupropion ER-naltrexone ER (Answer D): nausea occurs in 32% of treated patients compared with 6.7% of control patients.

Therefore, of the medications listed, the one with the least adverse effects is lorcaserin (Answer C),

making it the best choice for a patient such as the one described who is concerned about adverse effects.

EDUCATIONAL OBJECTIVE
Describe the adverse effect profile of currently available weight-loss medications and the indications for prescribing a weight-loss medication.

REFERENCE(S)
Apovian CM, Aronne LJ, Bessesen DH, et al; Endocrine Society. Pharmacological management of obesity: an Endocrine Society clinical practice guideline. *J Clin Endocrinol Metab.* 2015;100(2):342-362. PMID: 25590212

Yanovski SZ, Yanovski JA. Long-term drug treatment for obesity: a systematic and clinical review. *JAMA.* 2014;311(1):74-86. PMID: 24231879

Pi-Sunyer X, Astrup A, Fujioka K, et al; SCALE Obesity and Prediabetes NN8022-1839 Study Group. A randomized, controlled trial of 3.0 mg of liraglutide in weight management. *N Engl J Med.* 2015;373(1):11-22. PMID: 26132939

Yanovski SZ, Yanovski JA. Naltrexone extended-release plus bupropion extended-release for treatment of obesity. *JAMA.* 2015;313(12):1213-1214. PMID: 25803343

2 **ANSWER: A) Dietary modification**
Gastric bypass surgery has a dramatic effect on carbohydrate metabolism. Forty to fifty percent of patients who have diabetes mellitus preoperatively do not require medication for diabetes after surgery. Diabetes resolves in many of these individuals within weeks of the operation. It appears that the exposure of the distal bowel to food results in exaggerated secretion of GLP-1, which may facilitate the improvement in glucose control seen after surgery. Postprandial hypoglycemia is an uncommon late complication of gastric bypass surgery that is increasingly recognized. It appears that

in some individuals, perhaps in response to ongoing stimulation by GLP-1, β-cell proliferation occurs, resulting in islet hyperplasia associated with excessive insulin secretion and endogenous hyperinsulinemic hypoglycemia. Some patients develop multiple small insulinomas.

The management of this condition is controversial. While partial pancreatectomy (Answer B) was suggested in the initial series, other authors have suggested that many of these patients can be managed by reducing the intake of carbohydrates, consuming low–glycemic index carbohydrates, and always eating carbohydrates in the context of a mixed meal. Although acarbose (Answer D), octreotide (Answer C), calcium-channel blockers, and diazoxide have all been used as treatments, diet alone (Answer A) alleviates symptoms in 50% to 70% of affected individuals. Thus, dietary modification is the initial treatment choice.

It appears that the condition recurs in many individuals who have a subtotal pancreatectomy, and those who have more aggressive pancreatic surgery can develop pancreatic diabetes. For this reason, pancreatectomy is currently used only if other treatments fail and the patient remains debilitated by frequent episodes of hypoglycemia that limit functional capacity.

EDUCATIONAL OBJECTIVE
Manage hyperinsulinemic hypoglycemia that develops after gastric bypass surgery.

REFERENCE(S)

Service GJ, Thompson GB, Service FJ, Andrews JC, Collazo-Clavell ML, Lloyd RV. Hyperinsulinemic hypoglycemia with nesidioblastosis after gastric bypass surgery. *N Engl J Med.* 2005;353(3):249-254. PMID: 16034010

Rariy CM, Rometo D, Korytkowski M. Post-gastric bypass hypoglycemia. *Curr Diab Rep.* 2016;16(2):19. PMID: 26868861

3 ANSWER: D) Persons with prediabetes treated with lifestyle intervention

Surprisingly, good data from randomized controlled trials on the benefits of weight loss with a reduction in overall mortality are very limited. However, data from long-term follow-up of a trial in China similar to the Diabetes Prevention Program show a mortality benefit resulting from weight loss through lifestyle intervention in persons with prediabetes (Answer D). Overall, these data are consistent with the idea that while weight loss consistently produces improvements in markers of metabolic health, mortality benefits are most likely the result of marked weight loss in more obese patients or more modest weight loss earlier in the course of the development of metabolic disease.

No data are available that show mortality benefits with weight-loss medications (Answer A). While a number of studies demonstrate a mortality benefit related to gastric bypass surgery (Answer B), none of these are randomized controlled trials, which raises the question of potential selection bias. However, these data are growing and are fairly strong.

The Look AHEAD trial (Action for Health in Diabetes) was designed to test the idea that weight loss through lifestyle changes would reduce cardiovascular morbidity and mortality in persons with diabetes (Answer C). Participants in this trial lost more than 8% of their body weight over the first year of the study and sustained a 4.5% weight loss at 4 years. The effect of this weight loss was to improve a range of health parameters, including blood pressure, glucose levels, insulin levels, and serum lipid levels. Unfortunately, the trial was stopped early because of "futility." The statisticians determined that despite enrolling and retaining more than 5000 participants, the study did not have the power to show a beneficial effect of weight loss. The reason being that the observed event rates for prespecified cardiovascular endpoints were much lower than had been predicted, making the original power calculations inaccurate. The low event rates were most likely due to the high-quality medical care that the participants were receiving, including good blood pressure control, statin use, and generally high levels of physical activity, even in those randomly assigned to the control arm.

EDUCATIONAL OBJECTIVE
Summarize the data from randomized controlled trials of the effect of weight-loss interventions on mortality.

REFERENCE(S)

Look AHEAD Research Group, Wing RR, Bolin P, et al. Cardiovascular effects of intensive lifestyle intervention in type 2 diabetes [published correction appears in *N Engl J Med*. 2014;370(19):1866]. *N Engl J Med*. 2013;369(2):145-154. PMID: 23796131

Brancati FL, Evans M, Furberg CD, et al; Look AHEAD Study Group. Midcourse correction to a clinical trial when the event rate is underestimated: The Look AHEAD (Action for Health in Diabetes) Study. *Clin Trials*. 2012;9(1):113-124. PMID: 22334468

Wing RR, Lang W, Wadden TA, et al; Look AHEAD Research Group. Benefits of modest weight loss in improving cardiovascular risk factors in overweight and obese individuals with type 2 diabetes. *Diabetes Care*. 2011;34(7):1481-1486. PMID: 21593294

Li G, Zhang P, Wang J, et al. Cardiovascular mortality, all-cause mortality, and diabetes incidence after lifestyle intervention for people with impaired glucose tolerance in the Da Qing Diabetes Prevention Study: a 23-year follow-up study. *Lancet Diabetes Endocrinol*. 2014;2(6):474-480. PMID: 24731674

Arterburn DE, Olsen MK, Smith VA, et al. Association between bariatric surgery and long-term survival. *JAMA*. 2015;313(1):62-70. PMID: 25562267

4   ANSWER: C) Change from gabapentin to topiramate

Drug-induced weight gain is a common clinical problem. A number of drug classes can cause this problem, including antidiabetes medications, antipsychotic agents, antidepressant agents, mood stabilizers, glucocorticoids, and progestational agents, to name just a few. Several management options are available for patients who have drug-induced weight gain. One is to reduce the dosage of the offending medication or to reconsider the value of that medication and to potentially stop it. Alternatively, a behavioral weight-management program can be instituted. Finally, the problematic medication can be stopped and an alternative medication can be prescribed. For example, a GLP-1 agonist or an SGLT-2 inhibitor can be used in place of, or in addition to, a sulfonylurea.

Among available antidepressant medications, bupropion (Answer A) is the most likely to produce weight loss. The weight loss with bupropion is in the 3% to 5% range. Fluoxetine can produce weight loss in some patients, but the effect is inconsistent. Topiramate (Answer C) is a medication that is FDA approved for epilepsy and migraine headaches. Although there are a number of studies in which it was used specifically for weight loss, it is not FDA approved for weight loss. However, there is strong evidence that it produces a 6% to 8% weight loss that is sustained at 1 year. While both bupropion and topiramate can produce weight loss, topiramate produces more weight loss on average than does bupropion. A number of clinical trials have examined the efficacy of low-carbohydrate diets (Answer B). These studies show that although weight loss over the initial 6 months may exceed that seen with other diet types, weight loss at 1 year is no different than that seen with other diet types, averaging 3% to 4%.

EDUCATIONAL OBJECTIVE
Identify medications used for other conditions that can promote weight gain and suggest alternatives that are weight neutral or produce weight loss.

REFERENCE(S)

Rosenstock J, Hollander P, Gadde KM, Sun X, Strauss R, Leung A; OBD-202 Study Group. A randomized, double-blind, placebo-controlled, multicenter study to assess the efficacy and safety of topiramate controlled release in the treatment of obese type 2 diabetic patients. *Diabetes Care*. 2007;30(6):1480-1486. PMID: 17363756

Eliasson B, Gudbjörnsdottir S, Cederholm J, Liang Y, Vercruysse F, Smith U. Weight loss and metabolic effects of topiramate in overweight and obese type 2 diabetic patients: randomized double-blind placebo-controlled trial. *Int J Obes (London)*. 2007;31(7):1140-1147. PMID: 17264849

Apovian CM, Aronne LJ, Bessesen DH, et al; Endocrine Society. Pharmacological management of obesity: an Endocrine Society clinical practice guideline. *J Clin Endocrinol Metab*. 2015;100(2):342-362. PMID: 25590212

5. ANSWER: C) Thiamine

The symptoms displayed by this patient are characteristic of Wernicke encephalopathy, which is caused by a deficiency of thiamine (Answer C). Thiamine deficiency causes neuronal death due to metabolic dysfunction of astrocytes within the central nervous system. The classic triad of this condition is confusion, ataxia, and nystagmus. A wide range of other abnormalities can be seen, including cranial nerve dysfunction, peripheral neuropathies, seizures, and psychosis. Because thiamine is a water-soluble vitamin, body stores can be depleted within days to weeks of inadequate intake. The condition typically presents 4 to 12 weeks after bariatric surgery but can occur as early as 2 weeks and as late as 18 months after surgery. Although most commonly reported following gastric bypass surgery, Wernicke encephalopathy can occur after any type of bariatric surgery. The most common antecedent is persistent vomiting, which then severely limits thiamine intake. Other less common precipitating factors are intravenous glucose or parenteral nutrition administration without thiamine supplementation. The condition is important to recognize, as treatment with parenteral thiamine (100 mg daily for 7 to 14 days, or 500 mg 3 times daily for 3 days) must be administered to prevent serious morbidity.

Although vitamin B_{12} deficiency (Answer A) can cause neurologic symptoms and signs, body stores of B_{12} are sizable, so deficiency does not usually occur until 6 to 24 months after bariatric surgery. Folate deficiency (Answer B) is uncommon and typically presents as anemia. Zinc deficiency (Answer D) is rare. It is associated with skin and hair findings and is primarily seen after biliary pancreatic diversion.

EDUCATIONAL OBJECTIVE
Differentiate among the vitamin deficiencies that can occur after gastric bypass surgery.

REFERENCE(S)

Aasheim ET. Wernicke encephalopathy after bariatric surgery, a systematic review. *Ann Surg.* 2008;248(5):714-720. PMID: 18948797

Serra A, Sechi G, Singh S, Kumar A. Wernicke encephalopathy after obesity surgery: a systematic review. *Neurology.* 2007;69(6):615. PMID: 17679686

Mechanick JI, Kushner RF, Sugerman HJ, et al; American Association of Clinical Endocrinologists; Obesity Society; American Society for Metabolic & Bariatric Surgery. American Association of Clinical Endocrinologists, The Obesity Society, and American Society for Metabolic & Bariatric Surgery medical guidelines for clinical practice for the perioperative nutritional, metabolic, and nonsurgical support of the bariatric surgery patient [published correction appears in *Obesity (Silver Spring).* 2010;18(3):649]. *Obesity (Silver Spring).* 2009;17(Suppl 1):S1-S70. PMID: 19319140

6. ANSWER: B) Ventral tegmentum and the nucleus accumbens

For many years, researchers investigating the role of the brain in regulating hunger and satiety focused on the hypothalamus. The arcuate nucleus of the hypothalamus (Answer D) has neurons that respond to leptin, insulin, ghrelin, and a number of metabolites and is central to what has been termed homeostatic feeding. Homeostatic feeding could be considered to be the regulation of hunger and satiety in response to the energy imbalance produced by underfeeding and overfeeding. The lateral hypothalamic area contains neurons that are downstream of neurons in the arcuate nucleus and is important in regulating physical activity, as well as relaying information about food intake to other brain regions.

The medial and lateral prefrontal cortex (Answer A) is involved in the control of impulsivity and regulation of behavior and is probably important in a person's ability to "fight the urge" to overeat. Brodmann area 17 in the occipital lobe (Answer C) is the primary visual processing area in the cortex, also known as "visual one" or V1, which may have a role in processing visual food cues such as response to pictures of food in advertising material.

The nucleus of the solitary tract and the dorsal vagal nucleus (Answer E) are in the brainstem and are crucial in relaying information from the gastrointestinal tract to the brain and also are important in organizing some of the mechanics of food intake and digestion.

Because of the failure of medications that act through hypothalamic neurotransmitters to produce weight loss in humans, researchers have begun to look towards other brain regions in their attempt to understand why obesity is so common. The patient described in this vignette is not eating because of hunger (homeostatic feeding), but rather reports eating because of a craving. The brain regions important in this type of feeding, so called nonhomeostatic or hedonic feeding, are the ventral tegmentum and nucleus accumbens (Answer B) where reward appears to be sensed. The neurotransmitter dopamine acting in these brain regions is most likely involved in mediating the rewarding aspects of food intake.

EDUCATIONAL OBJECTIVE
List the functions of several brain regions that are important in regulating food intake.

REFERENCE(S)
Morton GJ, Meek TH, Schwartz MW. Neurobiology of food intake in health and disease. *Nat Rev Neurosci.* 2014;15(6):367-378. PMID: 24840801

Rangel A. Regulation of dietary choice by the decision-making circuitry. *Nat Neurosci.* 2013;16(12):1717-1724. PMID: 24270272

Tanaka SC, Doya K, Okada G, Ueda K, Okamoto Y, Yamawaki S. Prediction of immediate and future rewards differentially recruits cortico-basal ganglia loops. *Nat Neurosci.* 2004;7(8):887-893. PMID: 15235607

Berthoud HR. The neurobiology of food intake in an obesogenic environment. *Proc Nutr Soc.* 2012;71(4):478-487. PMID: 22800810

7 ANSWER: C) Diabetes mellitus
Because a laparoscopic banding procedure does not bypass any intestinal segment and does not cause malabsorption, it is not associated with vitamin or mineral deficiencies (Answers A, B, D, and E). The sleeve gastrectomy can be associated with B_{12} deficiency, but it is not as common after this procedure as it is with gastric bypass. Roux-en-Y gastric bypass is associated with thiamine deficiency, B_{12} deficiency, and, less commonly, zinc deficiency that typically causes a rash and diarrhea. In this patient, the longstanding, poorly controlled

diabetes (Answer C) is the most likely primary cause of her peripheral neuropathy.

EDUCATIONAL OBJECTIVE
Identify the common vitamin deficiencies that occur after bariatric surgical procedures.

REFERENCE(S)
Mechanick JI, Kushner RF, Sugerman HJ, et al; American Association of Clinical Endocrinologists; Obesity Society; American Society for Metabolic & Bariatric Surgery. American Association of Clinical Endocrinologists, The Obesity Society, and American Society for Metabolic & Bariatric Surgery medical guidelines for clinical practice for the perioperative nutritional, metabolic, and nonsurgical support of the bariatric surgery patient [published correction appears in *Obesity (Silver Spring).* 2010;18(3):649]. *Obesity (Silver Spring).* 2009;17(Suppl 1):S1-S70. PMID: 19319140

8 ANSWER: B) Phentermine-topiramate for potential birth defects
Lorcaserin is a selective 5-HT2C receptor agonist. Previous serotonin agonists fenfluramine and dexfenfluramine were associated with cardiac valve problems. However, lorcaserin is specific for a serotonin receptor subtype that is not found in the heart. Studies conducted for up to 2 years in several thousand participants showed no evidence of valvular problems. Although the US FDA has a postmarketing program looking for cardiac valve problems with lorcaserin use, there is no Risk Evaluation and Mitigation Strategy (REMS) in place (thus, Answer A is incorrect).

Phentermine is a sympathomimetic amine. It is a stimulant and should be avoided in those with a history of drug addiction and bipolar disease. However, phentermine is an old medication and is not subject to REMS (thus, Answer C is incorrect).

Although orlistat theoretically could cause deficiency of fat-soluble vitamins, the evidence that this is a significant problem is minimal (thus, Answer D is incorrect). In patients who take warfarin, however, the INR should be followed if orlistat therapy is initiated. Orlistat can decrease blood levels of cyclosporine.

Liraglutide, 3.0 mg daily, (Answer E) did have a REMS program related to risk of medullary thyroid cancer due to associated risk in animal studies that has not been observed in humans to date and for acute pancreatitis. More than half of reported cases of acute pancreatitis were due to gallstone pancreatitis, but cholecystitis is not part of the REMS program.

Exposure to topiramate in the first trimester of pregnancy has been associated with an increased risk of cleft lip and cleft palate. For this reason, phentermine-topiramate is under a REMS program (thus, Answer B is correct). Women of reproductive age who are prescribed phentermine-topiramate should have a negative pregnancy test before starting the medication and this should be repeated monthly as long as the patient is taking the medication.

EDUCATIONAL OBJECTIVE
List the common adverse effects of weight-loss medications.

REFERENCE(S)
Colman E, Golden J, Roberts M, Egan A, Weaver J, Rosebraugh C. The FDA's assessment of two drugs for chronic weight management. *N Engl J Med*. 2012;367(17):1577-1579. PMID: 23050510

Qsymia [package insert]. Mountain View, CA: VIVUS, Inc; 2012-2013. Also available at: https://qsymia.com/patient/include/media/pdf/prescribing-information.pdf.

9 **ANSWER: B) Phentermine-topiramate ER, 15 mg/92 mg daily**
Phentermine-topiramate ER (Answer B) is currently the most effective weight-loss medication available. It results in an 8% to 10% placebo-subtracted weight loss. Phentermine alone (Answer C) yields a 3% to 5% weight loss, which is similar to the weight loss observed with orlistat (Answer E), although some studies show even lower efficacy of this pancreatic lipase inhibitor. Lorcaserin (Answer A) results in 4% to 5% placebo-subtracted weight loss. Although the weight loss is not dramatic, some patients lose more than this and it has relatively few adverse effects. Liraglutide (Answer D) is not currently approved by the US FDA for weight loss. At the 3 mg dosage, it results in 4%

to 6% weight loss, but nausea is a common adverse effect. When considering any weight-loss medication, it is important to remember that the weight loss prompted by a drug is additive to the weight loss induced by lifestyle changes and also that weight loss in any particular patient may vary widely from these average ranges.

EDUCATIONAL OBJECTIVE
Describe the relative effectiveness of commonly prescribed weight-loss medications.

REFERENCE(S)
Yanovski SZ, Yanovski JA. Long-term drug treatment for obesity: a systematic and clinical review. *JAMA*. 2014;311(1):74-86. PMID: 24231879

Garvey WT, Ryan DH, Look M, et al. Two-year sustained weight loss and metabolic benefits with controlled-release phentermine/topiramate in obese and overweight adults (SEQUEL): a randomized, placebo-controlled, phase 3 extension study. *Am J Clin Nutr*. 2012;95(2):297-308. PMID: 22158731

Fidler MC, Sanchez M, Raether B, et al; BLOSSOM Clinical Trial Group. A one-year randomized trial of lorcaserin for weight loss in obese and overweight adults: the BLOSSOM trial. *J Clin Endocrinol Metab*. 2011;96(10):3067-3077. PMID: 21795446

Astrup A, Rössner S, Van Gaal L, et al; NN8022-1807 Study Group. Effects of liraglutide in the treatment of obesity: a randomised, double-blind, placebo-controlled study [published correction appears in *Lancet*. 375(9719):984]. *Lancet*. 2009;374(9701):1606-1616. PMID: 19853906

10 **ANSWER: C) Food impaction**
Although it is natural and appropriate to assume that the surgeon who performed her procedure is responsible for complications of the surgery, endocrinologists who follow these patients should be aware of the common mechanical complications that occur because patients may not have access to their surgeon or they may not relate a symptom to their previous surgery. A range of mechanical complications can occur with gastric banding. If the band is tightened too much, the patient may have difficulty swallowing. If the patient tries to eat food too fast without cutting it into

small enough pieces, the food can be impacted at the level of the band, as is the case in this vignette (Answer C).

A "slipped band" (Answer E) occurs when the stiches or staples securing the band in place fail and the band migrates either proximally up the esophagus or distally to the lower stomach. A slipped band typically presents with nausea and vomiting and may have associated abdominal pain or reflux symptoms. The symptoms described in the vignette occurred while the patient was eating, which is more typical of food impaction. Gastric band erosion (Answer B) typically occurs in the first year after surgery, but can present 2 to 5 years after implantation. Band erosion may present as unexplained weight regain with abdominal pain, or may present with signs of infection as the gastric wall is perforated at the site of the erosion with gastric contents tracking along the filling catheter to the subcutaneous port site. Anastomotic problems only occur following gastric bypass surgery because this surgery involves anastomoses between the stomach and intestine and different segments of the intestine. An anastomotic ulcer (Answer A) can present as pain, bleeding, or symptoms of obstruction due to edema around the ulcer resulting in a restriction in the orifice between intestinal segments. An anastomotic leak (Answer D) typically occurs 5 to 7 days postoperatively when the patient has already been discharged from the hospital. The mechanism is thought to be ischemia at an anastomotic junction. The patient may have tachycardia, tachypnea, abdominal pain, fever, and, importantly, shoulder pain. The shoulder pain is referred pain from subdiaphragmatic irritation caused by gastric contents spilling into the peritoneal cavity.

EDUCATIONAL OBJECTIVE
Describe the clinical presentations of common mechanical complications of bariatric surgical procedures.

REFERENCE(S)
Brown WA, Egberts KJ, Franke-Richard D, Thodiyil P, Anderson ML, O'Brien PE. Erosions after laparoscopic adjustable gastric banding: diagnosis and management. *Ann Surg.* 2013;257(6):1047-1052. PMID: 23673685

Wayman CS, Nord JH, Combs WM, Rosemurgy AS. The role of endoscopy after vertical banded gastroplasty. *Gastrointest Endosc.* 1992;38(1):44-46. PMID: 1612378

Al Harakeh AB. Complications of laparoscopic Roux-en-Y gastric bypass. *Surg Clin North Am.* 2011;91(6):1225-1237. PMID: 22054150

11 ANSWER: B) Liraglutide, 3 mg daily
Patients are fortunate that a number of US FDA–approved weight-loss medications are now available. The range of options makes it important for clinicians to tailor the specific weight-loss medication that they prescribe to the unique needs of each patient. The patient in this vignette qualifies for a weight-loss medication because her BMI is greater than 30 kg/m². However, she has a number of medical conditions that complicate the choice.

Orlistat (Answer A) would not be ideal because it can alter the levels of fat-soluble vitamins including vitamin K, which could affect the degree of anticoagulation that she is getting from her usual dose of warfarin. There are concerns about using liraglutide (Answer B) and naltrexone-bupropion (Answer D) in patients with known cardiovascular disease or uncontrolled hypertension because these medications can increase pulse rate due to sympathomimetic effects. Fortunately, this patient does not have either of these conditions. However, naltrexone-bupropion is relatively contraindicated because bupropion can lower the seizure threshold. Phentermine-topiramate (Answer C) is FDA approved for weight loss, but topiramate as a single agent is not. The recent Endocrine Society guidelines specifically recommend that it not be used for weight loss, as there are other medications that are FDA approved. Phentermine-topiramate should be used with caution in women of reproductive age because it has been associated with birth defects. Women taking this combination should have a documented negative pregnancy test before starting the medication and then pregnancy tests every month while taking it. Of the listed medications, the best choice for this patient is liraglutide (Answer B).

EDUCATIONAL OBJECTIVE
List the contraindications for specific weight-loss medications.

REFERENCE(S)

Apovian CM, Aronne LJ, Bessesen DH, et al; Endocrine Society. Pharmacological management of obesity: an Endocrine Society clinical practice guideline. *J Clin Endocrinol Metab.* 2015;100(2):342-362. PMID: 25590212

Yanovski SZ, Yanovski JA. Long-term drug treatment for obesity: a systematic and clinical review. *JAMA.* 2014;311(1):74-86. PMID: 24231879

Yanovski SZ, Yanovski JA. Naltrexone extended-release plus bupropion extended-release for treatment of obesity. *JAMA.* 2015;313(12):1213-1214. PMID: 25803343

12 **ANSWER: A) Liraglutide, 3.0 mg daily**
This patient needs to lose weight to improve his fatty liver disease and optimize his candidacy for liver transplant in the future. He would benefit from a lower-fat and controlled-carbohydrate diet, but he will not likely be able to lose weight through increasing physical activity given his sedentary lifestyle and severe obesity (BMI >50 kg/m²), which makes the addition of medical therapy desirable at this point. Liraglutide, 3.0 mg daily (Answer A), is associated with an average weight loss of 6% to 7% over one year. In addition, liraglutide has been associated with an improved lipid profile, including a 13% reduction in triglycerides. A small randomized, placebo-controlled trial of liraglutide 1.8 mg daily, vs placebo for 48 weeks in patients with biopsy-proven nonalcoholic steatohepatitis showed that 39% (9/23) of patients in the liraglutide group vs 9% (2/23) of patients in the placebo group had resolution of steatohepatitis as determined by liver biopsy (LEAN trial 2016). Although both liraglutide and lorcaserin improve glycemic control, none of the other agents listed (Answers B, C, D, E) are associated with a significant reduction in triglycerides, which would benefit this patient who has obesity, hypertriglyceridemia, and fatty liver disease.

EDUCATIONAL OBJECTIVE
Select appropriate medical therapy for weight loss on the basis of a patient's individual characteristics and risk profile.

REFERENCE(S)

Armstrong MJ, Gaunt P, Aithal GP, et al. Liraglutide safety and efficacy in patients with non-alcoholic steatohepatitis (LEAN): a multicentre, double-blind, randomized, placebo-controlled trial phase 2 study. *Lancet.* 2016;387(10019):679-690. PMID: 26608256

Apovian CM, Aronne LJ, Bessesen DH, et al; Endocrine Society. Pharmacological management of obesity: an endocrine Society clinical practice guideline. *J Clin Endocrinol Metab.* 2015;100(2):342-362. PMID: 25590212

Yanovski SZ, Yanovski JA. Long-term drug treatment for obesity: a systematic and clinical review. *JAMA.* 2014;311(1):74-86. PMID: 24231879

Garvey WT, Ryan DH, Look M, et al. Two-year sustained weight loss and metabolic benefits with controlled-release phentermine/topiramate in obese and overweight adults (SEQUEL): a randomized, placebo-controlled, phase 3 extension study. *Am J Clin Nutr.* 2012;95(2):297-308. PMID: 22158731

Smith SR, Weissman NJ, Anderson CM, et al; Behavioral Modification and Lorcaserin for Overweight and Obesity Management (BLOOM) Study Group. Multicenter, placebo-controlled trial of lorcaserin for weight management. *N Engl J Med.* 2010;363(3):245-256. PMID: 20647200

le Roux CW, Astrup A, Fujioka K, et al; SCALE Obesity Prediabetes NN8022-1839 Study Group. 3 years of liraglutide versus placebo for type 2 diabetes risk reduction and weight management in individuals with prediabetes: a randomised, double-blind trial. *Lancet.* 2017;389(10077):1399-1409. PMID: 28237263

Pi-Sunyer X, Astrup A, Fujioka K, et al; SCALE Obesity and Prediabetes NN8022-1839 Study Group. A randomized, controlled trial of 3.0 mg of liraglutide in weight management. *N Engl J Med.* 2015;373(1):11-22. PMID: 26132939

Yanovski SZ, Yanovski JA. Naltrexone extended-release plus bupropion extended-release for treatment of obesity. *JAMA.* 2015;313(12):1213-1214. PMID: 25803343

13
ANSWER: D) Kidney stones

Obesity increases the risk of both chronic kidney disease and kidney stones (Answer D). However, the risk of having a kidney stone approximately doubles in the first 6 months after bariatric surgery. A 6-year follow-up study after multiple types of bariatric surgery found new stone formation in 11% of patients who underwent bariatric surgery compared with 4.3% of nonsurgical control patients. Although there is increased risk for sleeve gastrectomy, Roux-en-Y gastric bypass, and biliopancreatic diversion/duodenal switch, the risk was higher for the malabsorptive procedures. After bariatric surgery, patients excrete increased amounts of oxalate in their urine, which form calcium oxalate stones predominantly, although other types of stones have been reported including hydroxyapatite and struvite stones. Patients can help to prevent stone formation by drinking plenty of water, following a low-oxalate diet, and decreasing animal protein intake.

Glucose and lipid metabolism improves after bariatric surgery (thus, Answers A and C are incorrect). Menstrual and reproductive function improves after bariatric surgery (thus, Answer B is incorrect). Onycholysis (Answer E), painless separation of the nail from the nailbed, is a common condition usually associated with thyroid disease, psoriasis, infections, or trauma, but it has no clear association with bariatric surgery and weight loss.

EDUCATIONAL OBJECTIVE
Describe common complications of bariatric surgery, including the increased risk for kidney stones.

REFERENCE(S)
Lieske JC, Mehta RA, Milliner DS, Rule AD, Bergstralh EJ, Sarr MG. Kidney stones are common after bariatric surgery. *Kidney Int.* 2015;87(4):839-845. PMID: 25354237

14
ANSWER: A) Ghrelin

Many gut hormones act through the circulation and peripheral nervous system (vagal afferents) on the central nervous system pathways, particularly in the hypothalamus and arcuate nucleus, to regulate appetite. Ghrelin (Answer A) is the only hormone listed as an answer choice that stimulates appetite through the NPY-Agouti-related peptide (AgRP) orexigenic neuronal pathways. Ghrelin is secreted by the stomach and rises in the morning after awakening and at regular intervals before each meal stimulating nutrient intake. Blocking the effects of ghrelin through blocking its receptor should decrease hunger, although such a compound has not been successfully developed to assist with weight loss.

All of the hormones listed (GLP-1 [Answer B], cholecystokinin [Answer C], peptide YY [Answer D], leptin) stimulate satiety via anorexigenic signaling via the POMC/CART neuronal pathways. As nutrients pass through the gut, GLP-1 is released from the small intestine, cholecystokinin from the duodenum, and peptide YY from the large intestine. Leptin is secreted by adipose tissue and circulating levels are directly proportional to adipose tissue mass signaling adequate fuel stores. Antagonizing the effect of satiety hormones would only serve to make patients hungrier and consume more food.

EDUCATIONAL OBJECTIVE
Describe the various hormones affecting appetite regulation and weight.

REFERENCE(S)
Schwartz MW, Woods SC, Porte D Jr, Seeley RJ, Baskin DG. Central nervous system control of food intake. *Nature.* 2000;404(6778):661-671. PMID: 10766253

Morton GJ, Meek TH, Schwartz MW. Neurobiology of food intake in health and disease. *Nat Rev Neurosci.* 2014;15(6):367-378. PMID: 24840801

Sohn JW, Elmquist JK, Williams KW. Neuronal circuits that regulate feeding behavior and metabolism. *Trends Neurosci.* 2013;36(9):504-512. PMID: 23790727

Shah M, Vella A. Effects of GLP-1 on appetite and weight. *Rev Endocr Metab Disord.* 2014;15(3):181-187. PMID: 24811133

15
ANSWER: B) Kidney stones

Many diets can result in weight loss. Varying the macronutrient content has less effect on long-term weight loss than adherence to a reduced-calorie diet that allows weight loss of approximately 1 lb per week. Reducing caloric intake by 500 calories a day should result in meaningful weight loss over time. The low-carbohydrate, moderate-protein, high-fat ketogenic diet is based on restricting carbohydrates to 20 to 60 g daily while maintaining adequate protein intake and replacing carbohydrate calories with fat calories. This approach forces the body to switch from burning carbohydrates to breaking down fat (lipolysis) into fatty acids for fuel and generating ketone bodies causing ketosis. Both low-fat and low-carbohydrate dietary approaches with the same total daily caloric intake have been shown to result in a similar amount of weight loss at 1 year (11-13 lb [5-6 kg]).

The ketogenic diet is associated with typical adverse effects, including severe fatigue and headaches in the first few weeks, as well as bad breath from ketosis, constipation, and potentially significant increases in LDL cholesterol from the high-fat content. Cataract formation (Answer A) due to increased fat intake has not been reported in patients following a ketogenic diet. Eruptive xanthoma (Answer C) can occur with extremely high triglycerides (>1000 mg/dL), which is not likely on the ketogenic diet in the absence of an underlying genetic disorder causing hypertriglyceridemia. The low-carbohydrate ketogenic diet improves glycemic control, so glucosuria (Answer D) is not a common finding in the absence of diabetes. Drinking plenty of fluids is important, as dehydration is also common with the ketogenic diet and can contribute to kidney stone formation (Answer B). Kidney stone formation can occur due to the increase in production and build-up of uric acid. Also, the accompanying mild acidemia has been theorized to increase bone turnover, causing an increase in calcium excretion and potentially contributing to stone formation.

EDUCATIONAL OBJECTIVE
List the risks and benefits of common diet plans for weight loss, including the ketogenic diet.

REFERENCE(S)
Gardner CD, Trepanowski JF, Del Gobbo LC, et al. Effect of low-fat vs low-carbohydrate diet on 12-month weight loss in overweight adults and the association with genotype pattern or insulin secretion: the DIETFITS randomized clinical trial. *JAMA*. 2018;319(7):667-679. PMID: 29466592

16
ANSWER: C) Add evolocumab

This patient's clinical picture is consistent with familial hypercholesterolemia. Fenofibrate (Answer B) and niacin (Answer D) have not been shown to reduce cardiovascular event rates when added to statin therapy. However, data from the IMPROVE-IT trial recently demonstrated that ezetimibe (Answer A) added to a regimen of simvastatin, 40 mg daily, resulted in a modest but statistically significant 6.4% reduction in a composite cardiovascular endpoint. This might be a reasonable option. However, given this patient's dramatic elevation in LDL cholesterol, the best next step is to add evolocumab (Answer C), which is a monoclonal antibody that targets and degrades PCSK9.

PCSK9 circulates in the blood and alters the liver's handling of LDL cholesterol by stimulating degradation of LDL receptors, which allows less LDL to be cleared from the circulation. Persons with genetic mutations that lower PCSK9 levels have lower LDL-cholesterol levels because they have higher numbers of LDL receptors to clear LDL cholesterol from the circulation. A number of pharmaceutical approaches to lowering PCSK9 levels have been developed. Evolocumab was approved in August 2015. It is specifically approved for use in addition to diet and maximally tolerated statin therapy in adult patients with heterozygous or homozygous familial hypercholesterolemia. The other US FDA–approved medication in this class is alirocumab. An additional treatment option for patients with familial hypercholesterolemia is lipopheresis, although this is not widely available.

Switching from atorvastatin 80 mg daily to rosuvastatin 40 mg daily (Answer E) might lower LDL cholesterol to similar or slightly greater effect, but the lipid-lowering effect would be significantly less than that observed with evolocumab.

Summarize the utility of proprotein convertase subtilisin/kexin type 9 (PCSK9) inhibitors in the treatment of patients with familial hypercholesterolemia.

REFERENCE(S)

Cannon CP, Blazing MA, Giugliano RP, et al; IMPROVE-IT Investigators. Ezetimibe added to statin therapy after acute coronary syndromes. *N Engl J Med.* 2015;372(25):2387-2397. PMID: 26039521

Sabatine MS, Giugliano RP, Wiviott SD, et al; Open-Label Study of Long-Term Evaluation against LDL Cholesterol (OSLER) Investigators. Efficacy and safety of evolocumab in reducing lipids and cardiovascular events. *N Engl J Med.* 2015;372(16):1500-1509. PMID: 25773607

Ajufo E, Rader DJ. Recent advances in the pharmacological management of hypercholesterolaemia. *Lancet Diabetes Endocrinol.* 2016;4(5):436-446. PMID: 27012540

17 ANSWER: A) A statin

While there has been concern for some time about the potential risk of treating individuals who have abnormal liver function tests with lipid-lowering drugs, there is no evidence that these drugs cause severe or progressive hepatic damage or that they cannot be safely used in patients with chronic liver disease. The GREACE study (Greek Atorvastatin and Coronary Heart Disease Evaluation) demonstrated that in individuals with liver function tests less than 3 times the upper normal limit, there are no adverse effects of lipid-lowering drugs on liver function tests over time and there are significant benefits to lipid-lowering therapy in cardiovascular disease risk reduction.

Approximately 3 million persons in the United States have chronic hepatitis C viral infection and a larger but unquantified number of obese patients have nonalcoholic fatty liver disease or nonalcoholic steatohepatitis. Fibrates, metformin, and thiazolidinediones reverse nonalcoholic fatty liver disease/nonalcoholic steatohepatitis. Some patients with chronic liver disease have lipid or lipoprotein abnormalities that, in the big scheme of things, require therapy because they are potentially as important as or more important than the

liver disease. This patient has familial combined hyperlipidemia and a family history of coronary heart disease; he fits the criteria for a statin benefit group (no diabetes, aged 40-75 years, LDL cholesterol 70-189 mg/dL, + 7.5% risk of cardiovascular disease event in the next 10 years).

In the absence of serious or progressive liver disease, he first requires therapy with a statin (Answer A). While diet alone (Answer B) might provide modest reduction in cardiovascular disease risk, the benefit would be substantially lower than that resulting from statin therapy. Likewise, neither a fibrate (Answer C), ezetimibe (Answer D), nor niacin (Answer E) would provide the cardiovascular disease risk reduction comparable to that of a statin. Since a statin is safe to use in this patient and it has the greatest benefits, it is the treatment of choice.

EDUCATIONAL OBJECTIVE
Assess the risk of liver toxicity from statin use.

REFERENCE(S)

Athyros VG, Tziomalos K, Gossios TD, et al; GREACE Study Collaborative Group. Safety and efficacy of long-term statin treatment for cardiovascular events in patients with coronary heart disease and abnormal liver tests in the Greek Atorvastatin and Coronary Heart Disease Evaluation (GREACE) Study: a post-hoc analysis. *Lancet.* 2010;376(9756):1916-1922. PMID: 21109302

Khorashadi S, Hasson NK, Cheung RC. Incidence of statin hepatotoxicity in patients with hepatitis C. *Clin Gastroenterol Hepatol.* 2006;4(7):902-907. PMID: 16697272

Demyen M, Alkhalloufi K, Pyrsopoulos NT. Lipid-lowering agents and hepatotoxicity. *Clin Liver Dis.* 2013;17(4):699-714. PMID: 24099026

18 ANSWER: C) Oral contraceptive use

Hypertriglyceridemia has a number of causes including genetic mutations, medications, and other medical conditions. The described patient has both high triglycerides and high HDL-cholesterol levels. This can be observed in the setting of alcohol use or estrogen use. The history lists oral contraceptives (Answer C) as a medication, and this is the most likely culprit. The frank hypertriglyceridemia that this patient exhibits can occur in someone with an underlying predisposition to hypertriglyceridemia who then begins oral estrogens. This typically does not occur with transdermal estrogens, but it can occur with oral estrogens given for postmenopausal symptoms.

Lipoprotein lipase is the key enzyme in the catabolism of circulating triglyceride-rich lipoproteins VLDL and chylomicrons. Apolipoprotein C2 is a cofactor for lipoprotein lipase, so both lipoprotein lipase deficiency (Answer A) and apolipoprotein C2 deficiency (Answer B) can cause marked hypertriglyceridemia. Triglyceride levels in affected individuals are typically greater than 1000 mg/dL (>11.30 mmol/L) and can be 2000 to 3000 mg/dL (22.60-33.90 mmol/L). The enzyme cholesterol ester transfer protein (CETP) exchanges cholesterol esters in HDL for triglyceride in VLDL and chylomicrons, resulting in increased clearance of HDL cholesterol. This process is increased when triglyceride levels are high. This explains the common association between increased triglyceride levels and decreased HDL-cholesterol levels. CETP deficiency (Answer D) is associated with very high HDL-cholesterol levels but not hypertriglyceridemia. Lipoprotein lipase deficiency and apolipoprotein C2 deficiency cause high triglyceride levels, but because of CETP, HDL-cholesterol levels are typically low.

EDUCATIONAL OBJECTIVE
Identify the most likely cause of high triglycerides in a patient with high HDL-cholesterol levels.

REFERENCE(S)
Baksu B, Davas I, Agar E, Akyol A, Uluocak A. Do different delivery systems of estrogen therapy influence serum lipids differently in surgically menopausal women? *J Obstet Gynaecol Res.* 2007;33(3):346-352. PMID: 17578365

Brien SE, Ronksley PE, Turner BJ, Mukamal KJ, Ghali WA. Effect of alcohol consumption on biological markers associated with risk of coronary heart disease: systematic review and meta-analysis of interventional studies. *BMJ.* 2011;342:d636. PMID: 21343206

19   ANSWER: E) Change simvastatin to atorvastatin 80 mg daily

The 2013 American Heart Association guidelines on the treatment of blood cholesterol to reduce atherosclerotic cardiovascular risk focus on not only the decision of whom to treat with a statin but what the treatment goal is. The current American Heart Association guidelines suggest choosing low-, moderate-, or high-intensity statins based on the patient's level of risk given data from randomized controlled trials to define which specific statins and dosages constitute low-intensity treatment (<30% LDL reduction), moderate-intensity treatment (30%-50% LDL reduction), or high-intensity treatment (>50% LDL reduction). The older National Cholesterol Education Program Adult Treatment Panel III guidelines set the target as the absolute LDL-cholesterol level based on the patient's risk for cardiovascular disease.

The described patient is at high risk for future cardiovascular events because he has already had a myocardial infarction. Therefore, high-intensity statin therapy is warranted, which the new guidelines define as atorvastatin, 80 mg daily (Answer E). The dosage can be reduced to 40 mg daily if the patient does not tolerate the higher dosage. Atorvastatin, 20 mg daily (Answer D), is a moderate-intensity statin and is thus incorrect. His current treatment with simvastatin, 20 mg daily (Answer A), or a dosage increase to 40 mg daily (Answer B) would be considered moderate-intensity therapy and not appropriate for his level of risk. Adding ezetimibe (Answer C) to a statin would lower cardiovascular risk by approximately 15% based on the IMPOVE-IT trial, but it should be added to the highest-intensity statin for maximal effect. Thus, changing from a moderate- to a high-intensity statin would be the best next step.

EDUCATIONAL OBJECTIVE
Describe the targets of therapy in the new American Heart Association cholesterol guidelines.

REFERENCE(S)

Stone NJ, Robinson JG, Lichtenstein AH, Bairey Merz CN, Blum CB, Eckel RH, et al; American College of Cardiology/American Heart Association Task Force on Practice Guidelines. 2013 ACC/AHA guideline on the treatment of blood cholesterol to reduce atherosclerotic cardiovascular risk in adults: a report of the American College of Cardiology/American Heart Association Task Force on Practice Guidelines [published correction in *Circulation*. 2014;129(25 Suppl 2):S46-S48]. *Circulation*. 2014;129(25 Suppl 2):S1-S45. PMID: 24222016

Stone NJ, Robinson JG, Lichtenstein AH, Goff DC Jr, Lloyd-Jones DM, Smith SC Jr, et al; 2013 ACC/AHA Cholesterol Guideline Panel. Treatment of blood cholesterol to reduce atherosclerotic cardiovascular disease risk in adults: synopsis of the 2013 American College of Cardiology/American Heart Association cholesterol guideline. *Ann Intern Med*. 2014;160(5):339-343. PMID: 24474185

Cannon CP, Blazing MA, Giugliano RP, et al; IMPROVE-IT Investigators. Ezetimibe added to statin therapy after acute coronary syndromes. *N Engl J Med*. 2015;372(25):2387-2397. PMID: 26039521

20 ANSWER: A) Insulin and glucose

The treatment for triglyceride-induced pancreatitis varies. Usually intravenous fluids and lack of oral intake rapidly reduces triglyceride levels. Additional measures have also been used. An insulin and glucose drip (Answer A) prevents fatty acid release from adipose tissues because it inhibits hormone-sensitive lipase and adipose triglyceride lipase activity and is thought to prevent production of triglycerides by the liver. There is no obvious downside to this therapy provided the patient does not become hypoglycemic, so glucose is usually added. No randomized controlled trials have established the benefit of this therapy.

Fenofibrate (Answer B) lowers triglycerides when used over the long term, but it would be of limited utility to quickly lower triglycerides in the setting of acute pancreatitis. High-dosage statins decrease triglycerides in patients with more modest hypertriglyceridemia but have no role in triglyceride-lowering in acute pancreatitis. Because heparin (Answer C) releases lipoprotein lipase from the arterial walls and increases intravascular lipolysis, it has been suggested as a treatment. However, there is concern about the use of heparin because of pancreatic hemorrhage. Although estrogens increase hepatic triglyceride production, there is no role for hormonal therapies (Answer D) in acute pancreatitis. Metformin (Answer E) has no role in the treatment of acute pancreatitis. One therapy that is sometimes used in the outpatient setting is orlistat. Orlistat prevents gastrointestinal absorption of fat by inhibiting pancreatic lipase, thus creating a forced low-fat diet. It has no role in the treatment of acute pancreatitis while the patient is not eating. Finally, plasmapheresis to remove triglycerides from the blood has been used in acute hypertriglyceridemic pancreatitis. However, it is not usually necessary because triglyceride levels are rapidly reduced with the cessation of food intake.

EDUCATIONAL OBJECTIVE
Guide acute therapy for hypertriglyceridemia-induced pancreatitis.

REFERENCE(S)

Semenkovich CF, Goldberg AC, Goldberg IJ. Disorders of lipid metabolism. In: Melmed S, Polonsky KS, Larsen PR, Kronenberg HM, eds. *Williams Textbook of Endocrinology*. 12th ed. Philadelphia, PA: Elsevier Saunders; 2011:1633-1674.

Brunzell JD. Clinical practice. Hypertriglyceridemia. *N Engl J Med*. 2007;357(10):1009-1017. PMID: 17804845

Tolentino MC, Ferenczi A, Ronen L, Poretsky L. Combination of gemfibrozil and orlistat for treatment of combined hyperlipidemia with predominant hypertriglyceridemia. *Endocr Pract*. 2002;8(3):208-212. PMID: 12113634

21 ANSWER: B) Corneal arcus

Premature development of corneal arcus (Answer B) (under age 40 years per the Dutch Lipid Criteria for diagnosis of Familial Hyperlipidemia) is one of the signature signs of familial genetic hypercholesterolemia. The cardinal feature of the disorder on physical exam is tendon xanthoma affecting either the Achilles tendon or the tendons on the dorsum of the hands. The reason why lipid accumulates in the tendons is not completely understood, but it is thought to be secondary to recurrent inflammation and macrophage recruitment to where the tendon interacts with its overlying sheath. Tendon xanthomas are usually most prominent in the Achilles tendon. Some patients with familial hypercholesterolemia do not have tendon xanthomas but do have premature corneal arcus. In current practice, many patients with heterozygous familial hyperlipidemia do not exhibit these 2 signs, as they have been on lipid-lowering therapy for years before their specific genetic disorder is diagnosed.

Most often, patients with familial hypercholesterolemia have a heterozygous mutation in the gene encoding the LDL receptor. Defective apolipoprotein B, the ligand for the receptor, and a defect in an intracellular adaptor protein cause a similar phenotype. Persons who are heterozygous have total cholesterol levels of 350 to 600 mg/dL (9.06 to 15.54 mmol/L), LDL-cholesterol levels greater than 250 mg/dL (>6.48 mmol/L), premature coronary artery disease, and aortic stenosis.

This patient is being treated with atorvastatin, 80 mg daily; his off-therapy LDL-cholesterol concentration is most likely around 300 mg/dL (7.77 mmol/L). The homozygous form of this disease leads to atherosclerosis before age 20 years (sometimes before age 10 years). Liver transplant is often the treatment. Genetic testing does not alter therapy and is not usually performed.

Lipemia retinalis (Answer A) is the milky appearance of the retina and retinal vessels that accompanies severe hypertriglyceridemia. Eruptive xanthomas (Answer C) are acne-like papules that are found on extensor surfaces of the arms and on the back and buttocks. They are also a sign of severe hypertriglyceridemia. Palmar xanthomas (Answer D) are lipid depositions in the creases of the palms that occur with dysbetalipoproteinemia (formerly called type 3 hyperlipoproteinemia). Arthropathy (Answer E) is not a sign of a dyslipoproteinemia.

EDUCATIONAL OBJECTIVE
Identify physical findings of hyperlipidemias.

REFERENCE(S)
Semenkovich CF, Goldberg AC, Goldberg IJ. Disorders of lipid metabolism. In: Melmed S, Polonsky KS, Larsen PR, Kronenberg HM, eds. *Williams Textbook of Endocrinology*. 12th ed. Philadelphia, PA: Elsevier Saunders; 2011:1633-1674.

22 ANSWER: B) Add alirocumab

PCSK9 inhibitors, evolocumab and alirocumab (Answer B), are a new class of medications used to significantly lower LDL cholesterol and reduce cardiovascular disease. They are monoclonal antibodies that target and degrade the proprotein convertase subtilisin/kexin type 9 (PCSK9) protein. PCSK9 circulates in the blood and alters the liver's handling of LDL cholesterol. Both evolocumab and alirocumab are US FDA approved for clinical atherosclerotic cardiovascular disease and heterozygous familial hyperlipidemia. PCSK9 inhibitors have been studied in statin-intolerant patients (GAUSS-1 and GAUSS-2 studies), but statin intolerance alone is not currently an approved indication in the absence of clinical atherosclerotic cardiovascular disease or familial hyperlipidemia. Clinical trials have shown that LDL cholesterol is lowered approximately 60% by evolocumab and 55% to 60% by alirocumab, which would most likely reduce this patient's LDL cholesterol below 100 mg/dL (<2.59 mmol/L). The FOURIER trial showed that evolocumab reduced LDL cholesterol 59% in patients with known coronary disease and a baseline LDL-cholesterol level of ≥70 mg/dL or greater (≥1.81 mmol/L) who were taking a statin compared with placebo and lowered cardiovascular event rates by 15% over 3 years (hazard ratio, 0.85; 95% confidence interval, 0.79-0.92). Additionally, the study indicated there was added benefit at lower LDL-cholesterol levels than previously targeted.

In the ODYSSEY trial of alirocumab vs placebo after acute coronary syndrome, LDL cholesterol was lowered in the alirocumab group by 54.7% compared with LDL cholesterol in the placebo group at 48 months (mean LDL cholesterol 53.3 mg/dL vs 101.4 mg/dL, respectively). Risk of a major cardiovascular event was lowered by 15% (hazard ratio, 0.85; 95% confidence interval, 0.78-0.93; $P = .0003$) (preliminary results released at the

American College of Cardiology – 67th Scientific Sessions, March 2010).

The newer data regarding LDL-cholesterol lowering and associated lowering of cardiovascular disease risk will most likely shift the focus back to absolute LDL-cholesterol levels from the general group targets recommended in the 2013 American College of Cardiology/American Heart Association Cholesterol-Lowering Guidelines.

Niacin (Answer A) has been shown to lower LDL cholesterol in some trials in men, but it may also worsen this patient's glycemic control. Fenofibrate (Answer C) has not been shown to lower cardiovascular disease event rates. Lipopheresis (Answer D) has been used to clear LDL particles and reduce cardiovascular disease risk in some patients with heterozygous and homozygous familial hyperlipidemia, but it is invasive, not widely available, and would be an option only if all medications failed.

EDUCATIONAL OBJECTIVE
Explain the indications for treating patients who have hyperlipidemia with PCSK9 inhibitors.

REFERENCE(S)
Schwartz GG, Szarek M, Bhatt DL, et al. The ODYSESEY Outcomes Trial: topline results alirocumab in patients after acute coronary syndrome. American College of Cardiology, 67th Scientific Sessions. March 10, 2018. Available at: http://clinicaltrialresults.org/Slides/ACC2018/ODYSSEY_Steg.pdf

Sabatine MS, Giugliano RP, Keech AC, et al; FOURIER Steering Committee and Investigators. Evolocumab and clinical outcomes in patients with cardiovascular disease. *N Engl J Med.* 2017; 376(18):1713-1722. PMID: 28304224

Sabatine MS, Giugliano RP, Wiviott SD, et al; Open-Label Study of Long-Term Evaluation against LDL Cholesterol (OSLER) Investigators. Efficacy and safety of evolocumab in reducing lipids and cardiovascular events. *N Engl J Med.* 2015;372(16):1500-1509. PMID: 25773607

Ajufo E, Rader DJ. Recent advances in the pharmacological management of hypercholesterolemia. *Lancet Diabetes Endocrinol.* 2016;4(5):436-446. PMID: 27012540

Steg PG, et al. Joint ACC/JACC Late-Breaking Clinical Trials. Presented at: American College of Cardiology Scientific Session; March 10-12, 2018; Orlando, FL.

23 ANSWER: B) Switch metoprolol to amlodipine
Patients with collagen-vascular disease can develop severe hyperlipidemias. On occasion, these conditions are due to the production of antibodies that can inhibit lipoprotein lipase or heparin (and lipase binding to endothelium). Antibodies can also be directed to apolipoproteins: antibodies to apolipoprotein B lead to hypobetalipoproteinemia, and antibodies to apolipoprotein AI lead to low HDL-cholesterol levels. Several medications in this setting, as well as in patients without collagen-vascular disease, can exacerbate hypertriglyceridemia. One such class of medications is β-adrenergic blockers. Thus, substituting a calcium-channel blocker for metoprolol (Answer B) is correct.

Changing from one steroid to another (Answer A) should not affect hypertriglyceridemia. Although thiazide diuretics increase triglycerides, so does chlorthalidone (Answer C). Lisinopril (Answer D) does not affect triglyceride levels.

EDUCATIONAL OBJECTIVE
Advise patients on medications, such as β-adrenergic blockers, that increase triglyceride levels.

REFERENCE(S)
Stone NJ. Secondary causes of hyperlipidemia. *Med Clin North Am.* 1994;78(1):117-141. PMID: 8283927

Dinu AR, Merrill JT, Shen C, Antonov IV, Myones BL, Lahita RG. Frequency of antibodies to the cholesterol transport protein apolipoprotein A1 in patients with SLE. *Lupus.* 1998;7(5):355-360. PMID: 9696140

24 ANSWER: B) Myositis
A number of medications increase risk of myositis (Answer B) with statins. This is thought to be due to reduced statin clearance by the liver. In this situation, the concern is that interaction with the protease inhibitor will increase risk of myositis, which might lead to statin discontinuation. Reintroduction of the statin at a lower dosage or after a change in HIV therapy is, however,

a possibility. The best-studied drug interaction is that with gemfibrozil, which leads to a marked increase in circulating statin levels. Cyclosporine, which is often used as a long-term treatment in transplant recipients, also increases myositis risk. Greater LDL-cholesterol reduction in patients such as this one may be achieved with the use of low statin dosages supplemented with other LDL-cholesterol reduction therapies such as ezetimibe. Resins are likely to increase the patient's triglyceride levels. Other drugs that increase myositis risk include ketoconazole and erythromycin (Answer D). Patients taking a short-term course of these drugs are advised to stop their statins.

Patients such as the one in this vignette often develop diabetes mellitus (Answer A). High-dosage statin therapy will probably increase this risk, but it would not be a reason to avoid lowering the LDL cholesterol in a patient with great cardiovascular disease risk. Statins do not inhibit antiviral agents (Answer C). Increased transaminases in patients taking statins are common (1% to 2% of patients). However, liver disease caused by statins is rare, and provided the increases in transaminase levels are less than 3 times the upper normal limit, it is acceptable to continue the lipid-lowering therapy (thus, Answer E is incorrect). For this reason, the US FDA has recently changed its guidelines on monitoring liver function in statin-treated patients—it now recommends checking liver enzymes "as clinically indicated."

EDUCATIONAL OBJECTIVE
Identify the potential interaction of statins with protease inhibitors, which may lead to an increased risk of myositis.

REFERENCE(S)

Venero CV, Thompson PD. Managing statin myopathy. *Endocrinol Metab Clin North Am.* 2009;38(1):121-136. PMID: 19217515

Thompson PD, Clarkson P, Karas RH. Statin-associated myopathy. *JAMA.* 2003;289(13):1681-1690. PMID: 12672737

Kirchner JT. Clinical management considerations for dyslipidemia in HIV-infected individuals. *Postgrad Med.* 2012;124(1):31-40. PMID: 22314112

25 ANSWER: B) Lipoprotein (a)

Additional biomarkers of increased cardiovascular risk beyond LDL cholesterol have been used to further quantify cardiovascular risk in patients who have persistent disease despite good response to lipid-lowering therapy, including apolipoprotein B (Answer A), non-HDL cholesterol (Answer D), lipoprotein (a) (Answer B), and high-sensitivity C-reactive protein (Answer C).

Lipoprotein (a) is highly atherogenic and is associated with increased risk of cardiovascular disease, particularly premature cardiovascular disease. Lipoprotein (a) is an LDL particle with a large protein, apo (a), attached covalently to apo B that can incorporate into the arterial wall and contribute to atherosclerosis. Lipoprotein (a) may be modestly elevated in familial hyperlipidemia, but very high levels are associated with a significant increase in atherosclerotic disease. Persons with a lipoprotein (a) level in the upper tertile have an increased risk of cardiovascular disease (odds ratio, 1.7; 95% confidence interval, 1.4-1.9) compared with persons whose level is in the lower tertile.

Apolipoprotein B is a lipoprotein found on all atherogenic lipid particles, including LDL and triglyceride-rich particles. Non-HDL cholesterol has been suggested as a marker of cardiovascular risk because it also includes non-LDL (triglyceride risk) atherogenic particles. Apolipoprotein B and non-HDL cholesterol predict risk with LDL cholesterol in patients with primarily elevated LDL cholesterol and elevated triglycerides as found in patients with type 2 diabetes. This patient does not have diabetes or elevated triglycerides, which suggest apolipoprotein B and non-HDL cholesterol are not likely to be additionally informative beyond his LDL cholesterol level. Apolipoprotein B elevation can support a diagnosis of familial hyperlipidemia and is associated with high risk of cardiovascular disease, but his baseline LDL-cholesterol level was not typical of a patient with familial hyperlipidemia.

Elevated high-sensitivity C-reactive protein is also associated with increased cardiovascular disease risk, particularly related to insulin resistance, but it is not likely to explain this patient's residual cardiovascular risk given he is normal weight and does not have diabetes.

The 2013 American College of Cardiology/American Heart Association Cholesterol Lowering

Guidelines do not currently recommend measurement of biomarkers such as apolipoprotein B, lipoprotein (a), and high-sensitivity C-reactive protein for the purpose of primary risk stratification in addition to the lipid profile, but these measures may be used in select cases. Newer guidelines suggest additional markers may be used in select cases to further risk stratify patients, although clear pharmacologic strategies to lower cardiovascular disease risk by targeting lipoprotein (a) reduction are still lacking, although the particle is effectively removed by apheresis.

EDUCATIONAL OBJECTIVE
Describe the epidemiologic evidence for new lipid biomarkers of cardiovascular risk beyond the traditional lipid profile for risk stratification of residual cardiovascular disease.

REFERENCE(S)

Stone NJ, Robinson JG, Lichtenstein AH, et al; American College of Cardiology/American Heart Association Task Force on Practice Guidelines. 2013 ACC/AHA guideline on the treatment of blood cholesterol to reduce atherosclerotic cardiovascular risk in adults: a report of the American College of Cardiology/American Heart Association Task Force on Practice Guidelines [published correction appears in *Circulation*. 2014;129(25 Suppl 2):S46-S48]. *Circulation*. 2014;129(25 Suppl 2):S1-S45. PMID: 24222016

Danesh J, Collins R, Peto R. Lipoprotein(a) and coronary heart disease. Meta-analysis of prospective studies. *Circulation*. 2000;102(10):1082-1085. PMID: 10973834

Kamstrup PR, Benn M, Tybjaerg-Hansen A, Nordestgaard BG. Extreme lipoprotein(a) levels and risk of myocardial infarction in the general population: The Copenhagen City Heart Study. *Circulation*. 2008;117(2):176-184. PMID: 18086931

Nordestagarrd BG, Chapman MJ, Ray K, et al; European Atherosclerosis Society Consensus Panel. Lipoprotein(a) as a cardiovascular risk factor: current status. *Eur Heart J*. 2010;31(23):2844-2853. PMID: 20965889

26 ANSWER: D) Skin irritation/rash

The adverse event profile of PCSK9 inhibitor medications is favorable. In the FOURIER trial of evolocumab vs placebo, all adverse events were similar between evolocumab and placebo with the exception of injection site reactions that were uncommon but were slightly higher in the evolocumab group (2.1% vs 1.6%; $P < .001$), although allergic reactions were similar (3.1% vs 2.9%). Neurocognitive dysfunction (Answer A) was rare and similar between groups (1.6% vs 1.5%). Although there has been no evidence of cognitive dysfunction to date in clinical trials, there remains concern for patients who achieve very low levels of LDL cholesterol (eg, <30 mg/dL) on therapy. Liver function test elevation (Answer B) ≥3 times the upper normal limit was similar between groups (1.8% vs 1.8%). Myalgias (Answer C) (5.0 vs 4.8%), elevated creatine kinase (0.7% vs 0.7%), and rhabdomyolysis (0.1% vs 0.1%) were similar in treatment vs placebo groups, respectively.

In the ODYSSEY trial of alirocumab vs placebo after acute coronary syndrome, the only adverse event more common in the alirocumab group was injection site reactions on the skin (Answer D) (3.8% vs 2.1%, respectively; hazard ratio, 1.82; 95% confidence interval, 1.54-2.17) (preliminary results released at the American College of Cardiology – 67th Scientific Sessions, March 2010).

There is also concern for the development of new-onset diabetes with use of PCSK9 inhibitor therapy similar to what has been observed with statins. This is based on genetic epidemiology studies showing that loss-of-function mutations in the gene encoding PCSK9 are associated with lower LDL cholesterol and lower risk of cardiovascular disease but increased risk of type 2 diabetes. Increased risk of type 2 diabetes has not been demonstrated in clinical trials so far, but longer-term studies are needed to fully elucidate this risk.

EDUCATIONAL OBJECTIVE
Describe the adverse effect profile of the new class of cholesterol-lowering medications, PCSK9 inhibitors.

REFERENCE(S)

Sabatine MS, Giugliano RP, Keech AC, et al; FOURIER Steering Committee and Investigators. Evolocumab and clinical outcomes in patients with cardiovascular disease. *N Engl J Med.* 2017;376(18):1713-1722. PMID: 28304224

Sabatine MS, Giugliano RP, Wiviott SD, et al; Open-Label Study of Long-Term Evaluation against LDL Cholesterol (OSLER) Investigators. Efficacy and safety of evolocumab in reducing lipids and cardiovascular events. *N Engl J Med.* 2015;372(16):1500-1509. PMID: 25773607

Steg PG, et al. Joint ACC/JACC Late-Breaking Clinical Trials. Presented at: American College of Cardiology Scientific Session; March 10-12, 2018; Orlando, FL.

Schwartz GG, Szarek M, Bhatt DL, et al. The ODYSSEY Outcomes Trial: topline results alirocumab in patients After Acute Coronary Syndrome. American College of Cardiology – 67th Scientific Sessions, March 10, 2018. Available at: http://clinicaltrialresults.org/Slides/ACC2018/ODYSSEY_Steg.pdf

27 ANSWER: D) Continue atorvastatin and add fenofibrate

This patient has known cardiovascular disease in the context of type 2 diabetes and mixed hyperlipidemia, with both elevated LDL cholesterol and triglycerides. She is at very high risk for another cardiovascular event and will benefit from continuing the statin for cardiovascular risk reduction (thus, Answers A and C are incorrect). The most common inherited lipid disorder in type 2 diabetes is familial combined hyperlipidemia, which has a very variable clinical phenotype regarding LDL-cholesterol and triglyceride elevations, which can shift over time within the same patient. This patient most likely had a triglyceride concentration greater than 1000 mg/dL (>11.3 mmol/L), as she had several episodes of pancreatitis. Her current fasting triglyceride concentration of 760 mg/dL (8.59 mmol/L) while on a statin (≥500 mg/dL [≥5.65 mmol/L]) does put her risk for pancreatitis. The 2013 American College of Cardiology/American Heart Association Guidelines on the Treatment of Blood Cholesterol to Reduce Atherosclerotic Cardiovascular Risk in Adults recommend treating triglycerides as a secondary target when levels remain above 500 mg/dL. She would benefit from lipid-lowering therapy targeted at lowering triglycerides.

Both fibrates gemfibrozil and fenofibrate effectively lower triglycerides, but gemfibrozil is contraindicated due to concurrent use of a statin because of the increased risk of muscle-related adverse effects, including myositis and rhabdomyolysis (thus, Answers A and B are incorrect). Adding fenofibrate to a statin (Answer D) is the safer choice for additional triglyceride lowering. Niacin (Answer E) may help to lower triglycerides, but it would also likely worsen her diabetes and is therefore not the best choice.

EDUCATIONAL OBJECTIVE
Recommend when and how to treat hypertriglyceridemia in patients with cardiovascular disease.

REFERENCE(S)

Stone NJ, Robinson JG, Lichtenstein AH, et al; American College of Cardiology/American Heart Association Task Force on Practice Guidelines. 2013 ACC/AHA guideline on the treatment of blood cholesterol to reduce atherosclerotic cardiovascular risk in adults: a report of the American College of Cardiology/American Heart Association Task Force on Practice Guidelines [published correction appears in *Circulation.* 2014;129(25 Suppl 2):S46-S48]. *Circulation.* 2014;129(25 Suppl 2):S1-S45. PMID: 24222016

Stone NJ, Robinson JG, Lichtenstein AH, et al; 2013 ACC/AHA Cholesterol Guideline Panel. Treatment of blood cholesterol to reduce atherosclerotic cardiovascular disease risk in adults: synopsis of the 2013 American College of Cardiology/American Heart Association cholesterol guideline. *Ann Intern Med.* 2014;160(5):339-343. PMID: 24474185

Berglund L, Brunzell JD, Goldberg AC, et al; Endocrine Society. Evaluation and treatment of hypertriglyceridemia: an Endocrine Society clinical practice guideline. *J Clin Endocrinol Metab.* 2012;97(9):2969-2989. PMID: 22962670

28 ANSWER: B) Treat with rosuvastatin once weekly

Statin intolerance is a common clinical problem, and it is especially an issue in patients with underlying conditions that may predispose to muscularskeletal adverse effects. Aside from reviewing other medications that might interfere with statin metabolism (eg, gemfibrozil, cyclosporine, amiodarone), screening for hypothyroidism is also important, as it is in all patients with hypercholesterolemia. The only reasonable management option listed is to treat the patient with a once-weekly (or alternate day) statin (Answer B). This strategy might result in fewer muscle symptoms.

Coenzyme Q10 (Answer A) circulates in the blood associated with LDL cholesterol, and statin treatment reduces coenzyme Q10. Although coenzyme Q10 has been used for statin-induced myalgia, no data confirm that this supplement is beneficial. However, it also does not appear to have any downside risk, so it is often used. Red yeast rice extract (Answer C) has been used in several supplement formulations to lower cholesterol. One meta-analysis published in 2006 showed some moderate lipid-lowering effects with red yeast rice extracts, but there are no rigorous trials, cardiovascular outcome trials, or long-term safety data available to support its recommendation for patients with hyperlipidemia. Fish oil (Answer D) is used for hypertriglyceridemia, but it has no significant LDL-cholesterol–lowering effects. Although omega-3 fatty acids have been touted as anti-inflammatory agents, they also have no known benefit in this condition. Finally, statin antibodies (Answer E) are not a clinical entity.

EDUCATIONAL OBJECTIVE
Develop a management strategy for statin-induced myalgia.

REFERENCE(S)
Backes JM, Gibson CA, Ruisinger JF, Moriarty PM. The high-dose rosuvastatin once weekly study (The HD-ROWS). *J Clin Lipidol*. 2012;6(4):362-367. PMID: 22836073

Marcoff L, Thompson PD. The role of coenzyme Q10 in statin-associated myopathy: a systematic review. *J Am Coll Cardiol*. 2007;49(23):2231-2237. PMID: 17560286

29 ANSWER: A) Coronary calcium score

Of these options, the test with the best predictive value for cardiovascular disease events in middle-aged men is the coronary artery calcium score (Answer A) obtained using CT imaging. Coronary calcium is thought to indicate response to inflammation in the artery. Although no screening test is perfect, this test is meant to detect early disease and the 5-year risk of coronary events. Moreover, a positive score is associated with better adherence to lifestyle modification. However, in younger patients (eg, those with familial hypercholesterolemia), this imaging fails to detect disease because atherosclerotic plaques in these patients are often not calcified. Coronary calcium has also been used to indicate subclinical cardiovascular disease in younger patients with type 1 diabetes.

Although LDL particle size has been promoted as an independent risk factor, small, dense LDL is highly correlated with hypertriglyceridemia, low HDL cholesterol, and metabolic syndrome. Moreover, there are no guidelines for use of LDL particle size distribution (Answer B) to alter therapy. Measurement of apolipoprotein B (Answer C) provides similar data to that from assessment of non-HDL cholesterol. Antioxidant levels (Answer D) and vitamin E levels are not risk factor indicators. Palmitate (Answer E) is a saturated fatty acid that might be especially inflammatory, but its measurement has no role in cardiac risk assessment. Additional blood tests that might be performed with some justification include measurement of lipoprotein (a), C-reactive protein, and hemoglobin A_{1c}. White blood cell counts are a well-established indicator of cardiac risk, but variability precludes their use as a screening test.

This man does not require therapy for LDL-cholesterol reduction. Additional lipid-lowering therapies are not indicated unless there is concern for or evidence of vascular disease. With a family history of premature disease, one could argue that knowing whether he is at higher than expected risk would change this calculation.

EDUCATIONAL OBJECTIVE
Recommend the coronary artery calcium score as a possible tool to assess cardiovascular disease risk.

REFERENCE(S)

Guerci AD, Arad Y, Agatston A. Predictive value of EBCT scanning. *Circulation*. 1998;97(25):2583-2584. PMID: 9657482

Orakzai RH, Nasir K, Orakzai SH, et al. Effect of patient visualization of coronary calcium by electron beam computed tomography on changes in beneficial lifestyle behaviors. *Am J Cardiol*. 2008;101(7):999-1002. PMID: 18359321

30 ANSWER: C) Apolipoprotein E2/E2

The apolipoprotein (apo) E2/E2 phenotype (Answer C) is present in patients with dysbetalipoproteinemia, which is also referred to as type III hyperlipidemia, or broad-beta disease. Classic skin manifestations include tuberoeruptive lesions at the elbows and palmar xanthomas as observed in this patient. The apo E2/E2 phenotype occurs in about 1 per 100 persons, but the development of characteristic dyslipidemia is infrequent and usually appears later in life due to acquired medical conditions such as hypothyroidism, obesity, diabetes mellitus, or estrogen replacement therapy. The lipoprotein that accumulates is a remnant of triglyceride metabolism (beta VLDL) and is associated with an increased risk of atherosclerotic vascular disease. Although the calculated LDL-cholesterol level is increased in this patient, it is spurious due to accumulation of the beta VLDL. This remnant is cholesterol ester–enriched and has "balanced" concentrations of cholesterol and triglyceride, which accounts for the nearly equal serum cholesterol and triglyceride levels.

ABCA1 is a protein involved in moving cholesterol from peripheral tissues onto HDL particles. Deficiency of this protein (Answer A) results in the condition known as Tangier disease, characterized by very low HDL-cholesterol levels and the classic physical examination finding of orange tonsils, which this patient does not have. LDL-receptor deficiency (Answer B) results in the condition known as familial hypercholesterolemia. Patients with familial hypercholesterolemia have very high LDL-cholesterol levels, tendinous xanthomas, and premature coronary artery disease. Apolipoprotein C2 is a cofactor for lipoprotein lipase. Deficiency of apolipoprotein C2 (Answer D) therefore results in marked hypertriglyceridemia such as that seen in lipoprotein lipase deficiency. Overproduction of apolipoprotein B (Answer E) is the underlying problem in patients with familial combined hyperlipidemia. These individuals can have elevations in both triglycerides and LDL cholesterol such as that described in this patient, but this condition is not associated with the classic skin lesions (tuberoeruptive and palmar xanthomas) that are characteristic of dysbetalipoproteinemia.

EDUCATIONAL OBJECTIVE
Identify the clinical features of dysbetalipoproteinemia.

REFERENCE(S)

Garg A, Simha V. Update of dyslipidemia. *J Clin Endocrinol Metab*. 2007;92(5):1581-1589. PMID: 17483372

Walden CC, Hegele RA. Apolipoprotein E in hyperlipidemia. *Ann Intern Med*. 1994;120(12):1026-1036. PMID: 8185134

Marais AD, Solomon GA, Blom DJ. Dysbetalipoproteinaemia: a mixed hyperlipidaemia of remnant lipoproteins due to mutations in apolipoprotein E. *Crit Rev Clin Lab Sci*. 2014;51(1):46-62. PMID: 24405372

Pituitary Board Review

Laurence Katznelson, MD • Stanford University

1 **ANSWER: D) Perform a pituitary-directed MRI**

This patient responded nicely to bromocriptine and stopped it appropriately when she became pregnant. However, now at 37 weeks' gestation, she is having increasing headaches. This could be due to an increase in tumor size, preeclampsia, pregnancy-induced hypertension, anxiety, etc. In other words, the headaches themselves are nonspecific. A good first step in determining whether the headaches are caused by tumor growth is to obtain formal visual fields, which, in this patient, were normal. Then, before instituting a specific treatment (restarting bromocriptine [Answer A], delivering the baby [Answer B], or performing surgery [Answer C]), it would be important to determine whether, in fact, the tumor has substantially increased in size. MRI (Answer D) is considered safe during pregnancy. The MRI scan should be performed without gadolinium contrast given concern of gadolinium exposure on the developing fetus. Because serum prolactin increases during pregnancy, measuring prolactin (Answer E) is not useful for assessment of tumor status during pregnancy.

EDUCATIONAL OBJECTIVE
Manage prolactinoma during pregnancy.

REFERENCE(S)
Molitch ME. Prolactinoma in pregnancy. *Best Pract Res Clin Endocrinol Metab.* 2011;25(6):885-896. PMID: 22115164

DeWilde JP, Rivers AW, Price DL. A review of the current use of magnetic resonance imaging in pregnancy and safety implications for the fetus. *Prog Biophys Mol Biol.* 2005;87(2-3):335-353. PMID: 15556670

2 **ANSWER: B) Lanreotide depot monthly**

Somatostatin analogues are effective in managing acromegaly and are often used as first-line medical therapy. Therefore, lanreotide depot, a somatotatin analogue, given monthly (Answer B) would be the initial treatment choice in this patient. Pegvisomant (Answer D) is effective and, in the most recent Endocrine Society guidelines, was recommended to be considered as first-line medical therapy when administered as daily, not weekly, dosing. Repeated surgery (Answer C) is probably not indicated if the residual tumor is within the cavernous sinus and is hence not surgically accessible. Irradiation (Answer A) could certainly be done if cabergoline, somatostatin analogue, or daily pegvisomant is ineffective.

EDUCATIONAL OBJECTIVE
Manage persistent acromegaly after transsphenoidal surgery.

REFERENCE(S)
Katznelson L, Laws ER Jr, Melmed S, et al. Acromegaly: an endocrine society clinical practice guideline. *J Clin Endocrinol Metab.* 2014;99(11):3933-3951. PMID: 25356808

Giustina A, Chanson P, Kleinberg D, et al; Acromegaly Consensus Group. Expert consensus document: a consensus on the medical treatment of acromegaly. *Nat Rev Endocrinol.* 2014;10(4):243-248. PMID: 24566817

3 **ANSWER: A) Dopamine agonist**

Some points cannot be overemphasized, and this is one. No one can state, legitimately, that a sellar mass is a particular type of lesion. In a teenager, a cystic suprasellar mass, especially one with calcifications, is often a craniopharyngioma, but not always. A serum prolactin level greater than 200 ng/mL (>8.7 nmol/L) is too high to be considered secondary to stalk effect or medication use. The patient's serum prolactin concentration is the clue that the mass is more likely a lactotroph adenoma. In this case, a misdiagnosis led to transcranial surgery, permanent partial loss of vision, and permanent panhypopituitarism. As with all prolactinomas, a dopamine agonist (Answer A) should be the initial treatment. The other modalities listed are reserved for patients who do not respond to dopamine agonist therapy, for cases in which the lesion is largely cystic and there is visual field compromise, or for true craniopharyngiomas.

EDUCATIONAL OBJECTIVE
Distinguish between hyperprolactinemia resulting from hypothalamic/stalk dysfunction and tumor production.

REFERENCE(S)
Freda PU, Post KD. Differential diagnosis of sellar masses. *Endocrinol Metab Clin North Am.* 1999;28(1):81-117. PMID: 10207686

Lucas JW, Zada G. Imaging of the pituitary and parasellar region. *Semin Neurol.* 2012;32(4):320-331. PMID: 23361479

ANSWER: D) Lanreotide depot
4 This patient has hyperthyroidism, a large multinodular goiter, and the unexpected finding of a TSH value that is not suppressed—an indication that a TSH-secreting tumor is the cause of her hyperthyroidism.

Somatostatin inhibits both GH and TSH, and somatostatin analogues can inhibit TSH secretion from the tumor, as well as decrease tumor size. Given her history of coronary artery disease and congestive heart failure, control of the hyperthyroidism is the first step. Thus, lanreotide depot (Answer D) is the correct treatment to administer now. Lanreotide depot is generally successful at normalizing thyroid hormone levels and can reduce the size of the tumor (which is invading the cavernous sinus). Surgery to debulk the pituitary tumor may be considered on an elective basis when she is clinically stable.

Saturated solution of potassium iodide (Answer B) can decrease the thyroid hormone levels for a short time, but it cannot be relied on for sustained treatment of the hyperthyroidism and it will have no effect on the size of the TSH-secreting tumor. Cabergoline (Answer A) has not been shown to be effective for TSH-secreting tumors. The decision of whether she should undergo thyroidectomy (Answer E) for thyroid cancer at age 77 years can be deferred until after her hyperthyroidism, atrial fibrillation, and congestive heart failure are brought under control. Although radioactive iodine (Answer C) will treat her hyperthyroidism, it will take months to work and will not treat her TSH-secreting pituitary tumor.

EDUCATIONAL OBJECTIVE
Treat TSH-secreting tumors on the basis of the physiology and regulation of TSH secretion.

REFERENCE(S)
Teramoto A, Sanno N, Tahara S, Osamura YR. Pathological study of thyrotropin-secreting pituitary adenoma: plurihormonality and medical treatment. *Acta Neuropathol.* 2004;108(2):147-153. PMID: 15185102

Beck-Peccoz P, Persani L, Mannavola D, Campi I. TSH-secreting adenomas. *Best Pract Res Clin Endocrinol Metab.* 2009;23(5):597-606. PMID: 19945025

ANSWER: A) Another transsphenoidal
5 **operation performed by an experienced pituitary surgeon**
In patients truly cured of Cushing disease, ACTH and cortisol levels are very low because they have been suppressed by the previously high cortisol levels. If the postoperative cortisol level is greater than 10 μg/dL (275.9 nmol/L), the chance that the patient has been cured is less than 10% and it is rare to need steroid support postoperatively. Usually, unless the cortisol level falls to less than 5 μg/dL (137.9 nmol/L), the patient has residual disease. Consideration should be given to repeated surgery (Answer A) in a patient such as this.

This patient is not currently truly hypercortisolemic, so medical therapy (Answer C) is not indicated now. Radiosurgery (Answer D) would be indicated only if repeated surgery, and perhaps medical therapy, has failed. Cortisol levels are usually less than 5 μg/dL (<137.9 nmol/L) when patients are cured and hydrocortisone is generally needed for several months, initially for both maintenance therapy and stress management, and then later just for stress (thus, Answer B is incorrect). ACTH stimulation testing (Answer E) is not useful in the immediate postoperative period because the adrenal glands themselves are not suppressed and should respond vigorously to exogenous ACTH, thereby giving a falsely reassuring result.

EDUCATIONAL OBJECTIVE
Assess patients with Cushing disease postoperatively.

REFERENCE(S)

Esposito F, Dusick JR, Cohan P, et al. Clinical review: early morning cortisol levels as a predictor of remission after transsphenoidal surgery for Cushing's disease. *J Clin Endocrinol Metab.* 2006;91(1):7- 13. PMID: 16234305

Hameed N, Yedinak CG, Brzana J, et al. Remission rate after transsphenoidal surgery in patients with pathologically confirmed Cushing's disease, the role of cortisol, ACTH assessment and immediate reoperation: a large single center experience. *Pituitary.* 2013;16(4):452-458. PMID: 23242860

Salmon PM, Loftus PD, Dodd RL, et al. Utility of adrenocorticotropic hormone in assessing the response to transsphenoidal surgery for Cushing's disease. *Endocr Pract.* 2014;20(11):1159-1164. PMID: 24936567

6 ANSWER: D) *AIP* (aryl hydrocarbon receptor interacting protein)

A small number of germline mutations are implicated in somatotroph tumorigenesis. These include mutations in *AIP* (associated with isolated familial pituitary adenomas), *MEN1*, (associated with multiple endocrine neoplasia type 1), and *PRKAR1A* (associated with the Carney complex). Germline inactivating mutations in *AIP* (aryl hydrocarbon receptor interacting protein) predispose individuals to pituitary tumors, especially somatotropinomas. Overall, approximately one-third of families with familial acromegaly harbor a germline *AIP* mutation. Furthermore, as many as 20% of individuals younger than 18 years who have apparently sporadic pituitary macroadenomas harbor a pathogenic germline *AIP* mutation. Tumors associated with *AIP* mutations are large and are often diagnosed in childhood or early adulthood, hence the typical presentation with gigantism. Importantly, these mutations exhibit low penetrance, so the disorder may appear to skip generations or be noted in distant relatives. The patient described in this vignette fits the profile, and of the choices listed, a germline mutation in *AIP* (Answer D) would be the most likely culprit associated with his disease.

Pituitary adenomas occur in a subset of individuals with multiple endocrine neoplasia type 1; however, hyperparathyroidism is the most frequent and usually the earliest presenting manifestation of this syndrome. Even in the unlikely event that this patient is a de novo case, the absence of parathyroid or a second endocrine neoplasia renders this diagnosis even more unlikely. Thus, an *MEN1* mutation (Answer E) is unlikely.

Postzygotic activating mutations in the *GNAS* gene (Answer A) are responsible for the rare syndrome known as McCune-Albright syndrome, which consists of polyostotic fibrous dysplasia, cutaneous pigmentation ("coast of Maine"), precocious puberty, hyperthyroidism, Cushing syndrome, and/or acromegaly due to somatotroph hyperplasia. Somatic activating point mutations in *GNAS*, referred to as the *Gsp* oncogene, however, represent one of the most common molecular alterations identified in sporadic somatotroph adenomas and are present in about 30% of sporadic GH-secreting tumors.

The protein encoded by *PROP1* (Answer C) is a transcription factor important in the differentiation of the GH and prolactin cell line.

Germline mutations in the *TBX19* gene (Answer B), which encodes a transcription factor that is important for terminal differentiation of pituitary pro-opiomelanocortin–expressing cells, do not cause pituitary adenomas, but instead cause a neonatal-onset form of congenital isolated ACTH deficiency.

EDUCATIONAL OBJECTIVE
Identify the genes associated with familial pituitary adenoma syndromes.

REFERENCE(S)

Tichomirowa MA, Barlier A, Daly AF, et al. High prevalence of AIP gene mutations following focused screening in young patients with sporadic pituitary macroadenomas. *Eur J Endocrinol.* 2011;165(4):509- 515. PMID: 21753072

Georgitsi M, De Menis E, Cannavò S, et al. Aryl hydrocarbon receptor interacting protein (AIP) gene mutation analysis in children and adolescents with sporadic pituitary adenomas. *Clin Endocrinol (Oxf)*. 2008;69(4):621-627. PMID: 18410548

Vandeva S, Jaffrain-Rea ML, Daly AF, Tichomirowa M, Zacharieva S, Beckers A. The genetics of pituitary adenomas. *Best Pract Res Clin Endocrinol Metab*. 2010;24(3):461-476. PMID: 20833337

7 ANSWER: C) Another MRI in 6 months

This 81-year-old patient has known coronary artery disease and a 1.2-cm incidental macroadenoma. He may have mild hypopituitarism, as evidenced by his low testosterone level with normal gonadotropin levels, but those measurements could also be compatible with age. His morning cortisol and free T_4 levels are normal. Thus, there is no indication for surgery (Answer B) or irradiation (Answers D and E). Appropriate management would simply be to assess for a change in tumor size in 6 months with another MRI (Answer C). Tumors such as this one grow quite slowly (0.6 mm/year on average), so he is in no imminent danger from tumor growth. At age 81 years, with known coronary artery disease, he is at greater risk of an adverse effect of surgery or irradiation than an adverse effect of tumor growth. If the MRI had shown significant suprasellar extension with abutment of the optic chiasm, then visual field testing (Answer A) should have been performed; otherwise, it should not.

EDUCATIONAL OBJECTIVE
Manage a pituitary incidentaloma.

REFERENCE(S)
Molitch ME. Pituitary tumours: pituitary incidentalomas. *Best Pract Res Clin Endocrinol Metab*. 2009;23(5):667-675. PMID: 19945030

Freda PU, Beckers AM, Katznelson L, et al; Endocrine Society. Pituitary incidentalomas: an Endocrine Society clinical practice guideline. *J Clin Endocrinol Metab*. 2011;96(4):894-904. PMID: 21474686

8 ANSWER: D) Start hydrocortisone

This pregnant woman has pituitary enlargement presenting near term, and it is most likely to be lymphocytic hypophysitis. Her prepregnancy history, indicating that she was well and had no problems conceiving, makes it very unlikely that this mass is a prolactinoma. MRI shows diffuse pituitary enlargement, which is more compatible with hypophysitis than a tumor, and, had gadolinium been given, there would have been diffuse enhancement rather than focal enhancement. (No data show adverse effects of performing MRI scans or giving gadolinium during pregnancy, although it is recommended to withhold gadolinium during pregnancy.) One of the striking features of hypophysitis occurring during pregnancy is the high risk of ACTH deficiency. This patient had a morning serum cortisol level of 9.0 µg/dL (248.3 nmol/L), which does not seem very low. However, it should be remembered that cortisol production increases 3-fold during pregnancy and cortisol-binding globulin levels are also very high, resulting in normal morning cortisol levels well above 20 µg/dL (>551.8 nmol/L). Therefore, her cortisol level of 9.0 µg/dL is fairly low and giving hydrocortisone (Answer D) is the correct answer.

As previously mentioned, she is very unlikely to have a prolactinoma, and instituting bromocriptine (Answer A) or cabergoline (Answer B) is not indicated. Unless her headaches become uncontrollable with pain medication or she develops a visual field defect, there is no indication for surgery (Answer C). Although in hypophysitis, the pituitary size often decreases after delivery, it is a relatively gradual reduction and there is no indication for urgent cesarean delivery (Answer E).

EDUCATIONAL OBJECTIVE
Diagnose and treat lymphocytic hypophysitis in a pregnant woman.

REFERENCE(S)
Rivera JA. Lymphocytic hypophysitis: disease spectrum and approach to diagnosis and therapy. *Pituitary*. 2006;9(1):35-45. PMID: 16703407

Molitch ME. Pituitary disorders during pregnancy. *Endocrinol Metab Clin North Am*. 2006;35(1):99-116. PMID: 16310644

9 ANSWER: B) *PROP1* mutation

Mutations in the genes encoding a number of transcription factors, including *POU1F1* (formerly *PIT1*) and *PROP1*, can cause disruption in the development of many pituitary cell types during embryogenesis, resulting in multiple pituitary hormone deficiencies. Mutations in the *PROP1* gene (Answer B) result in a decrease in PROP 1, a transcription factor important for the development of the somatotroph, lactotroph, and thyrotroph lineages with deficiencies of their respective hormones. Some affected individuals also have delayed puberty. Combined pituitary hormone deficiency (GH, prolactin, TSH) has an incidence of about 1 in 8000 births, and 10% have an affected family member. Between 25% and 50% of these cases are due to *POU1F1* or *PROP1* mutations. In this patient, the history of previous GH and thyroid hormone treatment starting in childhood suggests a congenital combined pituitary hormone deficiency. In some children with PROP 1 deficiency, there is an early pituitary enlargement of uncertain cause, which results in sellar enlargement and subsequent loss of pituitary volume, leading to an empty sella. In most series, when patients with empty sellas have evaluations of pituitary function, between one-quarter and one-third have varying degrees of hypopituitarism.

Acute trauma causing pituitary infarction (Answer A) would show blood in the pituitary with pituitary enlargement rather than a small pituitary. Sarcoidosis (Answer C) and Langerhans cell histiocytosis (Answer D) are infiltrative diseases of the hypothalamus and pituitary stalk and might present with stalk thickening rather than an empty sella. Both usually also present with diabetes insipidus.

Hemochromatosis (Answer E) can cause iron deposition in the pituitary and usually affects the gonadotroph cells; it is not associated with an empty sella.

EDUCATIONAL OBJECTIVE
Perform the differential diagnosis of an empty sella.

REFERENCE(S)
Prince KL, Walvoord EC, Rhodes SJ. The role of homeodomain transcription factors in heritable pituitary disease. *Nat Rev Endocrinol.* 2011;7(12):727-737. PMID: 21788968

Mendonca BB, Osorio MG, Latronico AC, Estefan V, Lo LS, Arnhold IJ. Longitudinal hormonal and pituitary imaging changes in two females with combined pituitary hormone deficiency due to deletion of A301,G302 in the PROP1 gene. *J Clin Endocrinol Metab.* 1999;84(3):942-945. PMID: 10084575

Guitelman M, Garcia Basavilbaso N, Vitale M, et al. Primary empty sella (PES): a review of 175 cases. *Pituitary.* 2013;16(2):270-274. PMID: 22875743

10 ANSWER: D) Give hypertonic saline to raise the serum sodium by 6 mEq/L (6 mmol/L) over 6 hours

Even a standard dose of desmopressin can cause hyponatremia if a person continues to drink; usually progressive nausea limits the intake. Unfortunately, in this case, the patient is unconscious and cannot control her fluid intake. The treatment at this point is tricky. One cannot judge any mental symptoms from the hyponatremia because she is unconscious, but she is at high risk for developing brain edema and is at risk for seizures and brain herniation because of the presumed rapid development of the hyponatremia.

Therefore, hypertonic saline at a rate of 1 mL/kg per h should be given over a few hours to raise her serum sodium about 4 to 6 mEq/L (4-6 mmol/L) to remove her from acute danger (Answer D). Although desmopressin should be held initially, the urine output must be observed very carefully; when it wears off, she will start to excrete high volumes of dilute urine and might experience an overly rapid correction of the hyponatremia. Correcting the hyponatremia at rates higher than about 12 mEq/L (12 mmol/L) over 24 hours could put her at risk for central pontine myelinolysis. However, the degree of hyponatremia is severe and has developed rapidly, so one cannot simply change the D5W to saline and wait for the desmopressin to wear off (Answers A, B, and C). Therefore, her urine output and serum sodium must be monitored every 2 to 4 hours to avoid a correction that is too rapid. Waiting 12 hours is insufficiently close monitoring. Reinstitution of desmopressin when urine output increases may then be indicated, but not when she is first seen.

EDUCATIONAL OBJECTIVE
Treat the acute development of severe hyponatremia.

REFERENCE(S)

Verbalis JG, Goldsmith SR, Greenberg A, et al. Diagnosis, evaluation, and treatment of hyponatremia: expert panel recommendations. *Am J Med*. 2013;126(10 Suppl 1):S1-S42. PMID: 24074529

Sterns RH. Disorders of plasma sodium--causes, consequences, and correction. *N Engl J Med*. 2015;372(1):55-65. PMID: 25551526

11 ANSWER: C) Temozolomide

This patient has a rapidly enlarging macroprolactinoma that is unresponsive to cabergoline, surgery, and stereotactic radiosurgery. The tumor is certainly acting in a malignant fashion. However, distant metastases would have to be demonstrated for this to qualify as a true malignancy. About 75% of these very aggressive tumors and some true pituitary carcinomas respond to temozolomide (Answer C), an alkylating agent used primarily for the treatment of glioblastomas. However, even those who respond for a while to this agent may have, over time, a bad outcome. Additional radiotherapy (Answer A) or surgery (Answer B) is unlikely to help. There are no data published regarding the use of pasireotide (Answer D) to treat prolactinomas.

EDUCATIONAL OBJECTIVE
Recommend a treatment strategy for aggressive pituitary tumors and pituitary carcinomas.

REFERENCE(S)

Di Ieva A, Rotondo F, Syro LV, Cusimano MD, Kovacs K. Aggressive pituitary adenomas--diagnosis and emerging treatments. *Nat Rev Endocrinol*. 2014;10(7):423-435. PMID: 24821329

McCormack AI, Wass JA, Grossman AB. Aggressive pituitary tumours: the role of temozolomide and the assessment of MGMT status. *Eur J Clin Invest*. 2011;41(10):1133-1148. PMID: 21496012

Whitelaw BC, Dworakowska D, Thomas NW, et al. Temozolomide in the management of dopamine agonist-resistant prolactinomas. *Clin Endocrinol (Oxf)*. 2012;76(6):877-886. PMID: 22372583

12 ANSWER: B) Ipilimumab

Ipilimumab (Answer B) is a monoclonal antibody used in the treatment of patients with metastatic melanoma. Hypophysitis has been reported in 10% to 15% of treated patients; pituitary enlargement can occur within 2 months of treatment initiation, and corticotrophs and thyrotrophs are the most common cell types affected. This form of hypophysitis is different from lymphocytic hypophysitis that occurs peripartum in women. Ipilimumab is an immune checkpoint inhibitor that enhances immune response by working through the cytotoxic T-lymphocyte–associated antigen 4 (CTLA-4). Although prednisone (Answer A) can certainly suppress ACTH secretion, it does not cause pituitary enlargement. High-dosage steroids are not effective in treating this hypophysitis.

Temozolomide (Answer C) is an alkylating agent used in the treatment of gliomas and has been useful in the treatment of some patients with pituitary carcinomas and very aggressive macroadenomas. Sunitinib (Answer D) is a tyrosine kinase inhibitor that has been used to treat thyroid cancer, among other cancers, but it has not been implicated as a cause of hypophysitis.

EDUCATIONAL OBJECTIVE
Identify medications that can cause hypophysitis.

REFERENCE(S)

Corsello SM, Barnabei A, Marchetti P, De Vecchis L, Salvatori R, Torino F. Endocrine side effects Induced by immune checkpoint inhibitors. *J Clin Endocrinol Metab*. 2013;98(4):1361-1375. PMID: 23471977

Faje AT, Sullivan R, Lawrence D, et al. Ipilimumab-induced hypophysitis: a detailed longitudinal analysis in a large cohort of patients with metastatic melanoma. *J Clin Endocrinol Metab*. 2014;99(11):4078-4085. PMID: 25078147

Albarel F, Gaudy C, Castinetti F, et al. Long-term follow-up of ipilimumab-induced hypophysitis, a common adverse event of the anti-CTLA-4 antibody in melanoma. *Eur J Endocrinol*. 2015;172(2):195-204. PMID: 25416723

13 ANSWER: B) Glucagon stimulation test with measurement of GH

This middle-aged man with fatigue, weight gain, decreased libido, and erectile dysfunction has evidence of partial hypopituitarism, with decreased function in his hypothalamic-pituitary-thyroid and hypothalamic-pituitary-gonadal axes. His history of a severe headache a few months before the development of hypopituitarism and the MRI showing an empty sella suggest that the headache was due to an infarction of a preexisting, unsuspected pituitary adenoma.

Acceptable tests for diagnosing GH deficiency include a glucagon stimulation test (Answer B), a combined arginine–GH-releasing hormone stimulation test (not arginine alone [Answer A]), or an insulin tolerance test (not provided as an answer choice). An IGF-1 measurement alone (Answer C) is incorrect because the IGF-1 level can be normal even if an acceptable stimulation test documents GH deficiency. If 3 or more axes are deficient, then no stimulation test is needed. This patient has 2 deficient axes, so a stimulation test is necessary to determine whether he is GH deficient (thus, Answer D is incorrect).

EDUCATIONAL OBJECTIVE
Determine the most appropriate test to diagnose GH deficiency.

REFERENCE(S)
Toogood AA, Stewart PM. Hypopituitarism: clinical features, diagnosis, and management. *Endocrinol Metab Clin North Am.* 2008;37(1):235-261. PMID: 18226739

Yuen KC, Tritos NA, Samson SL, Hoffman AR, Katznelson L. American Association of Clinical Endocrinologists and American College of Endocrinology Disease State Clinical Review: update on growth hormone stimulation testing and proposed revised cut-point for the glucagon stimulation test in the diagnosis of adult growth hormone deficiency. *Endocr Pract.* 2016;22(10):1235-1244. PMID: 27409821

Molitch ME, Clemmons DR, Malozowski S, Merriam GR, Vance ML; Endocrine Society. Evaluation and treatment of adult growth hormone deficiency: an Endocrine Society clinical practice guideline. *J Clin Endocrinol Metab.* 2011;96(6):1587-1609. PMID: 21602453

14 ANSWER: D) Metastasis
The key feature in this patient is the rapid growth of the mass. This is most consistent with a metastasis (Answer D); none of the other listed entities (Answers A, B, and C) grow this rapidly (with the possible exception of a prolactinoma during pregnancy). The finding of diabetes insipidus is compatible with either a metastasis or a craniopharyngioma and is very uncommon in patients with pituitary adenomas. The diabetes insipidus occurs because of involvement of the posterior pituitary by the metastasis. The most common cancers causing such metastases are breast cancer in women and lung cancer in men. A sellar metastasis can be the first presentation of a cancer.

EDUCATIONAL OBJECTIVE
Differentiate metastases from other pituitary mass lesions.

REFERENCE(S)
Al-Aridi R, El Sibai K, Fu P, Khan M, Selman WR, Arafah BM. Clinical and biochemical characteristic features of metastatic cancer to the sella turcica: an analytical review. *Pituitary.* 2014;17(6):575-587. PMID: 24337713

15 ANSWER: A) Radiotherapy
Transsphenoidal surgery is the first-line treatment for clinically nonfunctioning pituitary adenomas, but tumor tissue that is left in the sellar area has the potential for subsequent regrowth. Although it is not recommended as routine for every case, radiotherapy may be used to reduce tumor mass or prevent remnant regrowth. There are no randomized controlled trials of radiotherapy vs other treatment options, but several retrospective series have shown that individuals who undergo postoperative radiotherapy for clinically nonfunctioning pituitary adenomas have a 50% lower rate of recurrence than those who are simply observed when there is residual tumor seen on MRI. Adjuvant medical therapy appears to have only modest effects on preventing nonfunctioning pituitary adenoma recurrence or regrowth after transsphenoidal surgery, with the best results from cabergoline (Answer C) and less satisfactory results with bromocriptine and somatostatin analogues (Answer B). Although GnRH antagonists (Answer D) make theoretical sense to try in patients with gonadotroph adenomas, in practice their use has not been shown to be beneficial. Thus, of the choices presented in this case scenario, radiotherapy (Answer A) would likely be the most effective therapeutic strategy to prevent further growth of the remnant nonfunctioning pituitary

adenoma after surgery. However, given that such growth is likely to be slow and given the possibility that a dopamine agonist might prevent regrowth, it is very reasonable to try a dopamine agonist in a patient such as this and hold off on radiotherapy unless there is clear evidence of regrowth.

EDUCATIONAL OBJECTIVE
Guide the long-term management of clinically nonfunctioning pituitary adenomas.

REFERENCE(S)

Molitch ME. Nonfunctioning pituitary tumors and pituitary incidentalomas. *Endocrinol Metab Clin North Am.* 2008;37(1):151-171. PMID: 18226735

Freda PU, Beckers AM, Katznelson L, et al; Endocrine Society. Pituitary incidentaloma: an Endocrine Society clinical practice guideline. *J Clin Endocrinol Metab.* 2011;96(4):894-904. PMID: 21474686

Greenman Y, Tordjman K, Osher E, et al. Postoperative treatment of clinically nonfunctioning pituitary adenomas with dopamine agonists decreases tumour remnant growth. *Clin Endocrinol (Oxf).* 2005;63(1):39-44. PMID: 15963059

16 ANSWER: E) Repeat the MRI in 6 months

This 75-year-old man with known coronary artery disease was found to have a 1.4-cm incidental macroadenoma with no suprasellar extension. He does have mild hypopituitarism, as evidenced by his low gonadotropin and testosterone levels, but his morning cortisol and free T_4 levels are normal. The low testosterone seen with aging is usually accompanied by normal or mildly elevated gonadotropins rather than low gonadotropins. Thus, there is no indication for surgery (Answer B) or irradiation (Answer C), and he should be assessed for change in tumor size in 1 year with a repeated MRI (Answer E). Such tumors grow quite slowly (0.6 mm/y on average), so he is in no imminent danger from tumor growth. It is much more likely that at age 75 and with known coronary artery disease that he would have an adverse effect from surgery or irradiation than from tumor growth. If the MRI showed clinically significant suprasellar extension with abutment of the optic chiasm, then visual field testing (Answer A) should be performed; otherwise, it should not. Although there are reports of tumor shrinkage with dopamine agonists (Answer D), these agents are not consistently found to be useful in reducing the size of nonfunctioning pituitary macroadenomas. Also, there is no indication to try to shrinkage the tumor at this time.

EDUCATIONAL OBJECTIVE
Manage pituitary incidentalomas.

REFERENCE(S)

Freda PU, Beckers AM, Katznelson L, et al; Endocrine Society. Pituitary Incidentaloma: an Endocrine Society clinical practice guideline. *J Clin Endocrinol Metab.* 2011;96(4):894-904. PMID: 21474686

Molitch ME. Nonfunctioning pituitary tumors. *Handb Clin Neurol.* 2014;124:167-184. PMID: 25248587

17 ANSWER: A) Measurement of HAMA (human anti-mouse antibodies)

The typical patient with hyperthyroidism, including Graves disease, has autonomous production of thyroid hormone by the thyroid with resultant suppression of TSH levels. In a hyperthyroid patient, when TSH levels are normal or elevated in the setting of elevated T_4 and T_3 levels, the most common cause is a TSH-producing tumor. Therefore, MRI is often done next. In this case, the MRI was normal. In patients with TSH-secreting tumors, there is commonly an imbalance in the secretion of α-subunit, resulting in a relative increase in α-subunit disproportionate to the TSH level (not β subunit [Answer C]). The free α-subunit test was not an answer choice in this vignette.

An alternative explanation for the elevated TSH level in a patient such as this one is that the TSH measurement is artifactually elevated due to the presence of heterophile antibodies. These antibodies are directed against specific animal immunoglobulins, usually human anti-mouse antibodies (HAMA) (Answer A). In this case, a commercial laboratory detected the presence of HAMA antibodies. When specific HAMA-blocking reagents were added, the TSH concentration was documented to be <0.01 mIU/L. The patient works in an animal lab and was exposed to mice, which may have elicited this response.

A T_3 suppression test (Answer B) is now rarely done in patients with toxic nodular goiters. Petrosal sinus sampling (Answer D) is done primarily to distinguish between pituitary vs ectopic ACTH secretion in patients with Cushing syndrome. However, ectopic TSH secretion outside the cranium has actually never been reported in TSH-dependent hyperthyroidism.

EDUCATIONAL OBJECTIVE
Evaluate patients with hyperthyroidism who have nonsuppressed TSH levels.

REFERENCE(S)

Beck-Peccoz P, Lania A, Beckers A, Chatterjee K, Werneau JL. 2013 European Thyroid Association guidelines for the diagnosis and treatment of thyrotropin-secreting pituitary tumours. *Eur Thyroid J*. 2013;2(2):76-82. PMID: 24783044

Després N, Grant AM. Antibody interference in thyroid assays: a potential for clinical misinformation. *Clin Chem*. 1998;44(3):440-454. PMID: 9510847

18 ANSWER: E) Measure 8-AM cortisol and ACTH levels

Mistakenly, this patient's hypercortisolism was assumed to be due to an adrenal adenoma. About 10% of adrenal incidentalomas are bilateral. Bilateral macronodular hyperplasia can occur in patients with Cushing disease (ie, from excessive pituitary secretion of ACTH). In studies in which abdominal CT scans were performed in all patients with Cushing disease, 5% to 17% of patients have bilateral macronodular hyperplasia and several cases have been reported in which there was marked asymmetry with a large nodule on one side and questionable activity on the other side. In patients with Cushing syndrome, an ACTH level should always be measured (Answer E). This patient's ACTH level was elevated and her Cushing disease was cured by resection of a pituitary adenoma with resultant improvement in her symptoms and hirsutism and a reduction in the adrenal nodule size.

An ACTH stimulation test with measurement of 17-hydroxyprogesterone (Answer A) is sometimes helpful when diagnosing 21-hydroxylase deficiency but not Cushing syndrome.

Adrenal-directed evaluations/treatment (Answers B and D) should be done only if the ACTH level is suppressed. Petrosal sinus sampling for ACTH (Answer C) is done in patients in whom it is difficult to distinguish between a pituitary or an ectopic source of ACTH.

EDUCATIONAL OBJECTIVE
Evaluate patients with Cushing syndrome.

REFERENCE(S)

Nieman LK, Biller BM, Findling JW, et al. The diagnosis of Cushing's syndrome: an Endocrine Society Clinical Practice Guideline. *J Clin Endocrinol Metab*. 2008;93(5):1526-1540. PMID: 18334580

Imaki T, Naruse M, Takano K. Adrenocortical hyperplasia associated with ACTH-dependent Cushing's syndrome: comparison of the size of adrenal glands with clinical and endocrinological data. *Endocr J*. 2004;51(1):89-95. PMID: 15004414

19 ANSWER: C) Add pegvisomant

Although studies do show that increasing the somatostatin analogue dosage or increasing the dose frequency, such as every 21 days (Answer A) may be beneficial, these regimens are not generally adopted. Cabergoline (Answer B) can be useful in the setting of modest acromegaly, and it may show benefit in combination with octreotide. However, this regimen is effective in less than half of patients and is unlikely to be effective in this patient with more active disease. Radiation therapy (Answer D) often takes a number of years to be effective and it is therefore unlikely to be effective within 6 months. The addition of weekly pegvisomant (Answer C) is the most effective regimen in this timeframe. Pasireotide (Answer E) is more effective than either octreotide or lanreotide, but not clearly as effective as the combination of a somatostatin analogue and weekly pegvisomant.

EDUCATIONAL OBJECTIVE
Recommend the best therapeutic approach in a patient with acromegaly who has had a partial response to adjuvant therapy with somatostatin analogue therapy.

REFERENCE(S)

Katznelson L, Laws ER Jr, Melmed S, et al; Endocrine Society. Acromegaly: an endocrine society clinical practice guideline. *J Clin Endocrinol Metab.* 2014;99(11):3933-3951. PMID: 25356808

Giustina A, Chanson P, Kleinberg D, et al; Acromegaly Consensus Group. Expert consensus document: a consensus on the medical treatment of acromegaly. *Nat Rev Endocrinol.* 2014;10(4):243-248. PMID: 24566817

Strasburger CJ, Mattsson A, Wilton P, et al. Increasing frequency of combination medical therapy in the treatment of acromegaly with the GH receptor antagonist pegvisomant. *Eur J Endocrinol.* 2018;178(4):321-329. PMID: 29371335

20   ANSWER: C) Transsphenoidal surgery

All of these treatment modalities can improve Cushing disease, and treatment during pregnancy is advocated because it results in better fetal outcomes. Transsphenoidal surgery (Answer C) has a cure rate of 80% to 90% in expert neurosurgical hands, with very low complication and fetal loss rates when done in the second trimester. Surgery should be strongly considered in this patient.

Ketoconazole (Answer A) now has a black box warning regarding liver function abnormalities; it has never been approved for use during pregnancy and is only modestly successful. Mifepristone (Answer B) was originally developed as a progesterone receptor blocker and is a potent abortifacient (RU486); therefore, its use in pregnancy is absolutely contraindicated. There is experience with only about 50 cases in which somatostatin analogues have been used to treat acromegaly during pregnancy, with relatively minor adverse effects. However, somatostatin analogues cross the placenta and have unknown effects on the fetus. There is no documented experience with pasireotide (Answer D) during pregnancy, and it would be expected to worsen glucose tolerance in this population susceptible to gestational diabetes. Although cabergoline (Answer E) is safe when stopped after conception, there is little experience when used throughout pregnancy, and its ability to normalize cortisol levels in Cushing disease is only modest. Neither pasireotide nor cabergoline is absolutely contraindicated during pregnancy.

EDUCATIONAL OBJECTIVE
Guide treatment of Cushing disease during pregnancy.

REFERENCE(S)

Marions L. Mifepristone dose in the regimen with misoprostol for medical abortion. *Contraception.* 2006;74(1):21-25. PMID: 16781255

Lindsay JR, Jonklaas J, Oldfield EH, Nieman LK. Cushing's syndrome during pregnancy: personal experience and review of the literature. *J Clin Endocrinol Metab.* 2005;90(5):3077-3083. PMID: 15705919

Cohen-Kerem R, Railton C, Oren D, Lishner M, Koren G. Pregnancy outcome following non-obstetric surgical intervention. *Am J Surgery.* 2005;190(3):467-473. PMID: 16105538

21   ANSWER: A) DDAVP, 0.1 mg orally as needed for polyuria and hypernatremia

This patient has acute onset of diabetes insipidus. In this setting, the cause of the diabetes insipidus is central, due to deficiency of vasopressin. The goal of therapy is to control the free water depletion, as well as maintain comfort, from polyuria. DDAVP should be administered in a short-acting regimen with avoidance of prescheduled dosing given the risk of hyponatremia from syndrome of inappropriate antidiuretic hormone secretion in the subsequent days as part of the triphasic response following surgery. Therefore, DDAVP should be administered as needed (0.1 mg orally, and higher doses of 0.2 to 0.3 mg may be necessary) (Answer A) or as subcutaneous aqueous DDAVP, 0.5 to 1.0 mcg (not offered as an option here). Scheduled dosing of 1 spray intranasally twice daily (Answer D) should be avoided. Infusion of normal saline (Answer B) will not address the underlying pathophysiology, and fluid restriction (Answer C) is contraindicated in these patients who are prone to dehydration.

EDUCATIONAL OBJECTIVE
Manage diabetes insipidus following pituitary surgery.

REFERENCE(S)

Woodmansee WW, Carmichael J, Kelly D, Katznelson L; AACE Neuroendocrine and Pituitary Scientific Committee. American

Association of Clinical Endocrinologists and American College of Endocrinology disease state clinical review: postoperative management following pituitary surgery. *Endocr Pract.* 2015;21(7):832-838. PMID: 26172128

Fleseriu M, Hashim IA, Karavitaki N, et al. Hormonal replacement in hypopituitarism in adults: an Endocrine Society clinical practice guideline. *J Clin Endocrinol Metab.* 2016;101(11):3888-3921. PMID: 27736313

22 ANSWER: C) Start tolvaptan

Tolvaptan (Answer C) is an oral vasopressin receptor antagonist that is given intravenously for 1 to 4 days, and it is very effective in the treatment of moderate to severe hyponatremia following pituitary surgery. A vasopressin receptor antagonist may facilitate recovery from syndrome of inappropriate antidiuretic hormone secretion in this setting. If fluid restriction is to be successful, it should be to less than 1000 mL/24 h. A 1500-mL limit (Answer A) is too high. Demeclocycline (Answer B) causes partial nephrogenic diabetes insipidus and may be useful for patients with chronic, symptomatic hyponatremia; it is generally not used when hyponatremia develops acutely. Although furosemide (Answer D) causes an increase in urinary excretion of water in excess of sodium, correction of hyponatremia is minimal with its use.

EDUCATIONAL OBJECTIVE
Manage moderate to severe hyponatremia in the postoperative setting following transsphenoidal surgery.

REFERENCE(S)
Verbalis JG, Goldsmith SR, Greenberg A, et al. Diagnosis, evaluation, and treatment of hyponatremia: expert panel recommendations. *Am J Med.* 2013;126(10 Suppl 1):S1-S42. PMID: 24074529

Jahangiri A, Wagner J, Tran MT, et al. Factors predicting postoperative hyponatremia and efficacy of hyponatremia management strategies after more than 1000 pituitary operations. *J Neurosurg.* 2013;119(6):1478-1483. PMID: 23971964

23 ANSWER: B) GH deficiency

Hypopituitarism occurs following both penetrating and blunt head trauma in approximately 25% of individuals (range 15%-68%). The pathophysiology of hypopituitarism in patients with traumatic brain injury includes direct injury to the gland, vasospasm of the hypothalamo-hypophyseal blood supply, and compression of the hypothalamus and pituitary gland by edema, hemorrhage, or elevated intracranial pressure. Genetic factors, including certain apolipoprotein E haplotypes may influence this risk. Also, there are studies showing that antipituitary and antihypothalamic antibodies are found in patients with traumatic brain injury, although the pathogenic role is unclear. Autopsy series have shown necrotic glands in up to 80% of fatal cases. GH deficiency (Answer B) is the most common deficiency found, and this has critical implications, as GH deficiency may impact full convalescence.

All patients with moderate to severe traumatic brain injury should be evaluated for hypopituitarism during the acute and chronic course of their recovery. Immediately following the traumatic brain injury, emphasis on care during the first 2 weeks after traumatic brain injury should be on the adrenal axis and posterior pituitary function. In the subsequent months after injury, the entire anterior and posterior pituitary hormonal axes should be assessed. In addition, symptomatic patients with mild traumatic brain injury (including those with repetitive mild traumatic brain injury) and impaired quality of life are also at risk for hypopituitarism and neuroendocrine testing should be considered. Testing for chronic hypopituitarism following traumatic brain injury is usually performed at least 6 to 12 months following the event. Hormone replacement should be administered accordingly.

This patient does not have evidence for testosterone deficiency (Answer A), adrenal insufficiency (Answer C), or hypothyroidism (Answer D). There is no clear clinical implication of hypoprolactinemia (Answer E).

EDUCATIONAL OBJECTIVE
Diagnose hypopituitarism after head trauma and review its manifestations.

REFERENCE(S)
Tritos NA, Yuen KC, Kelly DF; AACE Neuroendocrine and Pituitary Scientific Committee. American Association of Clinical

Endocrinologists and American College of Endocrinology Disease State Clinical Review: A Neuroendocrine Approach to Patients with Traumatic Brain Injury. Endocrine practice: official journal of the American College of Endocrinology and the American Association of Clinical Endocrinologists. *Endocr Pract.* 2015;21(7):823-831. PMID: 26172127

Klose M, Feldt-Rasmussen U. Chronic endocrine consequences of traumatic brain injury - what is the evidence? *Nat Rev Endocrinol.* 2018;14(1):57-62. PMID: 28885623

Giuliano S, Talarico S, Bruno L, Nicoletti FB, Ceccotti C, Belfiore A. Growth hormone deficiency and hypopituitarism in adults after complicated mild traumatic brain injury. *Endocrine.* 2017;58(1):115-123. PMID: 27878771

24 ANSWER: C) Refer for transsphenoidal surgery

Most patients with prolactinomas respond very well to cabergoline, and the overall success rate in normalizing prolactin levels with cabergoline is higher than it is for bromocriptine. A few studies have shown that more than 50% of patients whose prolactin levels do not normalize on bromocriptine therapy will do so when switched to cabergoline. For this patient, neither bromocriptine nor cabergoline at routine dosages was able to significantly reduce her prolactin level. Further increasing the cabergoline dosage (Answer A) is unlikely to be more effective. Transsphenoidal surgery (Answer C) can provide a long-term cure in about 60% of patients with microprolactinomas and should be strongly considered in this patient who has not had a clear and successful response to a dopamine agonist. Clomiphene (Answer D) would be an option for a patient interested in fertility, but attempt at prolactin control in this patient is the priority. Radiation therapy (Answer B) is indicated for management of prolactinomas that are growing despite dopamine agonist therapy, are treatment resistant, and cannot be managed surgically. The risk of hypopituitarism following radiation therapy is substantial, making fertility management more complex. Therefore, radiation therapy is not recommended.

EDUCATIONAL OBJECTIVE
Manage a patient with a prolactinoma unresponsive to dopamine agonist therapy.

REFERENCE(S)
Gillam MP, Molitch ME, Lombardi G, Colao A. Advances in the treatment of prolactinomas. *Endocr Rev.* 2006;27(5):485-534. PMID: 16705142

Melmed S, Casanueva FF, Hoffman AR, et al; Endocrine Society. Diagnosis and treatment of hyperprolactinemia: an Endocrine Society clinical practice guideline. *J Clin Endocrinol Metab.* 2011;96(2):273-288. PMID: 21296991

25 ANSWER: A) Perform pituitary MRI

In pregnancy, estrogen stimulation may increase the size of pituitary tumors. Therefore, a noncontrast MRI (Answer A) should be performed in this patient given her headaches. Because she has worsening of what may be signs and symptoms of acromegaly, consideration of medical therapy may be important. In this setting, the general guideline is to administer short-acting octreotide (Answer B) with the goal of controlling symptoms, although it would be important to document whether there has been change in tumor size first. GH and IGF-1 measurements (Answer D) are not useful as biochemical assessments in a pregnant patient given the overlap with normal, so it is not necessary to measure these hormones. There are limited data with pegvisomant (Answer C), and it is not generally recommended for management in pregnancy.

EDUCATIONAL OBJECTIVE
Manage acromegaly in pregnant women.

REFERENCE(S)
Katznelson L, Laws ER Jr, Melmed S, et al; Endocrine Society. Acromegaly: an Endocrine Society clinical practice guideline. *J Clin Endocrinol Metab.* 2014;99(11):3933-3951. PMID: 25356808

Jallad RS, Shimon I, Fraenkel M, Medvedovsky V, Akirov A, Duarte FH, Bronstein MD. Outcome of pregnancies in a large cohort of women with acromegaly. *Clin Endocrinol (Oxf).* 2018;88(6):896-907. PMID: 29574986

Diabetes Mellitus, Section 2 Board Review

Michelle F. Magee, MD • Georgetown University

31 ANSWER: A) Sitagliptin

Research experience with incretin therapy in the hospital has shown improved glycemic control with a low risk of hypoglycemia, counteracting the hyperglycemic effects of stress hormones and improving cardiac function in patients with heart failure and acute ischemia. A few randomized controlled trials in general medicine and surgical patients have shown that a DPP-4 inhibitor alone or in combination with basal insulin is well tolerated and results in similar glycemic control and rates of hypoglycemia. The US FDA suggests not using saxagliptin and alogliptin in patients with congestive heart failure, so sitagliptin (Answer A) would be preferred in this patient.

A review of pharmacotherapy for hyperglycemia in noncritically ill, hospitalized patients reported that GLP-1 receptor agonists show promise in the hospital setting. They should, however, be avoided in patients in whom gastrointestinal disturbances are an issue.

Metformin use (Answer B) in this patient is contraindicated because he has advanced heart failure. Pioglitazone (Answer C) may lead to fluid retention and exacerbation of congestive heart failure. Also, because the time to onset of action is in the range of 2 to 3 weeks, it would not lead to short-term improvement in glycemic control in this hospital setting. Use of SGLT-2 inhibitors (Answer D) is associated with risk for ketoacidosis, urosepsis, urinary tract infections, and renal injury. Thus, their use cannot be recommended in the hospital setting until safety and effectiveness are established.

EDUCATIONAL OBJECTIVE
Recommend appropriate noninsulin agents for patients with diabetes mellitus in the inpatient setting.

REFERENCE(S)

Lansang MC, Umpierrez GE. Inpatient hyperglycemia management: a practical review for primary medical and surgical teams. *Cleve Clin J Med.* 2016;83(Suppl 1):S34-S43. PMID: 27176681

Pasquel FJ, Gianchandani R, Rubin DJ, et al. Efficacy of sitagliptin for the hospital management of general medicine and surgery patients with type 2 diabetes (Sita-Hospital): a multicentre, prospective, open-label, non-inferiority randomised trial. *Lancet Diabetes Endocrinol.* 2017;5(2):125-133. PMID: 27964837

U.S. Food and Drug Administration. FDA Drug Safety Communication: FDA adds warnings about heart failure risk to labels of type 2 diabetes medicines containing saxagliptin and alogliptin. April 5, 2016. Available at: http://www.fda.gov/Drugs/DrugSafety/ucm486096.htm. Accessed for verification May 11, 2018.

Mendez CE, Umpierrez GE. Pharmacotherapy for hyperglycemia in noncritically ill hospitalized patients. *Diabetes Spectr.* 2014;27(3):180-188. PMID: 26246777

32 ANSWER: C) Acarbose

Late postbariatric hypoglycemia is seen most commonly in patients who have undergone Roux-en-Y gastric bypass. Spikes in glucose due to rapid gastric emptying, vigorous insulin secretion, reduced insulin clearance and insulin-independent glucose uptake, and high levels of GLP-1 all contribute to the phenomenon. If medical nutrition therapy with a low–glycemic index meal plan does not enable control of the hypoglycemia, other medications can be added to the regimen. α-Glucosidase inhibitors (Answer C) slow postprandial glucose absorption and reduce postmeal blood glucose spikes and insulin secretion. Slow introduction and escalation in dosage can help to avoid the adverse effects of gastrointestinal discomfort.

Octreotide (Answer A), which reduces incretin and insulin secretion, can also be administered; however, its use may be limited by high cost and adverse effects, including diarrhea, steatorrhea, and acute hypoglycemia, most likely due to inhibition of insulin secretion. Diazoxide (Answer B) reduces insulin secretion, so it may also be used, but it can lead to fluid retention and headaches. Reports on the efficacy of GLP-1 receptor agonists (Answer D) in this setting have been variable.

Note: Image in stem reproduced with permission from: Patti M. Hypoglycemia after bariatric surgery. Meet the Professor Endocrine Case Management. Washington, DC: Endocrine Society. 2018: 13.

EDUCATIONAL OBJECTIVE
Explain the rationale and strategies for management of late postbariatric hypoglycemia.

REFERENCE(S)

Goldfine AB, Patti ME. How common is hypoglycemia after gastric bypass? *Obesity.* 2016;24(6):1210-1211. PMID: 27225595

Suhl E, Anderson-Haynes SE, Mulla C, Patti ME. Medical nutrition therapy for post-bariatric hypoglycemia: practical insights. *Surg Obes Relat Dis.* 2017;13(5):888-896. PMID: 28392017

Patti ME. Hypoglycemia after bariatric surgery. Meet the Professor Endocrine Case Management. Presented at ENDO in Chicago, Illinois. March, 2018.

33 ANSWER: C) Reduce his daily insulin glargine dose

The blood glucose results show that the patient is overinsulinized. Despite reasonable glucose levels before the evening meal and at bedtime on the evening that nothing-by-mouth status is implemented, his overnight and fasting blood glucose levels are low. He has also been having numerous low blood glucose readings at home, which also suggests that his basal insulin dose is too high. His glargine dose should be reduced (Answer C) to prevent severe hypoglycemia overnight and between meals. Reducing the dose will decrease the likelihood of further severe hypoglycemia episodes.

This patient most likely has absolute insulin deficiency due to pancreatic insufficiency. This is evidenced by his labile glycemic control, which

may be due to a combination of lack of insulin secretory reserve and suboptimal glucagon secretion as a result of his chronic pancreatitis. Therefore, insulin should not be completely withheld (Answer A) or he would be at risk for diabetic ketoacidosis. An insulin drip on general medicine and surgery units for a single blood glucose value over 200 mg/dL (Answer D) would not generally be indicated. Finally, compared with the usual insulin dose, on average an approximately 25% reduction in basal insulin dose the evening before a procedure is more likely to achieve blood glucose levels in the target range with decreased risk for hypoglycemia, so a 75% reduction in the glargine dose (Answer B) is greater than would be recommended.

EDUCATIONAL OBJECTIVE
Determine when basal insulin dosing is inappropriately high.

REFERENCE(S)

Demma LJ, Carlson KT, Duggan EW, Morrow JG 3rd, Umpierrez G. Effect of basal insulin dosage on blood glucose concentration in ambulatory surgery patients with type 2 diabetes. *J Clin Anesth.* 2017;36:184-188. PMID: 28183563

34 ANSWER: C) Diabetes-related mononeuritis affecting the third cranial nerve

In oculomotor (third) nerve palsy, the involved eye is deviated "down and out" (ie, infraducted and abducted). Diabetic mononeuropathy (Answer C) is one of the less common forms of neuropathy. Patients with diabetes can develop diplopia from isolated oculomotor (third), trochlear (fourth), or abducens (sixth) nerve palsies. Ophthalmoplegia, despite being a rare entity in diabetes mellitus, is associated with anxiety for the patient and is a diagnosis that is made after other pathologies have been excluded. In a 10-year series of more than 6000 patients hospitalized with diabetes, 0.4% were diagnosed with ophthalmoplegia, among whom isolated third nerve palsies accounted for most (59.3%), with sixth nerve palsies and multiple palsies accounting for the remainder. The mean age in this series was 65 ± 10 years, mean duration of diabetes was 16 ± 10 years, and most patients had type 2 diabetes. Most had poorly controlled diabetes with a mean hemoglobin A_{1c} level of 8.8% ± 2.5%.

Those with sixth nerve palsies had higher rates of coexistence of diabetic retinopathy and cardiovascular disease risk factors.

Among all cases of ocular misalignment from cranial nerve palsies, third nerve palsies are important because a subset is caused by life-threatening aneurysms. In a recent series of 145 patients from the Rochester Epidemiology Project, the most common causes of acquired third nerve palsy were presumed microvascular (42%), trauma (12%), compression from neoplasm (11%), postneurosurgery (10%), and compression from aneurysm (6%).

No specific treatment of nerve palsy–induced diplopia in patients with diabetes has been established. Management is expectant and the patient should be reassured.

Unilateral endocrine ophthalmopathy (Answer A) with entrapment of ocular muscles can cause diplopia, but one would not expect its onset to be sudden, and other features such as proptosis, chemosis, and conjunctival injection are common accompaniments. In addition, a characteristic appearance of the extraocular muscles on CT (enlargement of the extraocular muscle bellies with sparing of their tendinous insertions [frequently: inferior rectus > medial rectus > superior rectus]) associated with endocrine ophthalmopathy was not seen in this patient. It is not usual for pituitary adenomas (Answer B) to cause isolated third nerve impingement. As these neoplasms grow, they are more likely to cause visual field defects due to pressure on the optic nerve, rather than impinging on the oculomotor nerves. This patient does not have loss of vision due to optic nerve compression, just isolated third cranial nerve oculomotor deficits. He also does not have a reversible ischemic neurologic deficit (Answer D) as an etiology for his oculomotor palsy by definition because the deficit is still persistent after several days.

EDUCATIONAL OBJECTIVE
Diagnose third cranial nerve palsy.

REFERENCE(S)
Fang C, Leavitt JA, Hodge DO, et al. Incidence and etiologies of acquired third nerve palsy using a population-based method. *JAMA Ophthalmol.* 2017;135(1):23-28. PMID: 2789302

Greco D, Gambina F, Maggio F. Ophthalmoplegia in diabetes mellitus: a retrospective study. *Acta Diabetol.* 2009;46(1):23-26. PMID: 18758685

35 ANSWER: D) Insulin detemir, 30 units twice daily plus 18 units regular insulin every 6 hours

Very few studies directly address insulin management with enteral nutrition. In the one randomized controlled trial that has, SSRI was compared with SSRI plus insulin glargine and by the end of the study, 48% of the participants required addition of basal insulin to the regimen (thus, Answer D is correct and Answer C is incorrect). The basal insulin dose apportioned in Answer D (total of 60 units daily) is about 40% of her current total daily insulin requirement and represents a conservative estimate of her daily basal requirement. This approach will help to prevent hypoglycemia should her tube feedings be interrupted. Additionally, regular insulin every 4 hours is likely to lead to stacking and hypoglycemia.

Rapid-acting insulin every 6 hours (Answer A) would most likely not meet all insulin requirements, as this patient has a high total daily insulin requirement and needs basal insulin to enable glycemic control. Allocating all of the insulin to basal insulin plus correction doses as needed (Answer B) would place her at high risk for hypoglycemia should the tube feedings be interrupted.

An approach that matches insulin administered to the type and dose of enteral nutrition should be used to meet the patient's basal and nutrition needs.

The Endocrine Society Clinical Guidelines outline an approach to regimens that can be used.

Method of Enteral Nutrition Administration	Potential Approach to Insulin Therapy
Continuous enteral nutrition	• Basal insulin once daily (glargine or detemir) or twice daily (detemir or NPH) • Short- or rapid-acting insulin every 4 hours (rapid) or every 6 hours (regular)
Cycled feeding	• Basal insulin (glargine, detemir, or NPH) with short- or rapid-acting insulin at the start of enteral nutrition
Bolus feeding	• Short- or rapid-acting insulin before each bolus

In this case, both the nutritional and basal insulin needs were being met with intravenous insulin.

Answer D allocates 40% of her daily requirement to basal insulin and approximately 50% to nutritional insulin. The 40% allocation is conservative to help ensure that hypoglycemia will not occur if the enteral nutrition is interrupted. The insulin drip was stopped 30 minutes after the first doses of glargine and regular insulin had been administered to prevent rebound hyperglycemia. The 80% to 90% apportioning of her total daily dose into basal plus bolus insulin also anticipates a falling insulin requirement as she continues to recover as a hypoglycemia prevention strategy.

On this regimen, her follow-up blood glucose values were as follows:

- 177 mg/dL (9.8 mmol/L) 10:53 PM
- 156 mg/dL (8.7 mmol/L) 06:18 PM
- 250 mg/dL (13.9 mmol/L) 11:42 AM

As she slowly recovered, her daily insulin requirement declined and she was discharged to a rehabilitation facility on a regimen of insulin glargine, 10 units in the morning, and insulin lispro, 8 units before meals.

EDUCATIONAL OBJECTIVE
Create a physiologic basal-bolus subcutaneous insulin regimen for a patient being treated with continuous enteral feedings.

REFERENCE(S)
Korytkowski MT, Salata RJ, Koerbel GL, et al. Insulin therapy and glycemic control in hospitalized patients with diabetes during enteral nutrition therapy: a randomized controlled clinical trial. *Diabetes Care*. 2009;32(4):594-596. PMID: 19336639

Umpierrez GE, Hellman R, Korytkowski MT, et al. Richard HellmanManagement of hyperglycemia in hospitalized patients in non-critical care setting: an Endocrine Society Clinical Practice Guideline. *J Clin Endocrinol Metab*. 2012;97(1);16-38. PMID: 22223765

36 ANSWER: A) Exenatide twice daily
The short-acting GLP-1 receptor agonists exenatide twice daily (Answer A) and lixisenatide more effectively reduce postprandial hyperglycemia than the long-acting GLP-1 receptor analogues. However, their use may be associated with more nausea. The long-acting GLP-1 receptor analogues—albiglutide, dulaglutide (Answer D), exenatide LAR (Answer B), and liraglutide (Answer C)—have less impact on postprandial glucose.

EDUCATIONAL OBJECTIVE
Identify which GLP-1 receptor agonist has the most impact on postprandial hyperglycemia.

REFERENCE(S)
Buse JB, Rosenstock J, Sesti G, et al. Liraglutide once a day versus exenatide twice a day for type 2 diabetes: a 26-week randomised, parallel-group, multinational, open-label trial (LEAD-6). *Lancet*. 2009;374(9683):39-47. PMID: 19515413

Meier JJ. GLP-1 receptor agonists for individualized treatment of type 2 diabetes mellitus. *Nat Rev Endocrinol*. 2012;8(12):728-742. PMID: 22945360

37 ANSWER: D) Insulin degludec; give it at his convenience once daily
The duration of action of insulin degludec (Answer D) is longer than 42 hours; the half-life is approximately 25 hours and it reaches steady state in 2 to 3 days. It may be given safely and effectively with a minimum of 8 hours and maximum of 40 hours between doses. This makes it well suited to being used during travel, as long as the patient takes it once daily.

NPH insulin at bedtime, given at the same time when traveling (Answer A), is an impractical regimen as it difficult to give it at the same time when crossing multiple time zones. Insulin detemir may be given once daily at bedtime, but reducing the dose by 50% when traveling (Answer B) will lead to hyperglycemia. The half-life of U300 insulin glargine (Answer C) is about 23 hours. It reaches a steady state in 4 days, and the duration of action is less than or equal to 36 hours. Data regarding U300 insulin support its safety and efficacy up to a ± 3-hour window for administration, so this also may not be ideal for dosing when traveling.

EDUCATIONAL OBJECTIVE
Optimize basal insulin therapy for travel across time zones.

REFERENCE(S)

Ritzel R, Rouseel R, Bolli GB, et al. Patient-level meta-analysis of the EDITION 1, 2 and 3 studies: glycaemic control and hypoglycaemia with new insulin glargine 300 U/ml versus glargine 100 U/mL in people with type 2 diabetes. *Diabetes Obes Metab.* 2015;17(9):859-867. PMID: 25929311

Matheiu C, Hollander P, Miranda-Palma B, et al. Efficacy and safety of insulin degludec in a flexible dosing regimen vs insulin glargine in patients with type 1 diabetes (BEGIN: Flex T1): a 26-week randomized, treat-to-target trial with a 26-week extension. *J Clin Endocrinol Metab.* 2013;98(3):1154-1162. PMID: 23393185

38 ANSWER: E) Continue the intravenous insulin drip, keep her on nothing-mouth-status, and re-check a basic metabolic panel in 4 hours

At this time, the patient's anion gap is not in fact closed. Her albumin is low, most likely due to her ongoing hyperemesis, so transition from the intravenous insulin drip to subcutaneous insulin (Answers A, B, and C) is not appropriate. Anion gap is underestimated in the setting of hypoalbuminemia; if albumin decreased by 1 g/L, then the anion gap decreases by 0.25 mmol. To overcome the effects of the hypoalbuminemia on the anion gap, the corrected anion gap can be used: anion gap + 0.25 × (40-albumin) expressed in g/L.

When corrected for hypoalbuminemia, this patient's anion gap at the time of the proposed transition was 14.5. If her anion gap had been closed and she met criteria for resolution of diabetic ketoacidosis (a serum glucose level <200 mg/dL [<11.1 mmol/L] and 2 of the following: serum bicarbonate >15 mEq/L [>15 mmol/L]; pH >7.3; anion gap <12 for 8 to 12 hours), transitioning to insulin detemir (Answer B) would be the only appropriate option. At this time, regular insulin (U100 and U500), insulin aspart, insulin lispro (U100 and U200), NPH, and insulin detemir all are pregnancy category B. Insulin glargine (Answer A) no longer has a pregnancy category, and its package insert states there are "no well-controlled clinical studies in pregnant women." Insulin degludec (Answer C) should only be used during pregnancy if "potential benefits justify the potential risk to the fetus." The patient continues to be nauseated, and she has ongoing abdominal pain, so it is not yet appropriate for her to eat (Answer D).

Ultimately, the patient's corrected anion gap closed, and her regimen was transitioned from intravenous insulin to subcutaneous insulin using detemir and aspart. The patient's pregnancy-related blood glucose goals for pregestational diabetes were met (fasting <90 mg/dL; 1-hour postprandial <130-140 mg/dL; 2-hour postprandial <120 mg/dL).

EDUCATIONAL OBJECTIVE
Recommend an in-hospital insulin regimen for a pregnant patient with diabetic ketoacidosis.

REFERENCE(S)

Gosmanov AR, Gosmanova EO, Dillard-Cannon E. Management of adult diabetic ketoacidosis. *Diabetes Metab Syndr Obes.* 2014;7:255-264. PMID: 25061324

American Diabetes Association. 13. Management of diabetes in pregnancy: *Standards of Medical Care in Diabetes-2018.* Diabetes Care. 2018;41(Suppl 1):S137-S143. PMID: 29222384

Blum AK. Insulin use in pregnancy: an update. *Diabetes Spectr.* 2016;29(2):92-97. PMID: 27182178

39 ANSWER: A) Replace the sliding scale with a fixed and reduced dose of insulin with each meal

This case highlights the issue of simplification strategies for older patients with diabetes. This patient is still overinsulinized. It is not clear what insulin doses he is taking with each meal. When there may be errors in the insulin scale being used, the strategies that can be undertaken, especially in older adults such as this patient, include avoid insulin sliding scales and replacing them with fixed-dose insulin (Answer A) before meals.

Simplification strategies should be applied when barriers to diabetes self-care are present in older adults and will be matched to the barrier identified during the needs assessment process. Some examples of solutions that may be considered under these circumstances include:

- Discontinuing meal-time injections and substituting a noninsulin agent that acts to address postprandial blood glucose excursions (eg, a meglitinide) for a patient who forgets to take meal-time insulin injections
- Changing the time of day basal insulin is administered to a time the patient thinks will be easier to remember (eg, with breakfast or the evening meal instead of bedtime if the patient has been missing injections due to falling asleep right after dinner)
- Stopping meal insulin scales and starting a fixed insulin meal dose (strategy used in this case) if the patient is having trouble with numbers (health numeracy)
- Engaging family members or caregivers to give injections and minimizing number of insulin injections daily by substituting noninsulin alternative antihyperglycemic agents for those patients who cannot self-administer insulin
- Maximizing use of once-daily and/or once-weekly antihyperglycemic agents when medication doses are being missed; for older patients with multiple medications, use of a pill box or multidose pill pack pharmacy program may also be helpful if medication adherence is an issue

The patient's C-peptide level is low, so replacing his meal-time insulin with an oral agent (Answer B) to simplify his regimen is not an option, as he will need meal-time insulin onboard to control postmeal glucose levels. This is, however, often a useful strategy in older adults with adequate β-cell reserve who forget to take their meal-time insulin doses, particularly when they are on low doses (ie, <10 units of insulin per dose). His total daily dose of insulin is 47 units, so a concentrated insulin such as U500 is not indicated (Answer C). Finally, active engagement of caregivers (Answer D) is required when cognitive function testing reveals that deficits are present, which was not the case in this man after his hypoglycemia was corrected.

The patient was advised to reduce his meal insulin dose to 9 units. His continuous glucose monitoring after this regimen change is shown (*see image*).

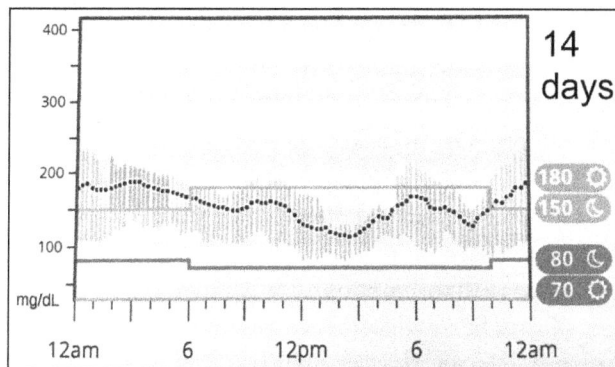

He found the continuous glucose monitoring so useful in helping to avoid hypoglycemic episodes that he obtained a personal continuous glucose monitor. At a future follow-up visit, he and his wife both observed that he was feeling a lot better, he was less tired, and his mind was sharper. Concerning the status of his diabetes, you deemed it appropriate for him to return to work.

EDUCATIONAL OBJECTIVE
Guide the strategy for simplification of the insulin regimen in older patients with hypoglycemia.

REFERENCE(S)
Munshi M. Cognitive dysfunction in older adults with diabetes: what a clinician needs to know. *Diabetes Care.* 2017;40(4):461-467. PMID: 28325796

Munshi, M, Slyne C, Segal AR, Saul N, Lyons C, Weinger K. Simplification of insulin regimen in older adults and risk of hypoglycemia. *JAMA Intern Med.* 2016;176(7):1023-1025. PMID: 27273335

Kirkman MS, Briscoe VJ, Clark N, et al. Diabetes in older adults. *Diabetes Care.* 2012;35(12):2650-2664. PMID: 23100048

Munshi MN, Segal AR, Suhl E, et al. Frequent hypoglycemia among elderly patients with poor glycemic control. *Arch Intern Med.* 2011;171(4):362-364. PMID: 21357814

Hay LC, Wilmshurst EG, Fulcher G. Unrecognized hypo- and hyperglycemia in well-controlled patients with type 2 diabetes mellitus: the results of continuous glucose monitoring. *Diabetes Technol Ther.* 2003;5(1):19-26. PMID: 12725703

40 **ANSWER: C) Hereditary spherocytosis**
Because of hemoglobin A_{1c}'s integral role in the diagnosis and treatment of diabetes, it is important to recognize clinical scenarios and interfering factors that yield false results. Hereditary spherocytosis (Answer C) has been documented as a cause of discrepancy between hemoglobin A_{1c} and glycemic control in patients with diabetes. This patient has a falsely low hemoglobin A_{1c} at this point in time, despite normal hemoglobin and hematocrit. It has varied over the years without apparent explanation based on fasting blood glucose levels. Given the relatively high frequency of mild hereditary spherocytosis, early testing should be considered in patients with an apparent discrepancy between hemoglobin A_{1c} and glucose meter readings, even in the absence of anemia. Alternative glycemic markers are necessary to monitor glucose control in affected patients.

This patient was referred to a hematologist and hereditary spherocytosis was diagnosed. Continuous glucose monitoring was recommended for ongoing management in view of her labile blood glucose values and the marked discrepancy between her hemoglobin A_{1c} and fructosamine levels.

Notable racial and ethnic differences (Answer B) can exist in hemoglobin A_{1c} readings for a given average glucose value. For example, persons of European ancestry have been reported to have hemoglobin A_{1c} levels approximately 0.1% to 0.4% lower for the same average glucose levels when compared with individuals of Hispanic, black, or Asian ancestry. The reasons for these differences are unclear. This patient's discrepant hemoglobin A_{1c} is marked and could not be explained on this basis.

Uremia (Answer A) and marked hypertriglyceridemia (usually with levels higher than 1750 mg/dL [>19.78 mmol/L]) may also falsely elevate hemoglobin A_{1c}; however, she is not uremic and her triglycerides are only mildly elevated (most likely due to her uncontrolled diabetes).

EDUCATIONAL OBJECTIVE
Identify hereditary spherocytosis as a cause of inaccurate hemoglobin A_{1c} results.

REFERENCE(S)
Radin MS. Pitfalls in hemoglobin A1c measurement: when results may be misleading. *J Gen Intern Med.* 2014;29(2):388-394. PMID: 24002631

41 **ANSWER: A) History of previous ulceration**
The lifetime risk of developing a foot ulcer in persons with diabetes mellitus is about 25%. Multiple factors are associated with an increased risk of ulceration, including previous ulceration or amputation, the presence of peripheral neuropathy with loss of protective sensation, foot deformity, and poorly controlled diabetes. All of the listed options are risk factors for the development of future ulcers, but the strongest predictive factor is a history of previous ulceration (Answer A), with an odds ratio of 56.8 and up to a 10-fold increased risk for amputation. Other factors are absent ankle reflexes (not knee reflexes [Answer C]) associated with neuropathy (odds ratio 6.48), abnormal monofilament testing (Answer D) (odds ratio 18.42), and male gender (odds ratio 2.15). Peripheral vascular disease (Answer B) is an important prognostic factor for delayed wound healing and amputations but not a strong independent predictor of foot ulceration.

EDUCATIONAL OBJECTIVE
Identify predictors of increased risk of foot ulcers.

REFERENCE(S)
Moura Neto A, Zantut-Wittmann DE, Fernandes TD, Nery M, Parisi MC. Risk factors for ulceration and amputation in diabetic foot: study in a cohort of 496 patients. *Endocrine.* 2013;44(1):119-124. PMID: 23124278

Boulton AJ, Armstrong DG, Albert SF, et al; American Diabetes Association; American Association of Clinical Endocrinologists. Comprehensive foot examination and risk assessment: a report of the task force of the foot care interest group of the American Diabetes Association, with endorsement by the American Association of Clinical Endocrinologists. *Diabetes Care.* 2008;31(8):1679-1685. PMID: 18663232

McNeely MJ, Boyko EJ, Ahroni JH, et al. The independent contributions of diabetic neuropathy and vasculopathy in foot ulceration. How great are the risks? *Diabetes Care.* 1995;18(2):216-219. PMID: 7729300

42 ANSWER: B) Insulin

Cystic fibrosis–related diabetes (CFRD) affects 40% to 50% of adults with CF. Its pathophysiology combines features of impaired insulin secretion and insulin resistance. According to the Cystic Fibrosis Foundation and American Diabetes Association guidelines, insulin (Answer B) is the recommended therapy for CFRD because of its ability to impact postprandial hyperglycemia and pulmonary function and because of its anabolic effects.

Data from several randomized controlled studies suggest that oral agents (such as glyburide [Answer C], metformin, and thiazolidinediones [Answer A]) are not as effective as insulin in improving nutritional status or blood glucose control in patients with CFRD.

Patients with CFRD generally have more rapid gastric emptying and lower levels of gastric inhibitory polypeptide and GLP-1 than patients with CF who do not have CFRD and control groups. Active GLP-1 is significantly decreased in patients with CF and CFRD compared with levels in healthy control patients ($P < .01$). Whether there is a role for incretin agents (Answer D) in CFRD treatment remains to be established.

EDUCATIONAL OBJECTIVE
Manage hyperglycemia in patients with cystic fibrosis–related diabetes.

REFERENCE(S)

Moran A, Pekow P, Grover P, et al; Cystic Fibrosis Related Diabetes Therapy Study Group. Insulin therapy to improve BMI in cystic fibrosis-related diabetes without fasting hyperglycemia: results of the cystic fibrosis related diabetes therapy trial. *Diabetes Care.* 2009;32(10):1783-1788. PMID: 19592632

Onady GM, Stolfi A. Insulin and oral agents for managing cystic fibrosis-related diabetes. *Cochrane Database Syst Rev.* 2016;4:CD004730. PMID: 27087121

Moran A, Brunzell C, Cohen RC, et al; CFRD Guidelines Committee. Clinical care guidelines for cystic fibrosis-related diabetes: a position statement of the American Diabetes Association and a clinical practice guideline of the Cystic Fibrosis Foundation, endorsed by the Pediatric Endocrine Society. *Diabetes Care.* 2010;33(12):2697-2708. PMID: 21115772

Ballmann M, Hubert D, Assael BM, et al; CFRD Study Group. Repaglinide versus insulin for newly diagnosed diabetes in patients with cystic fibrosis: a multicentre, open-label, randomised trial. *Lancet Diabetes Endocrinol.* 2018;6(2):114-121. PMID: 29199116

Kessler L. Treatment of cystic fibrosis related diabetes. *Lancet Diabetes Endocrinol.* 2018;6(3):167. PMID: 29475494

Kayani K, Mohammed R, Mohiaddin H. Cystic fibrosis-related diabetes. *Front Endocrinol (Lausanne).* 2018;9:20. PMID: 29515516

43 ANSWER: C) Progressively initiate more vigorous regular exercise

This relatively healthy woman with type 2 diabetes, who has no symptoms to suggest coronary heart disease, should be able to initiate regular exercise with slow progression as tolerated (Answer C). Although type 2 diabetes is associated with a 2-fold increased risk of coronary heart disease, national guidelines from the American Diabetes Association currently do not recommend the routine screening of asymptomatic patients with high cardiovascular disease risk because cardiac outcomes are not improved as long as cardiac risk factors are being treated. Randomized controlled trials have also found no clinical benefit of screening asymptomatic patients with type 2 diabetes and normal results from electrocardiography.

The modalities described in Answer A (exercise stress test) and Answer B (stress echocardiography) have some value in determining risk for cardiac events; however, screening asymptomatic patients with diabetes is not currently recommended. Exercise stress tests have comparable sensitivity and specificity in patients with and without diabetes (approximately 50% and 80%, respectively), and stress echocardiograms are even more accurate in predicting events. Cardiac rehabilitation (Answer D) is generally recommended for patients with recent interventions or other comorbidities.

Provide patients with diabetes mellitus exercise recommendations in the setting of managing cardiovascular disease risk.

REFERENCE(S)

American Diabetes Association. 9. Cardiovascular disease and risk management: standards of medical care in diabetes-2018. *Diabetes Care.* 2018;41(Suppl 1):S86-S104. PMID: 29222380

Patel NB, Balady GJ. Diagnostic and prognostic testing to evaluate coronary artery disease in patients with diabetes mellitus. *Rev Endocr Metab Disord.* 2010;11(1):11-20. PMID: 20225090

44 ANSWER: C) Screen for type 2 diabetes now with 75-g oral glucose tolerance testing; screen for gestational diabetes with 75-g oral glucose tolerance testing at 24 to 28 weeks' gestation

The correct answer is to screen for type 2 diabetes now with 75-g oral glucose tolerance testing. If this result is normal, she should be screened for gestational diabetes with 75-g oral glucose tolerance testing at 24 to 28 weeks' gestation (Answer C).

Given the increased risk of type 2 diabetes in this woman with a history of gestational diabetes, current American Diabetes Association guidelines recommend screening for undiagnosed type 2 diabetes at the time that pregnancy is established (thus, Answer A is incorrect). Hemoglobin A$_{1c}$ measurement, fasting plasma glucose measurement, and the 75-g oral glucose tolerance test may all be used as screening tests for type 2 diabetes; however, the oral glucose tolerance test is the most sensitive modality (thus, Answers B and D are incorrect).

The recurrence rate of gestational diabetes mellitus is high; at least 50% of future pregnancies will be affected. In a woman with a history of gestational diabetes, if type 2 diabetes is not present on testing when pregnancy is diagnosed, oral glucose tolerance testing should be repeated at the standard time of 24 to 28 weeks' gestation to screen for gestational diabetes. This could consist of a 2-step process (50-g oral glucose tolerance test and then, depending on threshold criteria, the 100-g oral glucose tolerance test) or a 1-step process (75-g oral glucose tolerance test). The 1-step process has significantly increased the number of women identified with gestational diabetes because it requires only 1 abnormal value rather than 2. However, because this increased identification has not clearly translated into improved maternal or neonatal outcomes, the 2-step approach to diagnosing gestational diabetes is still supported by several organizations, including the American College of Obstetrics and Gynecology.

Recommend a screening protocol for gestational diabetes mellitus.

REFERENCE(S)

American Diabetes Association. 13. Management of diabetes in pregnancy: standards of medical care in diabetes-2018. *Diabetes Care.* 2016;41(Suppl 1):S137-S143. PMID: 29222384

Committee on Practice Bulletins–-Obstetrics. Practice Bulletin No. 137: gestational diabetes mellitus. *Obstet Gynecol.* 2013;122(2 Pt 1):406-416. PMID: 23969827

45 ANSWER: B) Panretinal laser photocoagulation

Diabetic retinopathy, one of the most common microvascular complications in both type 1 and type 2 diabetes mellitus, is classified as nonproliferative when it consists of retinal microhemorrhages and hard exudates, the latter representing lipid deposition. With progressive ischemia, more ominous signs such as ischemic infarcts (cotton wool spots) and neovascularization occur. In the setting of neovascularization, classified as proliferative retinopathy, panretinal laser photocoagulation (Answer B) has been demonstrated to protect against vision loss.

Focal laser photocoagulation (Answer A) is typically used for isolated areas of neovascularization. Antivascular endothelial growth factor (anti-VEGF) drugs such as ranibizumab (Answer C) are used in refractory cases of diabetic retinopathy, although they are used more commonly in those with isolated macular edema. Vitrectomy (Answer D) is performed in patients with severe vision loss from severe proliferative diabetic retinopathy after vitreous hemorrhage and severe fibrous changes have developed. It is not a first-line therapy.

Recommend appropriate management of diabetic retinopathy.

REFERENCE(S)

Giuliari GP. Diabetic retinopathy: current and new treatment options. *Curr Diabetes Rev.* 2012;8(1):32-41. PMID: 22352446

46 **ANSWER: D) Diabetic radiculopathy**

Diabetic neuropathy has myriad manifestations and is generally more common in patients with long disease duration and poor glycemic control. Classification is subdivided into somatosensory, motor, and autonomic. The most common presentation involves damage to sensory nerve fibers and typically affects the distal extremities in a "stocking-glove" distribution. Affected patients describe numbness, paresthesias, and occasionally sharp, lancinating pains. Less common manifestations are acute sensory neuropathies characterized by sudden pain and dysesthesias in the distribution of one or more individual peripheral nerves or nerve roots. The patient in this vignette has left flank and left upper quadrant discomfort in the distribution of left nerve root T10. This may be seen in acute diabetic mononeuropathy or radiculitis (Answer D).

Autonomic dysfunction (Answer A) may affect one or several organ systems including the vasculature (orthostatic hypotension), the heart (silent ischemia, abnormal cardiac rhythms), the gastrointestinal tract (gastroparesis, constipation, diarrhea from bacterial overgrowth), and the urinary bladder (atonic bladder, chronic urinary tract infections, overflow incontinence). It does not cause pain syndromes. Herpes zoster (Answer B) can cause localized pain in a pattern similar to the one described here, but it does not cause dramatic tenderness. However, the pain can precede the typical rash but not usually for one week. Pancreatitis (Answer C) is unlikely without more nausea and pain in relation to eating. In this patient, the normal amylase and lipase values and negative CT scan also make this unlikely.

EDUCATIONAL OBJECTIVE

Diagnose rare syndromes of diabetic neuropathy.

REFERENCE(S)

Tesfaye S, Boulton AJ, Dyck PJ, et al; Toronto Diabetic Neuropathy Expert Group. Diabetic neuropathies; update on definitions, diagnostic criteria, estimation of severity, and treatments. *Diabetes Care.* 2010;33(10):2285-2293. PMID: 20876709

Casellini CM, Vinik AI. Clinical manifestations and current treatment options for diabetic neuropathies. *Endocr Pract.* 2007;13(5):550-566. PMID: 17872358

47 **ANSWER: B) Intravenous human regular insulin infusion titrated to maintain blood glucose between 140 and 180 mg/dL (7.8 and 10.0 mmol/L)**

This critically ill patient has severe hyperglycemia. The 2009 consensus statement from the American Association of Clinical Endocrinologists (AACE) and the 2015 American Diabetes Association (ADA) guidelines advise that hyperglycemic patients in the intensive care unit should receive intravenous insulin to control their glucose and that the glucose levels should be maintained between 140 and 180 mg/dL (7.8 and 10.0 mmol/L) (Answer B). This was based on the NICE-SUGAR study (Normoglycemia in Intensive Care Evaluation and Surviving Using Glucose Algorithm Regulation), which demonstrated no benefit from more stringent blood glucose control to less than 110 mg/dL (<6.1 mmol/L).

Insulin by intermittent subcutaneous injection (Answers A and D) has little role in the intensive care unit, since blood glucose control can be achieved more quickly and more reliably with intravenous administration. Achieving a lower target of 80 to 110 mg/dL (4.4 to 6.1 mmol/L) with intravenous insulin (Answer C) is now thought to yield no additional benefit, but, instead, it markedly increases the risk of severe hypoglycemia (more than 6-fold). A basal and prandial insulin regimen, such as insulin glargine and insulin aspart, is appropriate upon transfer out of the intensive care unit, but, as with regular insulin, it is not rapid enough in its action and is not as easily adaptable as an intravenous infusion.

REFERENCE(S)

Moghissi ES, Korytkowski MT, DiNardo M, et al; American Association of Clinical Endocrinologists; American Diabetes Association. American Association of Clinical Endocrinologists and American Diabetes Association consensus statement on inpatient glycemic control. *Diabetes Care*. 2009;32(6):1119-1131. PMID: 19429873

American Diabetes Association. 14. Diabetes care in the hospital: standards of medical care in diabetes-2018. *Diabetes Care*. 2015;41(Suppl 1):S144-S151. PMID: 29222385

48 **ANSWER: C) Pancreas transplant with or without a kidney transplant**

Necrobiosis lipoidica (Answer C) is rare condition that occurs in less than 1% of patients with diabetes. It is an inflammatory granulomatous skin disorder in which microangiopathy appears to have a role in pathogenesis. Among patients with necrobiosis lipoidica, 50% to 80% have diabetes. The lesions are classically seen overlying the anterior shin, characterized by a shallow depression into the dermis that is erythematous, often with a slightly yellow hue (due to lipid deposition) and with telangiectasias. Lesion size varies considerably, ranging between one and several centimeters in diameter, and lesions can grow over time and are frequently bilateral. They may be subject to ulceration.

Evidence for any specific treatment is limited to case reports and small clinical trials. Pancreas transplant with or without a kidney transplant (Answer C) resolves necrobiosis lipoidica. Kidney transplant alone (Answer A) does not. Antiplatelet therapy with dipyridamole (Answer B) alone does not lead to lesion resolution; however, dipyridamole combined with aspirin may improve necrobiosis lipoidica lesions, possibly due to lower thromboxane levels. Finally, glucocorticoids may be used to treat necrobiosis lipoidica. Systemic glucocorticoids may lead to complete closure of ulcerations except for atrophic ones. However, the impact on glycemia must be considered in taking this approach. Intralesional steroids (Answer D)

(injected into the borders of established lesion) and topical glucocorticoids, particularly for early lesions, may also be beneficial.

EDUCATIONAL OBJECTIVE
Identify dermopathies common to diabetes mellitus.

REFERENCE(S)

Feily A, Mehraban S. Treatment modalities of necrobiosis lipoidica: a concise systematic review. *Dermatol Reports*. 2015;7(2):5749. PMID: 26236446

Thiboutot DM. Clinical review 74: dermatological manifestations of endocrine disorders. *J Clin Endocrinol Metab*. 1995;80(10):3082-3087. PMID: 7559901

Heidenheim M, Jemec GE. Successful treatment of necrobiosis lipoidica diabeticorum with photodynamic therapy. *Arch Dermatol*. 2006;142(12):1548-1550. PMID: 17178979

49 **ANSWER: D) Result in improved glycemic control if used most days of the week, particularly in adults**

Studies of continuous glucose sensor systems have shown improvement in hemoglobin A_{1c} when compared with capillary self-monitored glucose values, both when used in combination with multiple daily insulin injections (mean difference, –0.2%) or in combination with starting insulin pump therapy (mean difference, –0.7%) (thus, Answer B is incorrect). Continuous glucose monitoring technology has been approved relatively recently by the US FDA as being accurate enough to be used for insulin dose adjustments (thus, Answer A is incorrect). Patients must, however, still use fingerstick blood glucose levels during the calibration period. Interstitial glucose readings usually lag behind capillary glucose levels by 7 to 15 minutes (thus, Answer C is incorrect), depending on the continuous glucose sensor system used and the rate of change of ambient plasma glucose levels (the faster the rate of change, the greater the lag).

EDUCATIONAL OBJECTIVE
Counsel patients regarding the expectations of the use of a continuous glucose monitoring system in glycemic management.

REFERENCE(S)

Langendam M, Luijf YM, Hooft L, Devries JH, Mudde AH, Scholten RJ. Continuous glucose monitoring systems for type 1 diabetes mellitus. *Cochrane Database Syst Rev.* 2012;1:CD008101. PMID: 22258980

Garg S, Zisser H, Schwartz S, et al. Improvement in glycemic excursions with a transcutaneous, real-time continuous glucose sensor: a randomized, controlled trial. *Diabetes Care.* 2006;29(1):44-50. PMID: 16373894

Juvenile Diabetes Research Foundation Continuous Glucose Monitoring Study Group, Tamborlane WV, Beck RW, et al. Continuous glucose monitoring and intensive treatment of type 1 diabetes. *N Engl J Med.* 2008;359(14):1464-1476. PMID: 18779236

Bergenstal RM, Tamborlane WV, Ahmann A, Buse JB, Dailey G, Davis SN, et al; STAR 3 Study Group. Effectiveness of sensor-augmented insulin-pump therapy in type 1 diabetes [published correction in *N Engl J Med.* 2010;363(11):1092]. *N Engl J Med.* 2010;363(4):311-320. PMID: 20587585

McQueen RB, Ellis SL, Maahs DM, Anderson HD, Nair KV, Campbell JD. Frequency of continuous glucose monitoring use and change in hemoglobin A1c for adults with type 1 diabetes in a clinical practice setting. *Endocr Pract.* 2014;20(10):1007-1015. PMID: 24793924

DeSalvo D, Buckingham B. Continuous glucose monitoring: current use and future directions. *Curr Diab Rep.* 2013;13(5):657-662. PMID: 23943230

Liebl A, Henrichs HR, Heinemann L, et al; Continuous Glucose Monitoring Working Group of the Working Group Diabetes Technology of the German Diabetes Association. Continuous glucose monitoring: evidence and consensus statement for clinical use. *J Diabetes Sci Technol.* 2013;7(2):500-519. PMID: 23567009

50 ANSWER: D) 76%

Vision loss from diabetes remains a major cause of blindness in the world. Numerous epidemiologic studies and clinical trials have documented the importance of glycemic control in patients with diabetes, including the Diabetes Control and Complications Trial (DCCT). Published in 1993, the DCCT was a landmark study that compared the effects of intensive vs conventional control on the onset and progression of diabetes-related complications over 6.5 years in more than 1400 patients with fairly early type 1 diabetes. The intensive control group showed a 76% reduction (Answer D) in the adjusted mean risk of the development of retinopathy compared with the control group. Also documented was a 54% slowing of progression of mild established retinopathy and a 47% reduction in the development of proliferative or severe proliferative retinopathy. Further, the occurrence of microalbuminuria was reduced by 39%, macroalbuminuria by 54%, and clinical neuropathy by 60%.

EDUCATIONAL OBJECTIVE
Counsel patients with type 1 diabetes mellitus regarding the magnitude of the potential impact of intensive control on the development of retinopathy.

REFERENCE(S)

Diabetes Control and Complications Trial Research Group, Nathan DM, Genuth S, etc. The effect of intensive treatment of diabetes on the development and progression of long-term complications in insulin-dependent diabetes mellitus. *N Engl J Med.* 1993;329(14):977-986. PMID: 8366922

51 ANSWER: C) 80-130 mg/dL (4.4-7.2 mmol/L)

Current American Diabetes Association guidelines recommend premeal blood glucose targets of 80 to 130 mg/dL (4.4 to 7.2 mmol/L) for individuals with type 2 diabetes (Answer C), rather than 70 to 130 mg/dL (3.9 to 7.2 mmol/L) (Answer B) or 90 to 140 mg/dL (5.0 to 7.8 mmol/L) (Answer D). A target of 60 to 120 mg/dL (3.3 to 6.7 mmol/L) (Answer A) would not provide a lower-limit buffer zone for preventing hypoglycemia.

Empirical evidence from the A1C-Derived Average Glucose study (ADAG) showed that the average fasting glucose levels associated with conventional hemoglobin A_{1c} targets are higher than those previously prescribed. The 80 to 130 mg/dL range is thought to allow clinicians and individuals to set realistic self-monitored blood glucose targets to reach individualized hemoglobin A_{1c} goals, without accruing increased risk of hypoglycemia.

EDUCATIONAL OBJECTIVE
Select appropriate premeal glucose targets for managing type 2 diabetes mellitus.

REFERENCE(S)
Nathan DM, Kuenen J, Borg R, Zheng H, Schoenfeld D, Heine RJ; A1c-Derived Average Glucose Study Group. Translating the A1C assay into estimated average glucose values [published correction appears in *Diabetes Care*. 2009;32(1):207]. *Diabetes Care*. 2008;31(8):1473-1478. PMID: 18540046

American Diabetes Association. 6. Glycemic targets: standards of medical care in diabetes-2018. *Diabetes Care*. 2018;41(Suppl 1):S55-S64. PMID: 29222377

52 **ANSWER: A) Both temperature and altitude**

Several physical factors influence the accuracy of blood glucose strips; the most common are altitude and temperature (thus, Answer A is correct and Answers B, C, and E are incorrect).

A group of mountain climbers tested blood glucose systems at 13,500 ft (4100 m). Glucose oxidase meters overestimated the glucose concentration by 6% to 15%. In another study, glucose oxidase meters overestimated values at low Po_2 levels and underestimated glucose values at high Po_2 levels. Glucose dehydrogenase-based systems are oxygen insensitive and are therefore not affected by altitude.

The effect of temperature is less predictable, and it can be either positive or negative at extreme cold temperatures. Temperature can affect readings indirectly as well, by influencing circulation to the skin (cold temperature), which may particularly affect results of alternate site testing.

No data are available on the effect of low barometric pressure (Answer D) on glucose meter readings.

EDUCATIONAL OBJECTIVE
Identify environmental factors that can affect the accuracy of some blood glucose meter readings.

REFERENCE(S)
Ginsberg BH. Factors affecting blood glucose monitoring: sources of errors in measurement. *J Diabetes Sci Technol*. 2009;3(4):903-913. PMID: 20144340

Olansky L, Kennedy L. Finger-stick glucose monitoring: issues of accuracy and specificity. *Diabetes Care*. 2010;33(4):948-949. PMID: 20351231

Schmid C, Baumstark A, Pleus S, Haug C, Tesar M, Freckmann G. Impact of partial pressure of oxygen in blood samples on the performance of systems for self-monitoring of blood glucose. *Diabetes Technol Ther*. 2014;16(3):156-165. PMID: 24205977

53 **ANSWER: D) Increase basal insulin to achieve overnight blood glucose levels between 60 and 99 mg/dL (3.3 and 5.5 mmol/L)**

During pregnancy, normalization of blood glucose levels reduces the risk of congenital malformations during the first 8 to 10 weeks and the risk of macrosomia and related comorbidities over the course of the pregnancy.

Optimal glycemic goals:

- Premeal, bedtime, and overnight = 60-99 mg/dL (3.3-5.5 mmol/L) (thus, Answer D is correct)
- Peak (1-hour) postprandial = 100-129 mg/dL (5.6-7.2 mmol/L)
- Mean daily = <110 mg/dL (<6.1 mmol/L)
- Hemoglobin A_{1c} = <6.0% (<42 mmol/mol)

The best way to do this is to increase her basal insulin to achieve overnight glucose levels between 60 and 99 mg/dL (3.3 and 5.5 mmol/L) (Answer D). Because her peak postprandial glucose measurements are within the target range on a fixed dose of prandial insulin, increasing prandial insulin doses (Answer C) is not indicated. Although blood pressure in pregnancy should be ideally maintained at 110-129/65-79 mm Hg, ACE inhibitors and angiotensin-receptor blockers (Answer B) are contraindicated during pregnancy. Antihypertensive agents that can be used in pregnancy include methyldopa, labetalol, diltiazem, clonidine, and prazosin. Statins (Answer A) are also contraindicated in pregnancy and should be discontinued as soon as pregnancy is documented. In pregnancy, there is increased red blood cell production and the red blood cell lifespan is shortened; hemoglobin A_{1c} can therefore be checked monthly during pregnancy. Thus, every 3 months (Answer E) is incorrect.

EDUCATIONAL OBJECTIVE
Make basic recommendations for management of glycemia and other comorbid conditions complicating a pregnancy to reduce the risk of congenital malformations and macrosomia.

REFERENCE(S)
American Diabetes Association. 13. Management of diabetes in pregnancy: standards of medical care in diabetes-2018. *Diabetes Care.* 2016;41(Suppl 1):S137-S143. PMID: 29222384

Kitzmiller JL, Block JM, Brown FM, et al. Managing preexisting diabetes for pregnancy: summary of evidence and consensus recommendations for care. *Diabetes Care.* 2008;31(5):1060-1079. PMID: 18445730

McCance DR. Pregnancy and diabetes. *Best Pract Res Clin Endocrinol Metab.* 2011;25(6):945-958. PMID: 22115168

54 ANSWER: A) He should consider a brief period of weightlifting before jogging to reduce the chance of hypoglycemia

With an adequate concentration of insulin on board, aerobic activity is most often associated with a slight increase, no change, or a mild decrease in blood glucose during or shortly after the activity. Anaerobic exercise, however, often induces a rise in blood glucose levels because of an associated increase in release of catecholamines (14- to 18-fold rise). Aerobic exercise is associated with a more modest rise (2- to 4-fold) in catecholamines. Hypoglycemia is certainly still possible with aerobic exercise such as jogging, especially if the jogging is strenuous, and there is no magic number for the ideal pre-jog glucose value that will guarantee against it (thus, Answer C is incorrect). Evidence has shown that including small amounts of anaerobic activity (eg, weightlifting) during aerobic exercise may reduce the drop in blood glucose levels associated with moderate-intensity aerobic exercise (thus, Answer A is correct). It should also be noted that following anaerobic exercise, a delayed drop in blood glucose can occur. This manifests as a reduction in mean interstitial glucose 4.5 to 6 hours after exercise. This blood glucose drop could increase the risk for hypoglycemia after weightlifting and for nocturnal hypoglycemia after weightlifting in the evening. This could be addressed by lowering the basal insulin delivery rate during the night.

Increasing his basal rate during jogging (Answer B) could heighten the risk for hypoglycemia by increasing the insulin onboard during the activity. Physical activity is recommended for patients with type 1 diabetes because regular exercise is associated with a longer life and a lower frequency of complications. Thus, avoiding aerobic activity to avoid hypoglycemia (Answer D) is incorrect.

EDUCATIONAL OBJECTIVE
Advise patients with type 1 diabetes mellitus about the effects of exercise on the risk of hypoglycemia.

REFERENCE(S)
Lumb AN, Gallen IW. Diabetes management for intense exercise. *Curr Opin Endocrinol Diabetes Obes.* 2009;16(2):150-155. PMID: 19300093

Yardley JE, Sigal RJ, Perkins BA, Riddell MC, Kenny GP. Resistance exercise in type 1 diabetes. *Can J Diabetes.* 2013;37(6):420-426. PMID: 24321724

Yardley JE, Kenny GP, Perkins BA. Resistance versus aerobic exercise: acute effects on glycemia in type 1 diabetes. *Diabetes Care.* 2013;36(3):537-542. PMID: 23172972

Cryer PE. Mechanisms of hypoglycemia-associated autonomic failure in diabetes. *N Engl J Med.* 2013;369(4):362-372. PMID: 23883381

Davis SN, Tate D, Hedrington MS. Mechanisms of hypoglycemia and exercise-associated autonomic dysfunction. *Trans Am Clin Climatol Assoc.* 2014;125:281-291. PMID: 25125745

55 ANSWER: D) Spot urine collection and measurement of albumin and creatinine

Abnormally high rates of albumin excretion are the earliest manifestation of diabetic nephropathy; albuminuria can be detected well before changes in creatinine clearance and pathologic proteinuria occur. Detection of microalbuminuria is the point in the course of nephropathy where treatment is most effective. Therefore, all patients with diabetes should have routine screening. Patients with type 2 diabetes should be screened for renal albumin excretion at the time of diabetes diagnosis because the actual onset and duration of disease are often hard to discern and most patients will have had at least several years of asymptomatic hyperglycemia. Screening for microalbuminuria can be done with a 24-hour urine collection, an overnight or 4-hour timed collection, or a spot collection with determination of the albumin-to-creatinine ratio (Answer D).

While a 24-hour collection (Answer A) is the most accurate way to quantify albumin excretion, there is a strong correlation between these values and the albumin-to-creatinine ratio. All of the measures require a specific assay for albumin because standard clinical laboratory measurements of urinary protein are not sensitive enough to detect microalbuminuria. Cystatin C or cystatin 3 (Answer C), a protein encoded by the *CST3* gene, is primarily used as a biomarker of kidney function. Its role in predicting new-onset or deteriorating cardiovascular disease is being studied. The principal advantage of cystatin C is for use in children and older adults, in whom the creatinine-based estimated glomerular filtration rate is less reliable, or in patients with conditions such as unusual muscle mass. Although estimation of the glomerular filtration rate (Answer B) is a useful means of monitoring renal function, it is not a sensitive index of diabetic nephropathy.

EDUCATIONAL OBJECTIVE
Screen for diabetic nephropathy.

REFERENCE(S)
Gross JL, de Azevedo MJ, Silveiro SP, Canani LH, Caramori ML, Zelmanovitz T. Diabetic nephropathy: diagnosis, prevention, and treatment. *Diabetes Care.* 2005;28(1):164-176. PMID: 15616252

56 ANSWER: B) Change from olanzapine to aripiprazole

The key features in this case are rapid weight gain and development of hypertriglyceridemia since initiation of olanzapine therapy. Atypical antipsychotic agents, such as olanzapine, are now frequently used to treat thought disorders because of a lower risk of extrapyramidal adverse effects than with traditional antipsychotic drugs. However, several compounds in this drug class have metabolic consequences, including weight gain, hyperlipidemia, insulin resistance, and impaired glucose metabolism. The drugs most frequently implicated are clozapine and olanzapine (thus, switching to clozapine [Answer A] would not make sense). Risperidone and quetiapine have intermediate effects, and aripiprazole (Answer B), ziprasidone, and amisulpride have little or no association with metabolic abnormalities. Although definitive epidemiologic data are not available, up to 30% to 40% of patients treated with clozapine and olanzapine are reported to develop weight gain and associated metabolic disorders. In this patient, the temporal association of olanzapine initiation and the onset of weight gain with subsequent hypertension and hypertriglyceridemia suggests that use of this medication is the proximate cause of his problems. Given that there are other antipsychotic drugs that have lesser metabolic effects, it is important to communicate with the physician treating the schizophrenia, discuss the likely role of olanzapine in this case, and explore alternative treatments.

Cushing syndrome is in the differential diagnosis of rapid weight gain and can be associated with hypertension and disordered lipid and glucose metabolism. However, this patient does not have cushingoid features on examination, making a biochemical workup unnecessary.

Although his triglyceride level is high, it is not in the range that causes concern for spontaneous pancreatitis (>1000 mg/dL [>11.30 mmol/L]). There is no urgency to lower his triglycerides with a fibrate (Answer C) as a means of primary prevention of coronary artery disease.

Although metformin (Answer D) effectively prevents the progression to diabetes in persons with prediabetes, a more direct solution to his impaired fasting glucose level is changing his psychotropic medication.

The combination of phentermine/topiramate (Answer E) has been approved to treat obesity. This medication has been reported to induce 5% to 10% weight loss, and this would most likely improve both the lipid disorder and impaired fasting glucose. However, the 2 components of this agent are centrally acting drugs and it has not been formally studied in persons with psychiatric disease. Trying to reduce body weight by other means is more prudent.

EDUCATIONAL OBJECTIVE
Manage the metabolic complications of atypical antipsychotic medications.

REFERENCE(S)

Newcomer JW. Metabolic considerations in the use of antipsychotic medications: a review of recent evidence. *J Clin Psychiatry*. 2007;68(Suppl 1): 20-27. PMID: 17286524

57 ANSWER: B) Macular edema

Macular edema (Answer B) is a common manifestation of retinal microvascular disease. The typical symptoms are consistent with those of this patient, with gradual onset of blurred vision occurring over months. She has known retinopathy, and it is not unusual for this to progress, even with stable findings on eye examinations in the past. Macular edema can be difficult to detect on office retinal exams, but it can be detected and staged by ophthalmologists using pupillary dilation, fluorescein angiography, and optical coherence tomography. In this regard, it is unfortunate that the patient is late on her annual ophthalmologic exam.

Once confirmed, macular edema is treated with intravitreous antivascular endothelial growth factor once monthly for a year. Until recently, focal laser therapy had been the treatment of choice. The diagnosis of macular edema associated with diabetic retinopathy is also impetus for better glucose control. Control of blood pressure and treatment of dyslipidemia can also prevent the progression of diabetic retinopathy.

Retinal detachment (Answer A) and vitreous hemorrhage (Answer C) usually present more acutely, rarely affect both eyes, and cause focal visual deficits rather than diffuse blurred vision. Mononeuritis (Answer E) can affect the cranial nerves, but it typically causes palsy or abnormal pupillary responses when associated with blurred vision; this condition, too, does not usually affect both eyes. Cataracts (Answer D) are common and cause blurred vision that develops gradually, not at the rapid pace described here.

EDUCATIONAL OBJECTIVE
Assess vision symptoms in patients with diabetes.

REFERENCE(S)

Diabetic Retinopathy Clinical Research Network, Elman MJ, Aiello LP, et al. Randomized trial evaluating ranibizumab plus prompt or deferred laser or triamcinolone plus prompt laser for diabetic macular edema. *Ophthalmology*. 2010;117(6):1064-1077. PMID: 20427088

VanderBeek BL, Shah N, Parikh PC, Ma L. Trends in the care of diabetic macular edema: analysis of a national cohort. *PLoS One*. 2016;11(2):e0149450. PMID: 26909797

Stitt AW, Lois N, Medina RJ, Adamson P, Curtis TM. Advances in our understanding of diabetic retinopathy. *Clin Sci (Lond)*. 2013;125(1):1-17. PMID: 23485060

58 ANSWER: E) Metformin

Metformin (Answer E) is the preferred initial therapy for type 2 diabetes and it should be used in this case. It is recommended that the metformin dosage be reduced by half once the glomerular filtration rate falls under 45 mL/min per m^2 and that the drug be stopped if the glomerular filtration rate falls below 30 mL/min per m^2.

Starting this patient on metformin as a first-line agent, 500 twice daily, and monitoring her hemoglobin A_{1c} response is the best practice. Given her age, tight glycemic control may not be indicated, and metformin should be adequate to prevent acute diabetic symptoms. Moreover, the drug is generally safe, inexpensive, and well-tolerated.

Pioglitazone (Answer B) is effective and generally well tolerated. However, the potential adverse effects of weight gain, edema, and bone loss are ones to avoid in this patient. DPP-4 inhibitors (Answer C) and GLP-1 receptor agonists (Answer D) are both likely to be effective in this patient, but they are expensive and have a relatively short history of use compared with that of metformin. α-Glucosidase inhibitors (Answer A) are safe but only reduce hemoglobin A_{1c} by approximately 0.5%; this treatment would be unlikely to help her reach her glycemic goal.

EDUCATIONAL OBJECTIVE
Explain the relationship between renal function and use of metformin.

REFERENCE(S)

Salpeter SR, Greyber E, Pasternak GA, Salpeter EE. Risk of fatal and nonfatal lactic acidosis with metformin use in type 2 diabetes mellitus. *Cochrane Database Systematic Rev*. 2010;(4):CD002967. PMID: 20393934

Lipska KJ, Bailey CJ, Inzucchi SE. Use of metformin in the setting of mild-to-moderate renal insufficiency. *Diabetes Care*. 2011;34(6):1431-1437. PMID: 21617112

59 ANSWER: B) Start diagnostic continuous glucose monitoring

This patient's hemoglobin A_{1c} level is higher than would be expected based on the reported home blood glucose readings. A hemoglobin A_{1c} value of 8.4% (68 mmol/mol) corresponds with an estimated average glucose value of 194 mg/dL (10.8 mmol/L). There is evidence that he is having nocturnal hypoglycemia. Continuous glucose monitoring (CGM) technology (Answer B) has been used as a tool to document the incidence and magnitude of both hypoglycemia and hyperglycemia in adults with diabetes. In adults with type 2 diabetes, even in those with apparently well-controlled diabetes, CGM has shown that hypoglycemia and excessive postprandial glycemic excursions are common. In older patients, CGM has demonstrated that hypoglycemia is extremely common and often asymptomatic, and even when the hemoglobin A_{1c} level is 8.0% or greater (≥64 mmol/mol), CGM has documented hypoglycemia rates to be as high as 65%. Ninety-five percent of these low values were not detected by traditional fingerstick blood glucose testing, nor by symptoms, which increases risk of harm to the patient. This patient does not monitor his blood glucose frequently, so it would be very helpful to start diagnostic CGM, which will determine the time(s) of day and to what degree hypoglycemia is present, if he has rebound hyperglycemia after such episodes, and his postprandial blood glucose trends. This will facilitate optimal adjustment of his insulin doses and provide insight into how his diet and physical activity are affecting his glycemic control.

Glycosylated albumin (Answer A) is similar to fructosamine, a measure of glycosylation of serum proteins, and it is a reasonable alternative to hemoglobin A_{1c} for assessing long-term glucose control with an advantage in cases where red blood cell turnover is altered. However, there is no reason to doubt the hemoglobin A_{1c} in this man, and measuring glycosylated albumin is only likely to validate that his overall glycemic control is poor.

Measuring C-peptide (Answer C) may detect residual β-cell function, but this man with long-standing diabetes who is taking 65 units of insulin daily will not be able to stop insulin therapy, so this information would not be clinically important now.

Finally, insulin antibodies (Answer D), which were relatively common when patients were treated with insulins extracted from bovine and porcine pancreas, caused both hyperglycemia and hypoglycemia by binding injected insulin and releasing it intermittently. However, antibodies in response to human insulins or analogues such as insulin glargine are very rare and there is not much evidence that this patient's blood glucose values are erratic, which is a hallmark of the clinical presentation when antibodies are present.

EDUCATIONAL OBJECTIVE
Interpret measures of glycemic control in the setting of type 2 diabetes mellitus.

REFERENCE(S)
American Diabetes Association. eAG/A1C Conversion Calculator. Available at: https://professional.diabetes.org/diapro/glucose_calc. Accessed for verification May 16, 2018.

Munshi MN, Segal AR, Suhl E, et al. Frequent hypoglycemia among elderly patients with poor glycemic control. *Arch Intern Med*. 2011;171(4):362-364. PMID: 21357814

Hay LC, Wilmshurst EG, Fulcher G. Unrecognized hypo- and hyperglycemia in well-controlled patients with type 2 diabetes mellitus: the results of continuous glucose monitoring. *Diabetes Technol Ther*. 2003;5(1):19-26. PMID: 12725703

Cheyne E, Kerr D. Making 'sense' of diabetes: using a continuous glucose sensor in clinical practice. *Diabetes Metab Res Rev*. 2002;18(Suppl 1):S43-S38. PMID: 11921429

Female Reproduction Board Review
Kathryn A. Martin, MD • Massachusetts General Hospital

ANSWER: C) Sleep study

Polycystic ovary syndrome is a common disorder that occurs in 6% to 8% of women. Affected patients usually present with hirsutism, acne, and irregular menses. Sixty percent of affected women become obese. In addition to being at increased risk for impaired glucose tolerance and type 2 diabetes mellitus with a risk 5 to 10 times that of age-matched control women, women with polycystic ovary syndrome are also at high risk for sleep apnea. Given this patient's history, the next step would be to do a sleep study (Answer C).

Although she has gained weight and reports fatigue, she has no other features to suggest hypercortisolism (Answer A). An oral glucose tolerance test (Answer B) is indeed the most sensitive test for the diagnosis of type 2 diabetes in women with polycystic ovary syndrome, but she has a normal hemoglobin A_{1c} value and her symptoms are most suggestive of sleep apnea. A serum total testosterone measurement (Answer D) is part of the evaluation for hirsutism and polycystic ovary syndrome, but it is unlikely to help determine the cause of her sleepiness.

EDUCATIONAL OBJECTIVE
Identify the high risk of sleep apnea associated with polycystic ovary syndrome.

REFERENCE(S)

McCartney CR, Marshall JC. Clinical practice. Polycystic ovary syndrome. *N Engl J Med*. 2016;375(1):54-64. PMID: 27406348

Legro RS, Arslanian SA, Ehrmann DA, et al; Endocrine Society. Diagnosis and treatment of polycystic ovary syndrome: an Endocrine Society Clinical Practice Guideline. *J Clin Endocrinol Metab*. 2013;98(12):4565-4592. PMID: 24151290

Ehrmann DA. Metabolic dysfunction in PCOS: relationship to obstructive sleep apnea. *Steroids*. 2012;77(4):290-294. PMID: 22178788

Tasali E, Chapotot F, Leproult R, Whitmore H, Ehrmann DA. Treatment of obstructive sleep apnea improves cardiometabolic function in young obese women with polycystic ovary syndrome. *J Clin Endocrinol Metab*. 2011;96(2):365-374. PMID: 21123449

ANSWER: B) Progestin-only pill

There are no contraindications to starting progestin-only contraceptives (Answer B) immediately after delivery in breastfeeding women, and it is thought that the benefits of contraception outweigh the theoretical concerns about any potential impact on lactation. Progestin-only methods other than the progestin-only pill would also be reasonable.

The risk of venous thromboembolism, which is high during pregnancy, remains high for the first 6 weeks postpartum, particularly in the first 3 weeks. Therefore, any form of hormonal contraception with estrogen (Answer A and C) is contraindicated in the early postpartum period. Ovulation resumes at a mean of 39 days postpartum in women who choose not to breastfeed. The first ovulation can occur before the first menses, so starting contraception is essential. For women who are breastfeeding, the return of ovulation is influenced by the frequency and duration of breastfeeding. Women who breastfeed resume ovulation less quickly; however, ovulation can occur before the first menses. Thus, recommending no contraception (Answer D) is incorrect.

EDUCATIONAL OBJECTIVE
Recommend the optimal contraceptive method in the immediate postpartum period.

REFERENCE(S)

Sultan AA, West J, Grainge MJ, et al. Development and validation of risk prediction model for venous thromboembolism in postpartum women: multinational cohort study. *BMJ*. 2016;355:i6253. PMID: 27919934

Tepper NK, Boulet SL, Whiteman MK, Monsour M, Marchbanks PA, Hooper WC, Curtis KM Postpartum venous thromboembolism: incidence and risk factors. *Obstet Gynecol*. 2014; 123(5):987.

Jackson E, Glasier A. Return of ovulation and menses in postpartum nonlactating women: a systematic review. *Obstet Gynecol*. 2011;117(3):657-662. PMID: 21343770

Pieh Holder KL. Contraception and breastfeeding. *Clin Obstet Gynecol*. 2015;58(4):928-935. PMID: 26457854

3 ANSWER: A) Normal FSH, high LH, high estradiol, and normal prolactin

This patient has amenorrhea due to uterine synechiae (retained products of conception/procedure/endometritis). She is having ovulatory cycles based on her history but is having no bleeding because of the scarring. These laboratory values are consistent with the late follicular phase or midcycle surge. Two weeks after her premenstrual symptoms, you would expect her to be nearing an LH surge, so both LH and estradiol would be high, FSH would be normal or suppressed, and prolactin would be normal (Answer A).

The pattern in Answer B is characteristic of primary ovarian insufficiency: high gonadotropins, low estradiol, and normal prolactin. There is no reason to suspect this and she has no suggestive symptoms. The pattern in Answer C represents a patient with infarction of the pituitary gland after postpartum hemorrhage (Sheehan syndrome): low gonadotropins, estradiol, and prolactin. While the postpartum bleeding might suggest this, she appears to be having ovulatory cycles. The pattern in Answer D is characteristic of hyperprolactinemia (high prolactin, low gonadotropins, and low estradiol). Again, this is not the correct diagnosis given her description of monthly symptoms that suggest ovulatory cycles.

EDUCATIONAL OBJECTIVE
Determine the most likely set of hormone patterns in a woman with amenorrhea due to uterine adhesions.

REFERENCE(S)

Zupi E, Centini G, Lazzeri L. Asherman syndrome: an unsolved clinical definition and management. *Fertil Steril*. 2015;104(6):1380-1381. PMID: 26484781

Diri H, Tanriverdi F, Karaca Z, et al. Extensive investigation of 114 patients with Sheehan's syndrome: a continuing disorder. *Eur J Endocrinol*. 2014;171(3):311-318. PMID: 24917653

4 ANSWER: D) Primary ovarian insufficiency

Antimullerian hormone is a marker of ovarian reserve and follicular number. Infertility specialists have used it extensively in clinical practice to evaluate older women with borderline elevated FSH levels to predict response to in vitro fertilization and to diagnose primary ovarian insufficiency (or in its early stages, diminished ovarian reserve/occult ovarian insufficiency). Antimullerian hormone levels are lower in women with impending primary ovarian insufficiency (with higher FSH levels) (Answer D). Another feature suggesting primary ovarian insufficiency in this patient is her short cycles (25 to 26 days) rather than the more typical 28 days.

A woman with polycystic ovary syndrome (Answer A) would have a high antimullerian hormone level and low FSH level. An FSH-secreting pituitary adenoma (Answer B) would be unusual in this age group and would more likely present with neurologic symptoms (headache and vision loss) than with infertility and shorter cycles. Importantly, women with hypothalamic amenorrhea (Answer C) also have a low antimullerian hormone level but a low-normal FSH level.

EDUCATIONAL OBJECTIVE
Explain the utility of measuring antimullerian hormone in women with amenorrhea.

REFERENCE(S)

Welt CK. Primary ovarian insufficiency: a more accurate term for premature ovarian failure. *Clin Endocrinol (Oxf)*. 2008;68(4):499-509. PMID: 17970776

Meczekalski B, Czyzyk A, Kunicki M, et al. Fertility in women of late reproductive age: the role of serum anti-Müllerian hormone (AMH) levels in its assessment. *J Endocrinol Invest*. 2016;39(11):1259-1265. PMID: 27300031

La Marca A, Ferraretti AP, Palermo R, Ubaldi FM. The use of ovarian reserve markers in IVF clinical practice: a national consensus. *Gynecol Endocrinol*. 2016;32(1):1-5. PMID: 26531067

Iliodromiti S, Anderson RA, Nelson SM. Technical and performance characteristics of anti-müllerian hormone and antral follicle count as biomarkers of ovarian response. *Hum Reprod Update*. 2015;21(6):698-710. PMID: 25489055

5 ANSWER: C) Hematocrit or hemoglobin measurement every 3 months

Testosterone administration at pharmacologic levels in women (or men) causes increased hematocrit and risk of polycythemia. This is a greater concern with parenteral testosterone administration, but it can be seen with the testosterone gels as well. Therefore, the current Endocrine Society guideline suggests that hematocrit or hemoglobin be measured at baseline and every 3 months for the first year, and then 1 to 2 times per year.

Serum testosterone measurements (Answer A) are also essential, but they should ideally be drawn midway between injections or at least 2 hours after application of a transdermal preparation. Hemoglobin A_{1c} measurement (Answer B) is not a component of the routine monitoring of hormone therapy for transgender men. Pap smears (Answer D) are performed if cervical tissue is present (many patients undergo hysterectomy and thus do not have cervical tissue). The schedule for cervical screening is the same as for women (every 3 years).

EDUCATIONAL OBJECTIVE
Identify the most important components of monitoring transgender men taking gender-affirming hormone therapy.

REFERENCE(S)

Hembree WC, Cohen-Kettenis PT, Gooren L, et al. Endocrine treatment of gender dysphoric/gender-incongruent persons: an Endocrine Society clinical practice guideline. *J Clin Endocrinol Metab*. 2017;102(11):3869-3903. PMID: 28945902

Gorton RN, Erickson-Schroth L. Hormonal and surgical treatment options for transgender men (female-to-male). *Psychiatr Clin North Am*. 2017;40(1):79-97. PMID: 28159147

Spack NP. Management of transgenderism. *JAMA*. 2013;309(5):478-484. PMID: 23385274

Deutsch MB, Feldman JL. Updated recommendations from the world professional association for transgender health standards of care. *Am Fam Physician*. 2013;87(2):89-93. PMID: 23317072

Fernandez JD, Tannock LR. Metabolic effects of hormone therapy in transgender patients. *Endocr Pract*. 2016;22(4):383-388. PMID: 26574790

6 ANSWER: A) Oral 17β-estradiol, 2 mg daily

This patient is an excellent candidate for estrogen. The results of the Women's Health Initiative are not relevant to her, as the mean age of the patients was 63 years and she is only 41. She should be approached like any woman with primary ovarian insufficiency and be treated with estrogen until the average age of menopause (50/51 years). She has severe symptoms that are interfering with her quality of life and her ability to function, so estrogen is indicated. Women with primary ovarian insufficiency are prescribed higher dosages of estrogen than other women. Progestin therapy is not indicated in a patient after hysterectomy, as its only role is to prevent endometrial hyperplasia. The best answer is oral 17β-estradiol, 2 mg daily (Answer A). She could also use unopposed transdermal estrogen, but it is not necessary (and was not offered as an option).

Two combination estrogen-progestin options are listed (Answers B and D) (one is an oral contraceptive), which she does not need. Venlafaxine (Answer C) is a nonhormonal alternative—this is an option for patients with breast cancer who cannot take estrogen, but she is an excellent candidate for estrogen.

EDUCATIONAL OBJECTIVE
Recommend the optimal approach to managing severe hot flashes in a 40-year-old woman after total hysterectomy and bilateral salpingo-oophorectomy.

REFERENCE(S)

Stuenkel CA, Davis SR, Gompel A, et al. Treatment of symptoms of the menopause: an Endocrine Society clinical practice guideline. *J Clin Endocrinol Metab*. 2015;100(11):3975-4011. PMID: 26444994

The NAMS 2017 Hormone Therapy Position Statement Advisory Panel. The 2017 hormone therapy position statement of The North American Menopause Society. Menopause. 2017;24(7):728-753. PMID: 28650869

Committee on Gynecologic Practice. Committee opinion No. 698: hormone therapy in primary ovarian insufficiency. *Obstet Gynecol*. 2017;129(5):e134-e141. PMID: 28426619

7 ANSWER: A) Transvaginal ultrasonography

Postmenopausal hirsutism or virilization of recent onset with a serum testosterone level greater than 150 ng/dL (>5.2 nmol/L) or a serum DHEA-S level greater than 700 to 800 µg/dL (18.9 to 21.7 µmol/L) suggests a neoplastic source of hyperandrogenism. Signs of virilization include deepening of the voice, increased muscle mass and clitoromegaly. Clitoromegaly is determined by clitoral length or by the clitoral index (length × width). A clitoral length greater than 10 mm or a clitoral index greater than 35 mm² is considered to be clitoromegaly. Virilization is only seen with more severe hyperandrogenemia (serum testosterone greater than 150 ng/dL [>5.2 nmol/L]). Postmenopausal women with polycystic ovary syndrome do not have serum testosterone levels in this range, nor are they virilized.

Women with ovarian hyperthecosis typically develop symptoms gradually, but some with severe hyperthecosis have a more rapid course with severe hyperandrogenemia that mimics androgen-secreting tumors. Women with androgen-secreting adrenal tumors often present with symptoms of Cushing syndrome in addition to virilization. Unlike ovarian tumors, adrenal androgen-secreting tumors often, but not always, cause elevation in serum levels of the adrenal androgen DHEA-S. However, DHEA-S can be normal in androgen-secreting adrenal tumors. Androgen-secreting ovarian tumors include Sertoli-Leydig–cell tumors, arrhenoblastomas, or hilus-cell tumors.

The first step in the evaluation of severe hyperandrogenism in postmenopausal women is transvaginal ultrasonography (Answer A) to look for a tumor or asymmetry of the ovaries, as the tumors are typically very small. If the ultrasound is negative, an adrenal CT (Answer D) should be performed, because there are occasional cases of adrenal tumors that secrete only testosterone. However, adrenal CT would not be the first test one would do. In addition, ultrasonography is a better imaging test for visualizing the ovaries than abdominal CT.

A dexamethasone suppression test (Answer B) is used in the workup of Cushing syndrome and might be indicated if an adrenal mass is detected. With adrenal Cushing syndrome, the presentation would be different from this patient's and the testosterone level would not be as high as it is in this vignette.

Combined ovarian and adrenal venous sampling (selective venous sampling) is performed on occasion for further evaluation in women with high serum testosterone concentrations (testosterone >150 ng/dL [>5.2 nmol/L]) and normal pelvic ultrasonography and adrenal imaging. It would not be the first step in the evaluation of this patient.

EDUCATIONAL OBJECTIVE
Evaluate postmenopausal hyperandrogenism.

REFERENCE(S)

Alpañés M, González-Casbas JM, Sánchez J, Pián H, Escobar-Morreale HF. Management of postmenopausal virilization. *J Clin Endocrinol Metab*. 2012;97(8):2584-2588. PMID: 22669303

Petersons CJ, Burt MG. The utility of adrenal and ovarian venous sampling in the investigation of androgen-secreting tumours. *Intern Med J*. 2011;41(1a):69-70. PMID: 21265966

Pugeat M, Déchaud H, Raverot V, Denuzière A, Cohen R, Boudou P; French Endocrine Society. Recommendations for investigation of hyperandrogenism. *Ann Endocrinol (Paris)*. 2010;71(1):2-7. PMID: 20096825

8. ANSWER: C) Oral contraceptive

Nonclassic congenital adrenal hyperplasia (CAH) is a cause of hyperandrogenic anovulation with a clinical presentation that is similar or identical to that of polycystic ovary syndrome (hirsutism with irregular menses). The incidence varies from 1 to 10 per 20,000 live births. Nonclassic CAH is more common in those of Italian, Hispanic, Ashkenazi Jewish, and Inuit descent. In women with nonclassic CAH, basal serum 17-hydroxyprogesterone concentrations (during the follicular phase of the menstrual cycle) are usually greater than 200 ng/dL (>6.1 nmol/L) (high-normal or high). The diagnosis of nonclassic 21α-hydroxylase deficiency can be confirmed in equivocal cases by documenting stimulated levels of 17-hydroxyprogesterone greater than 1000 to 1500 ng/dL (30.3 to 45.5 nmol/L) 30 to 60 minutes after ACTH stimulation.

Historically, dexamethasone (Answer A) (or other glucocorticoids) was used as first-line therapy for managing hirsutism in women with nonclassic CAH. While glucocorticoids suppress serum androgens more than combined estrogen-progestin contraceptives, oral contraceptives (Answer C) are more effective for reducing hirsutism as measured by Ferriman-Gallwey scores and this is the best option to manage this patient's oligomenorrhea and hirsutism.

Although metformin (Answer B) has not been systematically studied in women with nonclassic CAH, it could help restore ovulatory cycles. However, it is ineffective for treating hirsutism. Spironolactone (Answer D), an androgen receptor antagonist, can be added after 6 months if the improvement in her hirsutism in suboptimal. Spironolactone should not be used as monotherapy unless reliable contraception is used; if a patient inadvertently uses spironolactone during early pregnancy, there is a potential risk that a male fetus could become feminized.

EDUCATIONAL OBJECTIVE
Recommend the best treatment of nonclassic congenital adrenal hyperplasia.

REFERENCE(S)

Martin KA, Anderson RR, Chang J, et al. Evaluation and treatment of hirsutism in premenopausal women: an Endocrine Society clinical practice guideline. *J Clin Endocrinol Metab.* 2018;103(4):1233-1257. PMID: 29522147

Krone N, Rose IT, Willis DS, et al; United Kingdom Congenital Adrenal Hyperplasia Adult Study Executive (CaHASE). Genotype-phenotype correlation in 153 adult patients with congenital adrenal hyperplasia due to 21-hydroxylase deficiency: analysis of the United Kingdom Congenital Adrenal Hyperplasia Adult Study Executive (CaHASE) cohort. *J Clin Endocrinol Metab.* 2013;98(2):E346-E354. PMID: 23337727

Finkielstain GP, Kim MS, Sinaii N, et al. Clinical characteristics of a cohort of 244 patients with congenital adrenal hyperplasia. *J Clin Endocrinol Metab.* 2012;97(12):4429-4438. PMID: 22990093

Speiser PW, Azziz R, Baskin LS, et al; Endocrine Society. Congenital adrenal hyperplasia due to steroid 21-hydroxylase deficiency: an Endocrine Society clinical practice guideline [published correction appears in *J Clin Endocrinol Metab.* 2010;95(11):5137]. *J Clin Endocrinol Metab.* 2010;95(9):4133-4160. PMID: 20823466

9. ANSWER: B) Combined estrogen-progestin contraceptive

The best option in this healthy, 45-year-old perimenopausal woman at low risk for venous thromboembolism is a continuous low-dosage oral contraceptive (Answer B). It will provide contraception, as well as relief of her hot flashes and night sweats. In addition, it will suppress her hypothalamic-pituitary-ovarian axis (thereby controlling her cycles and bleeding). The 20-mcg oral contraceptives were originally developed for this population—they can be continued until the age of menopause if needed or desired. The rationale for giving the oral contraceptive in a continuous rather than cyclic regimen is to prevent hot flashes during the placebo week or pill-free interval.

The transdermal low-dosage estradiol patch and oral micronized progesterone (Answer A) is a possibility, but the estrogen dosage is low and may not relieve her symptoms. In addition, in a perimenopausal woman, continuous administration of progestin is likely to result in persistent breakthrough bleeding. A cyclic progestin regimen would be preferred. A levonorgestrel-releasing intrauterine device (Answer C) would manage her bleeding, but the gabapentin would not be nearly as effective as estrogen for her hot flashes. Medroxyprogesterone (Answer D) would provide some control of her bleeding, but no relief of her hot flashes.

EDUCATIONAL OBJECTIVE
Identify the best treatment options in a peri-menopausal woman with severe hot flashes (in the late transition).

REFERENCE(S)
Stuenkel CA, Davis SA, Gompel A, et al. Treatment of symptoms of the menopause: an Endocrine Society clinical practice guideline. *J Clin Endocrinol Metab*. 2015;100(11):3975-4011. PMID: 26444994

The NAMS 2017 Hormone Therapy Position Statement Advisory Panel. The 2017 hormone therapy position statement of The North American Menopause Society. *Menopause*. 2017;24(7):728-753. PMID: 28650869

Taylor HS, Manson JE. Update in hormone therapy use in menopause. *J Clin Endocrinol Metab*. 2011;96(2):255-264. PMID: 21296989

10 **ANSWER: D) Cardiac MRI**
Turner syndrome occurs in 1 in 2500 live births and is associated with growth failure, pubertal delay, and cardiac abnormalities. Current recommendations include comprehensive cardiovascular evaluation by a cardiology specialist, consisting of echocardiography in infants and children and MRI (Answer D) in older girls and women. Other initial testing should include renal ultrasonography; TSH to screen for autoimmune thyroiditis; screening for celiac disease and diabetes mellitus; and hearing, orthodontic, and psychosocial evaluations. Cardiac MRI is the most important test because congenital cardiac abnormalities are present in up to 50% of patients, and include coarctation of the aorta, bicuspid aortic valve, and partial anomalous pulmonary venous return. Cardiac MRI follow-up is recommended on a routine schedule based on the presence of abnormalities at baseline, as well as the aortic severity index.

There is no need to perform transvaginal ultrasonography (Answer A) unless Y-chromosomal material is present, in which case ultrasonography would be needed to assess for the risk of gonadoblastoma (5% to 30%). Patients with Turner syndrome are at increased risk for diabetes and screening (Answer B) is indicated, but cardiac MRI is the most important and urgent test to perform. Patients with Turner syndrome have an increased risk of autoimmune thyroid disease, but appropriate screening would be TSH and thyroid antibody assessment, not thyroid ultrasonography (Answer C).

EDUCATIONAL OBJECTIVE
Recommend appropriate evaluation for girls with gonadal dysgenesis.

REFERENCE(S)
Gravholt CH, Andersen NH, Conway GS, et al; International Turner Syndrome Consensus Group. Clinical practice guidelines for the care of girls and women with Turner syndrome: proceedings from the 2016 Cincinnati International Turner Syndrome Meeting. *Eur J Endocrinol*. 2017;177(3):G1-G70. PMID: 28705803

Davenport ML. Approach to the patient with Turner syndrome. *J Clin Endocrinol Metab*. 2010;95(4):1487-1495. PMID: 20375216

Ross JL, Quigley CA, Cao D, et al. Growth hormone plus childhood low-dose estrogen in Turner's syndrome. *N Engl J Med*. 2011;364(13):1230-1242. PMID: 21449786

Pinsker JE. Clinical review: Turner syndrome: updating the paradigm of clinical care. *J Clin Endocrinol Metab*. 2012;97(6):994-1003. PMID: 22472565

11 **ANSWER: D) Testosterone cypionate, 200 mg intramuscularly every 2 weeks**
Recently revised guidelines are available from the Endocrine Society for the treatment of persons with gender dysphoria/gender incongruence. Experts suggest evaluation by a mental health professional to confirm the diagnosis and ensure that any other mental health issues, if present, are well controlled. Traditionally, male dosages of intramuscular testosterone (Answer D) are administered to suppress the hypothalamic-pituitary-ovarian axis and menses and to induce virilization.

Medroxyprogesterone (Answer A) would suppress estrogen levels but would not facilitate masculinization. GnRH analogue therapy (Answer B) may be administered monthly or every 3 months depending on the formulation to induce and maintain complete suppression of the hypothalamic-pituitary-ovarian axis, and then low-dosage hormone therapy can be used; however, testosterone gel (25 mg daily) would be inadequate. Although use of a GnRH agonist is the most physiologic approach, this regimen is quite costly and is not available in many centers. DHEA at a dosage of 100 mg twice daily (Answer C) is a pharmacologic dosage of the prohormone, but it would not be enough to inhibit menses. In addition, it is not regulated in the United States, so dosage consistency is a problem. Also, spironolactone is an antiandrogen and is used for cross-gender hormone therapy in transgender females, not transgender males.

EDUCATIONAL OBJECTIVE
Recommend endocrine treatment options for masculinization in female-to-male transsexual patients.

REFERENCE(S)

Hembree WC, Cohen-Kettenis PT, Gooren L, et al. Endocrine treatment of gender-dysphoric/gender-incongruent persons: an Endocrine Society clinical practice guideline. *J Clin Endocrinol Metab*. 2017;102(11):3869-3903. PMID: 28945902

Spack NP. Management of transgenderism. *JAMA*. 2013;309(5):478-484. PMID: 23385274

Newfield E, Hart S, Dibble S, Kohler L. Female-to-male transgender quality of life. *Qual Life Res*. 2006;15(9):1447-1457. PMID: 16758113

Deutsch MB, Feldman JL. Updated recommendations from the world professional association for transgender health standards of care. *Am Fam Physician*. 2013;87(2):89-93. PMID: 23317072

12 ANSWER: A) Serum total testosterone
This patient is phenotypically female, with excellent breast development but an absent uterus and high LH and FSH levels. This is the presentation of a patient with complete androgen insensitivity syndrome, and the best next diagnostic test in addition to ordering karyotype analysis is to measure her serum testosterone level (Answer A). In androgen insensitivity syndrome, an individual with a 46,XY karyotype presents with a female phenotype because testosterone is unable to activate its receptor. This is confirmed by the absence of a cervix, as the mullerian ducts are needed for development of the upper one-third of the vagina, cervix, uterus, and fallopian tubes. The testosterone level distinguishes androgen insensitivity syndrome from the even more rare congenital absence of the uterus and vagina, (mullerian agenesis), which would present with absent menarche but normal pubertal development because of normal ovarian function. In androgen insensitivity syndrome, pubic and axillary hair is sparse because of lack of androgen in combination with estrogen action. Aromatization of testosterone in peripheral tissues results in high estrogen as well. Individuals with complete androgen insensitivity syndrome function as phenotypic females, although they are unable to bear children. The testes are often located in the groin and should be removed because of the potential for tumor formation (2%-5%).

Measuring estradiol (Answer B) would also be useful because it would be high-normal, but it would not give a definitive diagnosis. Measuring 17-hydroxyprogesterone (Answer C) is indicated in the evaluation of nonclassic congenital adrenal hyperplasia, which presents like polycystic ovary syndrome with oligomenorrhea and hyperandrogenic symptoms. Serum dihydrotestosterone (Answer D) can be useful in the diagnosis of 5α-reductase deficiency, but it would be less helpful in this clinical setting.

EDUCATIONAL OBJECTIVE
Review the differential diagnosis of primary amenorrhea associated an absent uterus and blind vaginal pouch.

REFERENCE(S)

Hughes IA, Davies JD, Bunch TI, Pasterski V, Mastroyannopoulou K, MacDougall J. Androgen insensitivity syndrome. *Lancet*. 2012;380(9851):1419-1428. PMID: 22698698

Tadokoro-Cuccaro R, Hughes IA. Androgen insensitivity syndrome. *Curr Opin Endocrinol Diabetes Obes*. 2014;21(6):499-503. PMID: 25354046

13 ANSWER: C) Oral contraceptive containing norethindrone

Contraception in women with polycystic ovary syndrome should be targeted not only to protect against unplanned pregnancy, but also to control the metabolic and hyperandrogenic phenotype (eg, an estrogen-progestin oral contraceptive [Answer C]). An intrauterine device is a consideration, but the levonorgestrel-releasing intrauterine device (Answer A) will not help her hyperandrogenism. There have been case reports of hair loss with this intrauterine device that are reversible with removal of the device. Increasing the metformin dosage will not provide any additional benefit for hirsutism, as no dosage has been found to be beneficial.

Oral contraceptives with a progestin associated with low venous thromboembolic risk such as norethindrone or levonorgestrel are preferred over those that may be associated with higher risk (such as third-generation progestins [eg, desogestrel, gestodene]). All oral contraceptives have an equivalent beneficial effect on hirsutism, using Ferriman-Gallwey scores as the patient-important outcome. Adding spironolactone (Answer B) or finasteride (Answer D) in a patient who is using barrier contraception is not optimal. Both drugs, if given inadvertently during early pregnancy, can cause feminization of a male fetus. Barrier contraception does not provide adequate pregnancy protection compared with an oral contraceptive.

EDUCATIONAL OBJECTIVE
Differentiate among contraceptive options for women with polycystic ovary syndrome.

REFERENCE(S)
Martin KA, Anderson RR, Chang RJ, et al. Evaluation and treatment of hirsutism in premenopausal women: an Endocrine Society clinical practice guideline. *J Clin Endocrinol Metab.* 2018 [Epub ahead of print] PMID: 29522147

Buzney E, Sheu J, Buzney C, Reynolds RV. Polycystic ovary syndrome: a review for dermatologists: Part II. Treatment. *J Am Acad Dermatol.* 2014;71(5):859.e1-859.e15. PMID: 25437978

Legro RS, Arslanian SA, Ehrmann DA, et al; Endocrine Society. Diagnosis and treatment of polycystic ovary syndrome: an Endocrine Society clinical practice guideline. *J Clin Endocrinol Metab.* 2013;98(12):4565-4592. PMID: 24151290

14 ANSWER: B) Pregnancy

It is always critical to exclude pregnancy (Answer B) in a woman of childbearing age who presents with irregular menses or amenorrhea. Pregnancy can be detected by an elevated serum hCG value before the time of a missed menses or in a urine pregnancy test soon afterward. During early pregnancy, the estrogen level rises and suppresses the gonadotropins.

The pattern of high LH, low FSH, and normal estradiol is seen in many women with polycystic ovary syndrome (Answer A). The extremely high estradiol and high prolactin rule out polycystic ovary syndrome. A patient with a prolactinoma (Answer C) would present with low FSH, low LH, and low estradiol because prolactin suppresses hypothalamic GnRH secretion. A high FSH, high LH, and low estradiol would be seen in a patient with primary ovarian insufficiency (Answer D).

EDUCATIONAL OBJECTIVE
Identify the laboratory changes seen in an amenorrheic patient who is pregnant.

REFERENCE(S)
Mesian S. The endocrinology of human pregnancy and fetoplacental neuroendocrine development. In: Strauss JF, Barbieri RL, eds. *Yen & Jaffe's Reproductive Endocrinology: Physiology, Pathophysiology, and Clinical Management.* 6th ed. Philadelphia, PA: Saunders; 2009:249-281.

15 ANSWER: C) Intrauterine adhesions (Asherman syndrome)

In the evaluation of amenorrhea, one considers whether the problem is due to a hormonal or mechanical problem, and then assesses the locus of the defect. This young woman had normal menarche and was able to conceive. She has no signs of hyperandrogenism. The most likely cause of her amenorrhea is intrauterine adhesions (Asherman syndrome) (Answer C) related to vigorous curettage of the endometrial lining after a miscarriage or with endometrial ablation.

Hyperprolactinemia due to mild thyroid dysfunction, medications, or tumors can suppress hypothalamic GnRH secretion and present as amenorrhea. However, in these situations, estradiol would be low (eg, 20 pg/mL rather than 70 pg/mL). A prolactinoma (Answer A) would be associated with elevated prolactin and low estradiol. Excessive stress, exercise, and low weight can result in amenorrhea (known as functional hypothalamic amenorrhea). However, functional hypothalamic amenorrhea (Answer B) would be associated with low estradiol. Primary ovarian insufficiency (Answer D) would be associated with high FSH and LH and low estradiol. In addition, the patient would most likely be experiencing hot flashes.

EDUCATIONAL OBJECTIVE
Determine the most likely cause of amenorrhea in a woman with normal hormone levels.

REFERENCE(S)
Zupi E, Centini G, Lazzeri L. Asherman syndrome: an unsolved clinical definition and management. *Fertil Steril.* 2015;104(6):1380-1381. PMID: 26484781

16 **ANSWER: B) Start escitalopram, 10 mg daily**

This patient has hot flashes and perimenopausal depression. Her hot flashes are now relieved with estrogen therapy, but she continues to have mood symptoms. Approximately 40% to 50% of perimenopausal women experience depression and/or anxiety symptoms during the menopausal transition. The symptoms are responsive to estrogen, but many women need both estrogen and an antidepressant (a selective serotonin reuptake inhibitor) (Answer B).

It is unlikely that a further increase in the estrogen dosage (Answer A) will help her mood symptoms since she has reached the therapeutic dosage for her hot flashes. An oral contraceptive (Answer C) is unlikely to be more helpful for her mood. Lastly, cognitive behavioral therapy (Answer D) has not been well studied in this population.

EDUCATIONAL OBJECTIVE
Identify and treat depression during the menopausal transition.

REFERENCE(S)
Stuenkel CA, Davis SA, Gompel A, et al. Treatment of symptoms of the menopause: an Endocrine Society clinical practice guideline. *J Clin Endocrinol Metab.* 2015;100(11):3975-4011. PMID: 26444994

Gordon JL, Girdler SS. Hormone replacement therapy in the treatment of perimenopausal depression. *Curr Psychiatry Rep.* 2014;16(12):517. PMID: 25308388

17 **ANSWER: D) No testing required**

Women older than 45 years who present with characteristic menopausal signs and symptoms are more likely to be in the menopausal transition than to have a new endocrine problem such as hyperprolactinemia or thyroid disease. Pregnancy must always be ruled out, but her hCG was negative. Although she has no hot flashes, her poor sleep and musculoskeletal symptoms are very suggestive of perimenopause, as these symptoms occur in up to 40% to 50% of women during the transition. While most perimenopausal women's sleep disturbances are related to hot flashes, others have poor sleep because of new-onset primary sleep disorders. Depression and anxiety can also contribute. Therefore, for women older than 45 years who present with irregular menstrual cycles with menopausal symptoms such as hot flashes, mood changes, joint aches, or sleep disturbances, biochemical evaluation or imaging is not necessary to make the diagnosis. Thus, no further testing is required (thus, Answer D is correct and Answers A, B, and C are incorrect). In fact, serum FSH measurement can be misleading because it is often normal (if measured after an ovulation or when serum estradiol is high). An endocrine evaluation should be performed for women younger than 45 years who present with oligomenorrhea, with or without menopausal symptoms.

EDUCATIONAL OBJECTIVE
Guide the evaluation and diagnosis of the menopausal transition.

REFERENCE(S)

Harlow SD, Gass M, Hall JE, et al; STRAW + 10 Collaborative Group. Executive summary of the Stages of Reproductive Aging Workshop + 10: addressing the unfinished agenda of staging reproductive aging. *J Clin Endocrinol Metab.* 2012;97(4):1159-1168. PMID: 22344196

Randolph JF Jr, Crawford S, Dennerstein L, et al. The value of follicle-stimulating hormone concentration and clinical findings as markers of the late menopausal transition. *J Clin Endocrinol Metab.* 2006;91(8):3034-3040. PMID: 16720656

18 ANSWER: B) Hysterectomy with bilateral oophorectomy

This 70-year-old woman has severe hyperandrogenism causing virilization (clitoromegaly) and endometrial hyperplasia due to peripheral conversion of androgens to estrogen. She has an extremely high testosterone level that is most likely due to an androgen-secreting ovarian or adrenal tumor. The negative adrenal CT and lack of coexisting hypercortisolism makes it most likely to be an ovarian source. Therefore, this patient should undergo a hysterectomy with bilateral oophorectomy (Answer B).

Some clinicians mistakenly assume that such a patient could be monitored with serial imaging (Answer A) if there is not a visible tumor on initial studies. However, with a testosterone level this high, a normal adrenal CT, and no evidence of hypercortisolism, she has an ovarian tumor and needs surgery. In premenopausal women who have not completed childbearing, the goal is to identify the affected ovary and perform unilateral oophorectomy. Ovarian venous sampling (Answer C) is a difficult procedure, and results are not reliable (it successfully predicts the side of the tumor in only about 60% of cases). In addition, in a 70-year-old patient, the potential risk of a sampling procedure outweighs moving forward with bilateral oophorectomy. A free testosterone concentration (Answer D) is neither necessary nor helpful.

EDUCATIONAL OBJECTIVE
Recommend the best management option for severe postmenopausal hyperandrogenism.

REFERENCE(S)

Outwater EK, Marchetto B, Wagner BJ. Virilizing tumors of the ovary: imaging features. *Ultrasound Obstet Gynecol.* 2000;15(5):365-371. PMID: 10976475

Demidov VN, Lipatenkova J, Vikhareva O, Van Holsbeke C, Timmerman D, Valentin L. Imaging of gynecological disease (2): clinical and ultrasound characteristics of Sertoli cell tumors, Sertoli-Leydig cell tumors and Leydig cell tumors. *Ultrasound Obstet Gynecol.* 2008;31(1):85-91. PMID: 18098335

19 ANSWER: D) No treatment necessary

No treatment is necessary for this patient now (Answer D), because it appears that she is recovering from her functional hypothalamic amenorrhea. Her laboratory values are consistent with a recent ovulation (she appears to be in the mid to late luteal phase and will have a period soon). The serum progesterone level of 7 ng/mL (22.3 nmol/L) confirms that she has ovulated. Progesterone levels are also high in pregnancy, but they are considerably higher than 7 ng/mL. Serum LH and FSH vary across the cycle, but are relatively low in the late luteal phase (just before the important small rise in serum FSH that is responsible for the recruitment of the cohort of follicles for the subsequent menstrual cycle). Serum estradiol concentrations peak just before the midcycle surge, but there is also a secondary rise in the luteal phase that corresponds with the rise in serum progesterone (both hormones secreted by the corpus luteum).

If there were no evidence of recovery, the next step would be to start a physiologic dosage of estrogen (Answer A), rather than a pharmacologic dosage (Answer C). Bisphosphonates (Answer B) should not be given in this setting. The best option is to reassure her that she is recovering and is likely to have a period.

EDUCATIONAL OBJECTIVE
Identify a postovulatory pattern of gonadotropin and gonadal steroid levels.

REFERENCE(S)

Perkins RB, Hall JE, Martin KA. Aetiology, previous menstrual function and patterns of neuro-endocrine disturbance as prognostic indicators in hypothalamic amenorrhoea. *Hum Reprod.* 2001;16(10):2198-2205. PMID: 11574516

Filicori M, Santoro N, Merriam GR, Crowley WF Jr. Characterization of the physiological pattern of episodic gonadotropin secretion throughout the human menstrual cycle. *J Clin Endocrinol Metab.* 1986;62(6):1136-1144. PMID: 3084534

20 ANSWER: B) Improved nutrition and weight gain

Evidence suggests that recovery of normal bone metabolism requires nutritional improvement, causing bone formation, and activation of the hypothalamic-pituitary-ovarian axis, decreasing bone resorption. The best strategy to improve bone density is to increase caloric intake, reduce exercise activity, or both (Answer B). This strategy should be tried before prescribing pharmacologic therapy. Physiologic estrogen (Answer A) could then be tried if improved nutrition was not successful. Oral contraceptive doses of estrogen (Answer C) are pharmacologic and not recommended for improving bone density in these patients. Bisphosphonates (Answer D) would not be used in this population.

EDUCATIONAL OBJECTIVE

Identify the best management strategy for patients with functional hypothalamic amenorrhea and low bone mineral density (osteoporosis).

REFERENCE(S)

Dominguez J, Goodman L, Sen Gupta S, et al. Treatment of anorexia nervosa is associated with increases in bone mineral density, and recovery is a biphasic process involving both nutrition and return of menses. *Am J Clin Nutr.* 2007;86(1):92-99. PMID: 17616767

Gordon CM, Ackerman KE, Berga SL, et al. Functional hypothalamic amenorrhea: an Endocrine Society clinical practice guideline. *J Clin Endocrinol Metab.* 2017;102(5):1413-1439. PMID: 28368518

Male Reproduction Board Review

Frances J. Hayes, MD • Massachusetts General Hospital

1 **ANSWER: A) Arrange for a sleep study**
Testosterone esters, including enanthate and cypionate, have been used for the treatment of male hypogonadism for more than 7 decades. They have the advantage of being the least expensive of the testosterone replacement modalities and they predictably restore testosterone levels to the normal range. However, they have unfavorable pharmacokinetics characterized by significant fluctuation in serum testosterone between peak and trough values. When administered by a deep intramuscular injection, testosterone is slowly released from this oily suspension into the circulation over a period of weeks. The esters are typically injected at 2-week intervals with levels reaching peak concentrations 24 to 48 hours after the injection followed by a gradual decline to the low-normal range before the next injection is due. When the interval between injections is extended to every 3 weeks, peak concentrations tend to be supraphysiologic and testosterone levels may fall to the hypogonadal range by the time the next injection is administered. Such wide excursions in serum testosterone concentrations can, in turn, cause undesirable swings in mood, libido, and energy levels. Given the pharmacokinetics of testosterone esters, they also tend to increase hematocrit more than transdermal testosterone preparations, especially when high dosages are given at less frequent intervals.

Increasing the testosterone dosage (Answer D) in a patient whose hematocrit is already high is not appropriate, especially given that the patient's testosterone level is in the desired range for a trough level (namely, the lower end of the normal range).

The pharmacokinetics of testosterone cypionate are similar to those of testosterone enanthate. Hence, switching esters (Answer B) will not address his problem.

Before initiating testosterone therapy, baseline hematocrit should be measured. Baseline hematocrit greater than 48% (and greater than 50% for men living at higher altitudes) is a relative contraindication to testosterone therapy because these men are more likely to develop a hematocrit level greater than 54% when treated with testosterone. The baseline hematocrit of 50% for this hypogonadal, nonsmoking patient is high. The Endocrine Society clinical practice guidelines recommend that the underlying cause of erythrocytosis be investigated before androgen therapy is prescribed. Given the patient's obesity and history of daytime somnolence, the possibility of obstructive sleep apnea should be considered and a sleep study should be arranged (Answer A).

Occasionally, phlebotomy (Answer C) may be necessary for testosterone therapy to be continued in a hypogonadal patient, but it is important to exclude other cause of erythrocytosis such as sleep apnea or chronic obstructive pulmonary disease before doing so.

EDUCATIONAL OBJECTIVE
Describe the pharmacokinetics of injectable testosterone esters and manage potential adverse effects.

REFERENCE(S)
Bhasin S, Brito JP, Cunningham GR, et al. Testosterone therapy in men with hypogonadism: an Endocrine Society clinical practice guideline. *J Clin Endocrinol Metab.* 2018;103(5):1715-1744. PMID: 29562364

Dobs AS, Meikle AW, Arver S, Sanders SW, Caramelli KE, Mazer NA. Pharmacokinetics, efficacy, and safety of a permeation-enhanced testosterone transdermal system in comparison with bi-weekly injections of testosterone enanthate for the treatment of hypogonadal men. *J Clin Endocrinal Metab.* 1999;84(10):3469-3478. PMID: 10522982

2 ANSWER: D) Refer him to a urologist

The diagnosis of hypogonadism made by the patient's primary care physician is correct based on the presence of symptoms of hypogonadism in association with 2 low morning testosterone levels. The issue at hand is whether the patient is an appropriate candidate for testosterone replacement. While the patient is eager to initiate testosterone therapy in the hope of improving his symptoms, it is the physician's responsibility to ensure that he is an appropriate candidate and that the risk-to-benefit ratio favors treatment. The Endocrine Society clinical practice guidelines recommend that clinicians assess prostate cancer risk in men being considered for testosterone therapy. As a general rule, it is recommended that patients who have a palpable prostate nodule or induration or PSA level greater than 4.0 ng/mL (>4.0 µg/L) need further urologic evaluation before testosterone therapy is initiated. However, in subgroups of men considered to be at increased risk for prostate cancer, such as African American patients or men with a first-degree relative with prostate cancer, the baseline PSA level at which referral to a urologist is recommended is greater than 3.0 ng/mL (>3.0 µg/L). Thus, in this man whose father had prostate cancer and who has 2 baseline PSA measurements greater than 3.0 ng/mL (>3.0 µg/L), referral to a urologist (Answer D) is the best next step in his management. Should findings from this urologic workup be reassuring, one could then proceed with testosterone replacement (Answer B).

While phosphodiesterase inhibitors (Answer A) would most likely help the patient's erectile dysfunction, they would not be an appropriate choice in this case as their use is contraindicated in patients taking nitrates given the risk of severe hypotension with this drug combination.

Testosterone therapy is not recommended in patients with untreated severe obstructive sleep apnea. However, this patient's sleep apnea is being treated with continuous positive airway pressure and appears to be well controlled based on the absence of daytime somnolence and the fact that his hematocrit is not elevated. Therefore, arranging a sleep study (Answer C) in a patient with an established diagnosis of obstructive sleep apnea and no symptoms would not yield any additional information.

EDUCATIONAL OBJECTIVE
List indications for urologic evaluation before initiating testosterone therapy.

REFERENCE(S)

Bhasin S, Brito JP, Cunningham GR, et al. Testosterone therapy in men with hypogonadism: an Endocrine Society clinical practice guideline. *J Clin Endocrinol Metab.* 2018;103(5):1715-1744. PMID: 29562364

Wittert G. The relationship between sleep disorders and testosterone. *Curr Opin Endocrinol Diabetes Obes.* 2014;21(3):239-243. PMID: 24739309

3 ANSWER: B) Refer him to a urologist

Although this patient's PSA level remains within the reference range and he has no lower urinary tract symptoms, he should be referred for urologic evaluation (Answer B) on the basis of the magnitude of its change. PSA levels are known to fluctuate in an individual and also have considerable test-retest variability. However, an increase of greater than 1.4 ng/mL (1.4 µg/L) (confirmed by a repeated test) over the course of a year in a man on testosterone therapy cannot be attributed to random variation alone. A systematic review of prostate risk during testosterone therapy found that the average increase in PSA after initiation of testosterone therapy is 0.3 ng/mL and 0.44 ng/mL in young and old men, respectively. A cutoff of 1.4 ng/mL has been adopted on the basis of the findings of a clinical trial that evaluated the effectiveness of finasteride vs placebo on lower urinary tract symptoms and prostate volume in men with benign prostatic hyperplasia. In that study, the upper limit of the 90% confidence interval for the change in PSA level in the placebo arm was 1.4 ng/mL (1.4 µg/L). Hence, on the basis of the findings of the finasteride study and the fact that the average increase in PSA levels on testosterone therapy is less than 0.5 ng/mL (0.5 µg/L) (regardless of patient age), the Endocrine Society's clinical practice guidelines recommend that patients with a PSA increase of greater than 1.4 ng/mL during testosterone therapy should be referred for urologic consultation. It is important to understand that this increase of 1.4 ng/mL in PSA concentration does not indicate prostate cancer, but only serves as a trigger for further evaluation. Simply providing reassurance and scheduling a follow-up visit without any action is inappropriate (Answer C).

This patient has experienced symptomatic improvement on his current testosterone dosage, and his on-treatment testosterone concentration is normal. Therefore, discontinuing treatment (Answer A) is not indicated at this time. Although this patient has an enlarged prostate on rectal examination, he does not have lower urinary tract symptoms. Therefore, treatment with a 5α-reductase inhibitor (Answer D) is not indicated.

EDUCATIONAL OBJECTIVE
Outline the appropriate prostate monitoring for middle-aged and older patients receiving testosterone replacement.

REFERENCE(S)
Bhasin S, Brito JP, Cunningham GR, et al. Testosterone therapy in men with hypogonadism: an Endocrine Society clinical practice guideline. *J Clin Endocrinol Metab.* 2018;103(5):1715-1744. PMID: 29562364

4 ANSWER: C) Reevaluate his hypothalamic-pituitary-gonadal axis in 6 to 12 months
Although the incidence of pituitary dysfunction after traumatic brain injury varies widely in published studies, it appears that pituitary dysfunction occurs commonly in men who experience moderate to severe traumatic brain injury. Low GH and testosterone concentrations are the most common abnormalities. However, it is unclear whether treatment with GH and/or testosterone is beneficial. Furthermore, longitudinal follow-up has demonstrated that many men recover function of these axes 3 to 12 months after the traumatic brain injury. In this man who appears to be recovering well from his brain injury, the best option is to reassess his gonadal axis 6 to 12 months after the initial injury (Answer C).

Treatment with hCG (Answer A) would raise his testosterone concentrations and stimulate spermatogenesis; however, he does not wish to start a family for at least 1 year so there is no urgency in starting treatment until it is clear that his hypothalamic-pituitary-gonadal axis has not recovered. Given that his libido is already beginning to improve and he has no problem with erections,

there is no indication to start testosterone (Answer B). A phosphodiesterase inhibitor (Answer D) would not be appropriate for a patient with low libido but normal erectile function.

EDUCATIONAL OBJECTIVE
Counsel a patient regarding the time course of secondary hypogonadism following traumatic brain injury.

REFERENCE(S)
Schneider HJ, Schneider M, Saller B, et al. Prevalence of anterior pituitary insufficiency 3 and 12 months after traumatic brain injury. *Eur J Endocrinol.* 2006;154(2):259-265. PMID: 16452539

Tanriverdi F, Senyurek H, Unluhizarci K, Selcuklu A, Casanueva FF, Kelestimur F. High risk of hypopituitarism after traumatic brain injury: a prospective investigation of anterior pituitary function in the acute phase and 12 months after trauma. *J Clin Endocrinol Metab.* 2006;91(6):2105-2111. PMID: 16522687

5 ANSWER: B) Low gonadotropins and low SHBG
This patient has glucocorticoid-induced hypogonadism. Glucocorticoid therapy in men can decrease serum testosterone levels because of combined effects on reduced GnRH secretion, as well as a direct effect on testosterone production from the testes. There is an inverse relationship between the dosage of glucocorticoids and serum testosterone levels, but in general, prednisone dosages of 7.5 mg daily or higher result in testosterone suppression. Glucocorticoid-induced suppression of gonadal hormones can occur as early as 3 days after initiating therapy. Although both primary and secondary forms of hypogonadism have been described, most studies report low or inappropriately normal gonadotropin levels in association with low serum testosterone, indicating a predominantly central process. Prednisone also lowers SHBG levels. Therefore, Answer B with low gonadotropins and low SHBG is the hormone profile most likely to characterize this patient's hypogonadism. The pattern in Answer A is incorrect because of the high SHBG level, and the patterns in Answers C and D are incorrect because they depict a predominantly gonadal defect.

Explain the suppressive effects of glucocorticoids on the hypothalamic-pituitary-gonadal axis in men.

REFERENCE(S)

Reid IR, Ibbertson HK, France JT, Pybus J. Plasma testosterone concentrations in asthmatic men treated with glucocorticoids. *Br Med J (Clin Res Ed)*. 1985;291(6495):574. PMID: 2931151

MacAdams MR, White RH, Chipps BE. Reduction of serum testosterone levels during chronic glucocorticoid therapy. *Ann Intern Med*. 1986;104(5):648-651. PMID: 3083749

6 ANSWER: A) Measure free testosterone

This patient's clinical presentation with decreased libido, erectile dysfunction, and fatigue is highly suggestive of hypogonadism. His physical examination also reveals gynecomastia. Despite this, 2 total testosterone values, both measured by liquid chromatography tandem mass spectrometry, are in the high-normal range. In such clinical scenarios, where the clinical phenotype is incongruent with biochemical results, clinicians should consider alterations in SHBG levels as a potential explanation. Certain clinical conditions are associated with elevated serum SHBG levels, including aging, liver disease, hyperthyroidism, medications (anticonvulsant drugs, estrogen), and HIV infection.

Thus, in cases such as this where the history is suggestive of hypogonadism and the patient has a disorder (in this case hepatitis) that is known to impact SHBG levels, measurement of free testosterone (Answer A) is required to diagnose androgen deficiency. Reliable methods of free testosterone measurement include (1) measurement by equilibrium dialysis (considered the gold standard, but is not routinely available in commercial laboratories); and (2) calculated free testosterone (derived from total testosterone and SHBG measurements using law of mass action equations). This patient's free testosterone level (measured by equilibrium dialysis) was low at 48 pg/mL (1.7 nmol/L) because of a markedly elevated SHBG level of 20.0 µg/mL (178 nmol/L), allowing a diagnosis of hypogonadism to be confirmed.

Referring this patient for psychiatric evaluation (Answer D) without taking further diagnostic steps would be inappropriate. Men with partial androgen insensitivity syndrome resulting from mutations in the gene encoding the androgen receptor (Answer C) can also present with symptoms and signs of hypogonadism in association with an elevated serum testosterone level. However, patients with partial androgen insensitivity syndrome tend to have additional clinical manifestations, including perineoscrotal hypospadias and infertility. Importantly, gonadotropin levels in such patients are elevated due to impaired testosterone negative feedback, unlike the gonadotropin profile of patients with HIV infection who typically have secondary hypogonadism. Epitestosterone is a biologically inactive 17-epimer of testosterone that is co-secreted by the Leydig cells of the testes. The urinary testosterone-to-epitestosterone ratio (Answer B) is measured in the evaluation of men suspected of androgen abuse. However, exogenous use of testosterone by this patient would be associated with suppressed gonadotropin levels.

EDUCATIONAL OBJECTIVE
Identify the biochemical profile of men with liver disease who experience alterations in the concentration of serum SHBG.

REFERENCE(S)

Bhasin S, Brito JP, Cunningham GR, et al. Testosterone therapy in men with hypogonadism: an Endocrine Society clinical practice guideline. *J Clin Endocrinol Metab*. 2018;103(5):1715-1744. PMID: 29562364

7 ANSWER: C) Adrenal hypoplasia congenita

The development of primary adrenal insufficiency in a patient with idiopathic hypogonadotropic hypogonadism should raise suspicion for adrenal hypoplasia congenita (Answer C), an X-linked recessive disease due to mutations in the *NR0B1* gene (also known as *DAX1*). The age at presentation and the severity of adrenal insufficiency are variable. Although adrenal insufficiency is most often diagnosed in childhood (some cases even presenting in the neonatal period), some patients present during adulthood (as in this vignette). Mutations in the *NR0B1* gene affect function of all levels of the hypothalamic-pituitary-gonadal axis, as well as the adrenal glands. There is a broad phenotypic spectrum for males with adrenal hypoplasia congenita. Unlike most patients with idiopathic hypogonadotropic hypogonadism, those with adrenal hypoplasia congenita fail to initiate spermatogenesis when treated with gonadotropin therapy due to the concomitant testicular defect.

Patients with partial hypopituitarism (Answer A) could present with hypogonadotropic hypogonadism and adrenal insufficiency but the latter would be secondary as opposed to primary. Autoimmune polyglandular endocrine deficiency syndromes (Answer B) could cause primary adrenal insufficiency but associated hypogonadism would be primary rather than secondary. Kallmann syndrome (Answer D) is the association of hypogonadotropic hypogonadism with anosmia. It is not the correct diagnosis for this patient as he has a normal sense of smell and it does not cause primary adrenal insufficiency.

EDUCATIONAL OBJECTIVE
Describe the clinical and biochemical presentation of adrenal hypoplasia congenita.

REFERENCE(S)
Jadhav U, Harris RM, Jameson JL. Hypogonadotropic hypogonadism in subjects with DAX1 mutations. *Mol Cell Endocrinol.* 2011;346(1-2):65-73. PMID: 21672607

Lin L, Achermann JC. Inherited adrenal hypoplasia: not just for kids! *Clin Endocrinol (Oxf).* 2004;60(5):529-537. PMID: 15104553

Reutens AT, Achermann JC, Ito M, et al. Clinical and functional effects of mutations in the DAX-1 gene in patients with adrenal hypoplasia congenita. *J Clin Endocrinol Metab.* 1999;84(2):504-511. PMID: 10022408

8 ANSWER: D) Serum prolactin measurement
This patient has secondary hypogonadism (low serum testosterone and inappropriately normal gonadotropin levels). Given that his testes are adult sized and he is normally virilized, he has acquired secondary hypogonadism after the onset of puberty. The differential diagnosis of postpubertal secondary hypogonadism includes a pituitary macroadenoma, Cushing syndrome, hyperprolactinemia, opioid use, and iron-overload syndromes (including hemochromatosis). Given the frequency with which hyperprolactinemia can cause hypogonadotropic hypogonadism, prolactin should be measured (Answer D) in all men with secondary hypogonadism.

In this patient, measurement of 24-hour urinary free cortisol (Answer A) is not indicated because of the absence of any features to suggest glucocorticoid excess (normal weight and blood pressure, no striae or evidence of proximal myopathy). The major indication for karyotype analysis in men with hypogonadism is to confirm a diagnosis of Klinefelter syndrome, the most common genetic cause of primary hypogonadism. Given that this patient does not have primary hypogonadism, screening for Klinefelter syndrome by karyotyping (Answer B) is not indicated.

Urine epitestosterone measurement (Answer C) is a test for exogenous testosterone abuse. Epitestosterone is produced by the testes, and the testosterone-to-epitestosterone ratio is elevated in patients who are taking exogenous testosterone. This patient is not abusing anabolic steroids as is evident from his physical examination and the fact that his gonadotropins are normal, not suppressed.

EDUCATIONAL OBJECTIVE
Measure prolactin in the evaluation of men with secondary hypogonadism.

REFERENCE(S)
Schlechte JA. Clinical impact of hyperprolactinaemia. *Baillieres Clin Endocrinol Metab.* 1995;9(2):359-366. PMID: 7625989

Bhasin S, Brito JP, Cunningham GR, et al. Testosterone therapy in men with hypogonadism: an Endocrine Society clinical practice guideline. *J Clin Endocrinol Metab.* 2018;103(5):1715-1744. PMID: 29562364

9 ANSWER: C) MRI of the sella
This patient has prepubertal hypogonadism as evidenced by his failure to develop secondary sexual characteristics or an increase in testicular size. Laboratory tests show profound secondary hypogonadism with otherwise normal pituitary function and prolactin levels. His presentation is thus consistent with idiopathic hypogonadotropic hypogonadism. However, before a definitive

diagnosis of idiopathic hypogonadotropic hypogonadism can be made, structural abnormalities in the hypothalamus or pituitary must be excluded. Therefore, MRI of the sella (Answer C) should be the next step in his evaluation.

Once a diagnosis of congenital hypogonadotropic hypogonadism has been made, targeted genetic testing can be considered. In the last decade, considerable advances have been made in unraveling the genetic basis of congenital hypogonadotropic hypogonadism and to date, mutations have been identified in approximately 40% of cases. While in familial cases the mode of inheritance can be used to guide genetic testing, most cases of congenital hypogonadotropic hypogonadism are actually sporadic, as in the patient described in this vignette. However, a careful clinical evaluation can be helpful in prioritizing genetic testing. In an analysis of 219 patients with Kallmann syndrome, the following clinical features were highly associated with specific gene defects: synkinesia (*KAL1*), dental agenesis (*FGF8/FGFR1*), digital bony abnormalities (*FGF8/FGFR1*), and hearing loss (*CHD7*). In this case, genetic testing for a *KAL1* mutation (Answer A) would not be the appropriate next step, as the diagnosis of idiopathic hypogonadotropic hypogonadism has not yet been confirmed. In any case, this patient would not be expected to harbor a *KAL1* mutation given his normal sense of smell, absence of cleft lip or palate, and absence of mirror movements.

A GnRH stimulation test (Answer B) would not be helpful, as it does not reliably differentiate among various etiologies of secondary hypogonadism, and even patients with a hypothalamic defect, as in this case, may not mount a gonadotropin response on initial exposure to stimulation with GnRH. Measurement of free testosterone (Answer D) would not provide any further insight in a patient who has eunuchoidism and prepubertal total testosterone levels.

EDUCATIONAL OBJECTIVE
Guide the appropriate workup in a patient with secondary hypogonadism.

REFERENCE(S)
Palmert MR, Dunkel L. Clinical practice. Delayed puberty. *N Engl J Med.* 2012;366(5):443-453. PMID: 22296078

Hayes FJ, Seminara SB, Crowley WF Jr. Hypogonadotropic hypogonadism. *Endocrinol Metab Clin North Am.* 1998;27(4):739-763. PMID: 9922906

Young J. Approach to the male patient with hypogonadotropic hypogonadism. *J Clin Endocrinol Metab.* 2012;97(3):707-718. PMID: 22392951

Costa-Barbosa FA, Balasubramanian R, Keefe KW, et al. Prioritizing genetic testing in patients with Kallmann syndrome using clinical phenotypes. *J Clin Endocrinol Metab.* 2013;98(5):E943-E953. PMID: 23533228

10 ANSWER: A) Measurement of transferrin saturation

This patient has secondary hypogonadism (symptoms and/or signs of hypogonadism, low serum testosterone, and low or inappropriately normal gonadotropin levels). Considering that his testes are adult size and he is normally virilized, one can conclude he has acquired secondary hypogonadism after the onset of puberty. The differential diagnosis of postpubertal, acquired secondary hypogonadism includes pituitary macroadenomas, Cushing syndrome, hyperprolactinemia, opioid use, and iron overload syndromes such as hemochromatosis. Hand arthralgias, chondrocalcinosis, hyperpigmentation, and secondary hypogonadism are the earliest manifestations of iron overload syndromes. In men, hereditary hemochromatosis often causes these sequelae in the third and fourth decades. Later in the disease course, patients may experience heart failure, cirrhosis, and diabetes mellitus. Acquired forms of iron overload syndromes (eg, due to multiple transfusions) also may cause disease earlier. Hemochromatosis is inherited in an autosomal recessive manner and has a prevalence of about 0.4% in populations of northern European descent, but it has much lower clinical penetrance, and disease severity is highly variable. Mutations in the *HFE* gene are responsible, and the most common genotype is homozygosity for the Cys282Tyr (C282Y) mutation. Assessment of transferrin saturation (Answer A) is the most useful initial test for hemochromatosis; a transferrin saturation less than 45% is enough to exclude the diagnosis. In the appropriate clinical setting, C282Y homozygosity suffices to diagnose hemochromatosis, but liver biopsy with iron staining remains the criterion standard for diagnosis.

Opioid abuse (Answer B) is a possibility in this man given his occupation and resultant access to opioids. However, opioids do not cause chondrocalcinosis and arthralgias. Cushing syndrome can be excluded as the etiology of secondary hypogonadism in this patient on the basis of his history and physical examination. Therefore, screening for Cushing syndrome with a dexamethasone suppression test (Answer C) is not indicated. Serial dilution of serum (Answer D) is done to assess for the "hook" effect when measuring prolactin in patients with marked hyperprolactinemia. This is unlikely in this man who has normal sellar imaging.

EDUCATIONAL OBJECTIVE
Diagnose hemochromatosis as a cause of secondary hypogonadism.

REFERENCE(S)

Bhasin S, Brito JP, Cunningham GR, et al. Testosterone therapy in men with hypogonadism: an Endocrine Society clinical practice guideline. *J Clin Endocrinol Metab*. 2018;103(5):1715-1744. PMID: 29562364

McDermott JH, Walsh CH. Hypogonadism in hereditary hemochromatosis. *J Clin Endocrinol Metab*. 2005;90(4):2451-2455. PMID: 15657376

Moyer TP, Highsmith WE, Smyrk TC, Gross JB Jr. Hereditary hemochromatosis: laboratory evaluation. *Clin Chim Acta*. 2011;412(17-18):1485-1492. PMID: 21510925

van Bokhoven MA, van Deursen CT, Swinkels DW. Diagnosis and management of hereditary haemochromatosis. *BMJ*. 2011;342:c7251. PMID: 21248018

11   ANSWER: D) Serum total testosterone measurement in 3 months

Severe systemic illness suppresses the hypothalamic-pituitary-gonadal axis and results in a hormonal profile of secondary hypogonadism. Testing for hypogonadism should ideally be done at a time representative of an individual's baseline health status. Measurement of serum testosterone and

gonadotropins should generally not be done in men with acute illness or an acute flare of chronic illness. For this man who was recently hospitalized for an exacerbation of chronic obstructive pulmonary disease, the best course of action would be to repeat the assessment of his gonadal access when he has fully recovered from the acute flare and he has returned to his baseline health (Answer D).

Serum iron studies (Answer B) and serum prolactin measurement (Answer C) are not indicated until hypogonadism has been confirmed, which is not the case here. Younger men with secondary hypogonadism should be tested for iron overload. The diagnostic value of assessing iron saturation in older men with secondary hypogonadism is much lower because most older men with hemochromatosis tend to present with cirrhosis or heart failure, not isolated hypogonadotropic hypogonadism. Assessment for hyperprolactinemia should be performed in all men with secondary hypogonadism. Free testosterone (Answer A) is helpful in diagnosing hypogonadism in situations where an altered SHBG level is suspected; however, this patient does not have any conditions that one would expect to alter SHBG concentrations.

EDUCATIONAL OBJECTIVE
Identify severe systemic illness as a cause of reversible suppression of the gonadal axis.

REFERENCE(S)

Bhasin S, Brito JP, Cunningham GR, et al. Testosterone therapy in men with hypogonadism: an Endocrine Society clinical practice guideline. *J Clin Endocrinol Metab*. 2018;103(5):1715-1744. PMID: 29562364

12   ANSWER: D) hCG and FSH injections

The 3 key elements of this case are: 1) the patient has secondary as opposed to primary hypogonadism; 2) the cause of his central defect is a pituitary rather than a hypothalamic lesion; and 3) his hypogonadism is congenital rather than acquired. In men with primary hypogonadism, fertility options are typically limited to assisted reproductive techniques such as intracytoplasmic sperm injection, use of donor sperm, or adoption. In contrast, men who have infertility due to secondary hypogonadism can have spermatogenesis induced with hormonal therapy in the form of either exogenous gonadotropins (hCG +/− FSH) or GnRH. Therefore, this patient with hypogonadotropic hypogonadism is an appropriate candidate for medical therapy, so intracytoplasmic sperm injection (Answer B) is incorrect.

The site of the defect in the hypothalamic-pituitary-gonadal axis dictates which form of medical therapy is most appropriate to stimulate spermatogenesis in a given patient. GnRH (Answer A) is administered subcutaneously through a portable infusion pump every 120 minutes. This therapy stimulates the gonadotrope cells of the anterior pituitary to make LH and FSH, which in turn, stimulate the testes to make testosterone and sperm. Thus, an intact pituitary gland is a prerequisite for GnRH to be effective in inducing spermatogenesis, so this option is incorrect for a patient who has hypopituitarism. By contrast, gonadotropin therapy is effective in patients with both pituitary and hypothalamic disease because gonadotropins act directly on the testes.

Gonadotropin therapy to induce spermatogenesis consists of subcutaneous administration of hCG alone (Answer C) or in combination with FSH (Answer D). hCG bears strong structural homology to LH, and acting through the LH receptor on Leydig cells it causes an increase in both intratesticular and systemic testosterone production. In men who become hypogonadal after normal puberty has been completed and thus have normal testicular size, treatment with hCG alone is adequate to stimulate spermatogenesis. However, patients who have congenital hypogonadotropic hypogonadism and prepubertal testes (<4 mL) need combination therapy with both hCG and FSH to stimulate growth of the seminiferous tubules. Thus, in this patient with congenital hypogonadism and 3-mL testes, combination therapy with hCG and FSH is correct.

EDUCATIONAL OBJECTIVE
Recommend appropriate treatment to restore fertility in a man with congenital hypogonadotropic hypogonadism.

REFERENCE(S)
Burris AS, Rodbard HW, Winders SJ, Sherins RJ. Gonadotropin therapy in men with isolated hypogonadotropic hypogonadism: the response to human chorionic gonadotropin is predicted by initial testicular size. *J Clin Endocrinal Metab.* 1988;66(6):1144-1151. PMID: 3372679

King TF, Hayes FJ. Long-term outcome of idiopathic hypogonadotropic hypogonadism. *Curr Opin Endocrinol Diabetes Obes.* 2012;19(3):204-210. PMID: 22499222

13 ANSWER: D) Sperm cryopreservation before chemotherapy

After 1 year of follow-up, azoospermia is seen in 90% of men with Hodgkin lymphoma who are treated with more than 3 courses of chemotherapy that includes an alkylating agent. In many of these patients, semen analysis is abnormal even before treatment and only approximately 30% of patients meet traditional criteria for sperm cryopreservation for intrauterine insemination. Nevertheless, cryopreservation of sperm (Answer D) remains the most reliable option for preserving male fertility in men about to undergo gonadotoxic chemotherapy with cyclophosphamide. Cryopreservation of human sperm does not decrease its capability for fertilization, and studies have demonstrated successful pregnancies with cryopreserved sperm. Optimal semen collection procedures for cryopreservation include obtaining at least 3 samples after abstinence for a minimum of 48 hours.

Leydig cells are less sensitive to the gonadal toxicity of chemotherapeutic agents than the germinal epithelium, which is why testosterone levels are generally preserved as in this vignette. While aromatase inhibitors (Answer A) can increase testosterone levels by blocking estrogen negative feedback leading to an increase in LH, increasing testosterone further within the normal range does not help preserve spermatogenesis.

Infertility related to chemotherapy is due to loss of spermatogonial stem cells, and the recovery of spermatogenesis occurs via recolonization of the seminiferous tubules by these stem cells. Currently, cryopreservation and subsequent transplant of spermatogonial stem cells (Answer C) is considered experimental.

It has been hypothesized that hormonal suppression and the resulting disruption of gametogenesis renders the gonad less sensitive to damage by the cytotoxic drugs. However, in clinical trials, hormonal suppression with GnRH agonists (Answer B) has not been shown to reliably afford gonadal protection, and its use has led to recovery of spermatogenesis in only 20% of patients.

EDUCATIONAL OBJECTIVE
Recommend the best strategy for fertility preservation in a man about to undergo treatment for Hodgkin lymphoma.

REFERENCE(S)
Howell SJ, Shalet SM. Spermatogenesis after cancer treatment: damage and recovery. *J Natl Cancer Inst Monogr*. 2005;34:12-17. PMID: 15784814

Jahnukainen K, Ehmcke J, Hou M, Schlatt S. Testicular function and fertility preservation in male cancer patients. *Best Pract Res Clin Endocrinol Metab*. 2011;25(2):287-302. PMID: 21397199

Levine J, Canada A, Stern CJ. Fertility preservation in adolescents and young adults with cancer. *J Clin Oncol*. 2010;28(32):4831-4841. PMID: 20458029

14 ANSWER: A) Y-Chromosome microdeletion

This patient has nonobstructive azoospermia based on a normal semen volume and presence of fructose in the ejaculate. He has normal LH and testosterone levels indicating normal Leydig-cell function but has an elevated FSH level due to lack of negative feedback from undetectable inhibin B indicating a selective defect in the seminiferous tubule compartment of the testis. This presentation is most likely due to a microdeletion in the Y-chromosome (Answer A), the second most common genetic cause of male infertility after Klinefelter syndrome. The male-specific region on the long arm of the Y chromosome has a locus known as the azoospermia factor (AZF) that contains genes needed for spermatogenesis. This AZF locus contains 3 regions: AZFa, AZFb, and AZFc. Deletions of the entire AZFa region result in complete atrophy of the tubular compartment, with only Sertoli cells seen on testicular biopsy, making

retrieval of sperm for intracytoplasmic sperm injection virtually impossible. Large deletions in the AZFb region also result in Sertoli-cell–only syndrome. Mutations in the AZFc region are the most common and account for 80% of Y-chromosome microdeletions. AZFc deletions are compatible with residual spermatogenesis, with oligospermia being a common presentation. These men may be candidates for intracytoplasmic sperm injection. Infertile men who do not have obstructive azoospermia, hypogonadotropic hypogonadism, or a karyotype abnormality should be tested for Y-chromosome microdeletions.

This patient does not have Klinefelter syndrome (Answer B) given his normal karyotype. Mutations in the *KISS1R* gene (Answer C) result in Kallmann syndrome, a condition characterized by congenital hypogonadotropic hypogonadism in association with anosmia or hyposmia. This patient's history of normal puberty, normal testes size, and elevated FSH levels are not consistent with this condition. Mutations in the cystic fibrosis transmembrane conductance regulator gene (*CFTR*) are a relatively frequent cause of infertility in men with obstructive azoospermia and are associated with congenital bilateral absence of the vas deferens. However, given that his vas deferens is palpable and that he has normal semen volume and fructose in the ejaculate, a *CFTR* mutation (Answer D) would not explain his presentation.

EDUCATIONAL OBJECTIVE
Recognize the presentation of Y-chromosome microdeletions and outline the differential diagnosis of nonobstructive azoospermia.

REFERENCE(S)
Vogt PH, Edelmann A, Kirsch S, et al. Human Y chromosome azoospermia factors (AZF) mapped to different subregions in Yq11. *Hum Mol Genet*. 1996;5(7):933-943. PMID: 8817327

Pryor JL, Kent-First M, Muallem A, et al. Microdeletions in the Y chromosome of infertile men. *N Engl J Med*. 1997;336(8):534-539. PMID: 9023089

Stahl PJ, Schlegel PN. Genetic evaluation of the azoospermic or severely oligozoospermic male. *Curr Opin Obstet Gynecol*. 2012;24(4):221-228. PMID: 22729088

15 ANSWER: B) Arrange for transrectal ultrasonography

The vas deferens is normally palpable as a thin ropelike structure within the spermatic cord. In this case, imaging using transrectal ultrasonography (Answer B) confirmed the clinical suspicion of bilateral absence of the vas deferens. This patient turned out to have a mutation in the *CFTR* gene, which is associated with cystic fibrosis. Congenital absence of the vas deferens, without the typical pulmonary and pancreatic manifestations of cystic fibrosis, is associated with compound heterozygosity for a classic (severe) *CFTR* mutation and a mild *CFTR* mutation. Given the autosomal recessive mode of inheritance of cystic fibrosis, screening of the female partner and genetic counseling are key components of the patient's management to determine the risk of transmitting this gene to offspring or of having a child with cystic fibrosis. When the records of his semen analyses were retrieved, they were consistent with an obstructive cause of azoospermia as evidenced by an ejaculate volume of 1 mL, absent fructose, and low pH (normal >7.2). The patient's initial low testosterone could be explained by his obesity and was not low enough to cause azoospermia.

Adding FSH injections (Answer A) would not be appropriate given his normal testicular size and endogenous FSH levels. Increasing his hCG dosage (Answer C) would not be appropriate given that his testosterone level is already near the upper end of the normal range. Clomiphene citrate (Answer D) would not be effective in a patient with obstructive azoospermia. Even in men with hypogonadotropic hypogonadism, clomiphene is not an approved medication to stimulate spermatogenesis and can have negative effects on bone health, libido, and body fat.

EDUCATIONAL OBJECTIVE
Explain the association between congenital bilateral absence of the vas deferens and infertility.

REFERENCE(S)

Anawalt BD. Approach to male infertility and induction of spermatogenesis. *J Clin Endocrinol Metab*. 2013;98(9):3532-3542.

Kolettis PN. The evaluation and management of the azoospermic patient. *J Androl*. 2002;23(3):293-305.

Finkelstein JS, Lee H, Burnett-Bowie SA, et al. Gonadal steroids and body composition, strength, and sexual function in men. *N Engl J Med*. 2013;369(11):1011-1022.

16 ANSWER: B) Klinefelter syndrome

On a statistical basis, the most common cause of congenital primary gonadal failure is Klinefelter syndrome (Answer B), which has an incidence of approximately 1 in 600. There is wide variability in the phenotypic spectrum depending largely on the degree of mosaicism. However, gynecomastia and small testes, as described in this vignette, are common presenting features. Gonadotropin concentrations are invariably elevated (FSH > LH) in men with Klinefelter syndrome (and other causes of primary hypogonadism) because of impaired negative feedback by both sex steroids and inhibin B. Most patients have testosterone values in the low-normal range or just below the lower end of normal. SHBG concentrations tend to be elevated in affected men because of increased estrogen production rates. Given that 98% or more of circulating testosterone is protein bound, the free testosterone fraction tends to be disproportionately lower than the total testosterone concentration in men with Klinefelter syndrome. The diagnosis is confirmed by obtaining a karyotype, which shows a 47,XXY pattern in more than 80% of cases. The karyotype of the patient in this vignette showed 47,XXY/46,XY mosaicism, which explains why his testes are larger than those in many patients with Klinefelter syndrome and why his testosterone level is still in the normal range.

Inactivating mutations in the gene encoding the FSH receptor (Answer A) are a rare cause of primary gonadal failure. Men harboring such mutations present with small testes and elevated FSH levels such as in the case described. However, unlike this patient, they have normal testosterone and LH levels and do not develop gynecomastia.

17α-Hydroxylase deficiency (Answer C) is a rare form of congenital adrenal hyperplasia that causes decreased production of glucocorticoids and sex steroids and increased synthesis of mineralocorticoid precursors due to loss-of-function mutations in the *CYP17* gene. Males with this disorder are undervirilized. The appearance of the external genitalia ranges from normal female to ambiguous to mildly underdeveloped male. The most commonly described phenotype is a small phallus, perineal hypospadias, and intra-abdominal or inguinal testes. Most patients with this disorder are hypertensive. The fact that the patient described in the vignette has scrotal testes with a normal phallus, no hypospadias, and normal blood pressure rules out this condition.

The incidence of mumps orchitis (Answer D) has declined dramatically since the introduction of the childhood vaccination program. However, in situations where parents decide not to have their children vaccinated, outbreaks of mumps can still occur. Orchitis is the most common complication of mumps in postpubertal men, affecting about 20% to 30% of cases. Thirty to fifty percent of affected testicles show some degree of atrophy. Mumps-associated orchitis results in severe pain, swelling, and tenderness at the affected site and is often associated with high fever, nausea, vomiting, and abdominal pain.

EDUCATIONAL OBJECTIVE
Construct the differential diagnosis of primary hypogonadism.

REFERENCE(S)
Groth KA, Skakkebæk A, Høst C, Gravholt CH, Bojesen A. Clinical review: Klinefelter syndrome--a clinical update. *J Clin Endocrinol Metab*. 2013;98(1):20-30. PMID: 23118429

Tapanainen JS, Aittomäki K, Min J, Vaskivuo T, Huhtaniemi IT. Men homozygous for an inactivating mutation of the follicle-stimulating hormone (FSH) receptor gene present variable suppression of spermatogenesis and fertility. *Nat Genet*. 1997;15(2):205. PMID: 9020851

Braunstein GD. Clinical practice: Gynecomastia. *N Engl J Med*. 2007;357(12):1229-1237. PMID: 17881754

17 ANSWER: C) Referral for surgical consultation

The pathophysiology of gynecomastia involves an imbalance between free estrogen and free androgen actions in the breast tissue. During mid-to-late puberty, relatively more estrogen may be produced by the testes and peripheral tissues before testosterone secretion reaches adult levels, resulting in the gynecomastia that commonly occurs during this period. Most adolescents presenting with isolated gynecomastia have physiologic pubertal gynecomastia, which generally appears at 13 or 14 years of age, lasts for 6 months or less, and then regresses. Although the diagnosis is evident in most cases, a thorough history that includes review of medications, environmental exposures, and illicit drug use and physical examination are necessary. The case described fits the diagnosis of pubertal gynecomastia, but unlike most cases, it has failed to regress and is causing significant psychological distress. Thus, while reassurance and observation (Answer B) constitute the best approach for younger patients with gynecomastia present for less than 1 year, it is not appropriate for this patient. Surgical resection (Answer C) should be considered for adolescents with physiologic gynecomastia that is greater than 4 cm in diameter, has not responded to medical therapy, persists for more than 1 year or after the patient is age 17 years, or is associated with embarrassment that interferes with normal daily activities.

This patient's examination findings do not suggest any features of malignancy such as nipple retraction, discoloration, or serosanguinous discharge. There is also no risk of malignant transformation of the breast tissue in pubertal gynecomastia. Therefore, mammography (Answer A) is not indicated. There is no medication approved by the US FDA for the treatment of pubertal gynecomastia. In general, pharmacologic approaches to gynecomastia are most effective during the phase of active proliferation and thus would not be expected to be beneficial in this patient in whom it has been present for 3 years. Even in adolescents with a short history of gynecomastia, aromatase inhibitors (Answer D) such as anastrozole have not been shown to be beneficial.

EDUCATIONAL OBJECTIVE
Diagnose and manage pubertal gynecomastia.

REFERENCE(S)

Braunstein GD. Clinical practice. Gynecomastia. *N Engl J Med.* 2007;357(12):1229-1237. PMID: 17881754

Guss CE, Divasta AD. Adolescent gynecomastia. *Pediatr Endocrinol Rev.* 2017;14(4):371-377. PMID: 28613047

Plourde PV, Reiter EO, Jou HC, et al. Safety and efficacy of anastrozole for the treatment of pubertal gynecomastia: a randomized, double-blind, placebo-controlled trial. *J Clin Endocrinol Metab.* 2004;89(9):4428-4433. PMID: 15356042

18 ANSWER: D) Testosterone abuse

This patient has tender gynecomastia. Breast tenderness suggests benign breast growth of recent onset (<6 months). He also has a high-normal testosterone concentration, and his high-normal calculated free testosterone concentration confirms that this is not strictly due to high SHBG concentrations, which can be seen in hepatitis and would decrease the free testosterone concentration. He also has high estradiol and low gonadotropin concentrations. This combination can be due to exogenous testosterone use or abuse (Answer D), endogenous or exogenous testosterone precursors (eg, dehydroepiandrosterone from an adrenal tumor), and endogenous or exogenous hCG (eg, hCG from a germ-cell tumor).

Although chronic hepatitis (Answer A) is commonly associated with elevated SHBG concentrations, the calculated free testosterone concentration remains normal unless the patient has underlying hypogonadism, so it would not explain this patient's hormone profile. An estrogen-secreting testicular tumor (Answer B) would cause elevated estradiol concentrations and suppressed gonadotropins but testosterone levels would not be high. Finasteride (Answer C) modestly raises serum testosterone concentrations by blocking the conversion of testosterone to dihydrotestosterone, but it would not cause suppressed gonadotropin concentrations.

EDUCATIONAL OBJECTIVE
Identify the clinical and biochemical features of exogenous testosterone abuse.

REFERENCE(S)

Amory JK, Wang C, Swerdloff RS, et al. The effect of 5alpha-reductase inhibition with dutasteride and finasteride on semen parameters and serum hormones in healthy men [published correction appears in *J Clin Endocrinol Metab.* 2007;92(11):4379]. *J Clin Endocrinol Metab.* 2007;92(5):1659-1665. PMID: 17299062

Braunstein GD. Clinical practice. Gynecomastia. *N Engl J Med.* 2007;357(12):1229-1237. PMID: 17881754

Anawalt BD. Gynecomastia. In: Jameson JL, De Groot LJ, eds. *Endocrinology: Adult and Pediatric.* 7th ed. Philadelphia, PA: Saunders Elsevier; 2015.

19 ANSWER: C) Testosterone plus an androgenic anabolic steroid plus an aromatase inhibitor

High doses of either exogenous testosterone or anabolic steroids suppress gonadotropins, so the degree of gonadotropin suppression does not help to distinguish between the 2 hormone regimens. However, the testosterone level is a useful discriminant, as androgenic anabolic steroids are not detected in a testosterone assay. Therefore, in this case, the patient's high testosterone level means an androgenic anabolic steroid plus an aromatase inhibitor (Answer D) is incorrect. The fact that the patient's estradiol level is low in the presence of a high testosterone level, which serves as the substrate for aromatase, indicates that the patient must also be taking an aromatase inhibitor (thus, Answer B is incorrect). This patient has a very low HDL-cholesterol level. While modest reductions in HDL cholesterol are typically seen with testosterone administration, high dosages of nonaromatizable androgens would be needed to suppress HDL cholesterol to 5 mg/dL, which is why Answer C, rather than Answer A, is correct.

EDUCATIONAL OBJECTIVE
Highlight the different hormonal profiles associated with testosterone and androgenic anabolic steroid use.

REFERENCE(S)

Pope HG Jr, Wood RI, Rogol A, Nyberg F, Bowers L, Bhasin S. Adverse health consequences of performance-enhancing drugs: an Endocrine Society scientific statement. *Endocr Rev.* 2014;35(3):341-375. PMID: 24423981

20 ANSWER: B) Start a GnRH agonist with a 0.05-mg estradiol patch

This patient has several risk factors for hypertriglyceridemia-induced pancreatitis, including familial hypertriglyceridemia, poorly controlled diabetes, and oral estrogen therapy. In male-to-female transgender patients, estrogen therapy is needed to develop female sexual characteristics. In patients with an intact hypothalamic-pituitary-gonadal axis, the estrogen dosage needed is supraphysiologic given the need to suppress testosterone secretion. However, combined use of a GnRH agonist with estrogen allows physiologic doses of estrogen to be used as testosterone secretion is already suppressed. Estrogen therapy can result in marked hypertriglyceridemia. However, the lipid effects of estrogen depend on the route of administration, with the transdermal route having less effect on HDL cholesterol and triglycerides than the oral route. Given this patient's history, the most appropriate hormone regimen would be a GnRH agonist and an initial low-dosage estrogen patch (Answer B), which can be titrated based on clinical response and triglyceride levels. Options that include oral estrogen such as conjugated equine estrogen (Answer A) and ethinyl estradiol (Answer D) are incorrect. Ethinyl estradiol has also been shown to increase the risk of venous thromboembolism significantly more than 17β-estradiol.

Given that the patient has been living as a woman for more than 2 decades, as well as the increased risk of depression and suicide in the transgender population, withholding further hormone therapy (Answer C) is likely to negatively affect her mental health. In addition, estrogen therapy was not her only risk factor for hypertriglyceridemia.

EDUCATIONAL OBJECTIVE
Guide the hormonal care of a transgender patient with hypertriglyceridemia.

REFERENCE(S)

Hembree WC, Cohen-Kettenis PT, Gooren L, et al. Endocrine treatment of gender-dysphoric/gender-incongruent persons: an Endocrine Society clinical practice guideline. *J Clin Endocrinol Metab.* 2017;102(11):3869-3903. PMID: 28945902

Aljenedil S, Hegele RA, Genest J, Awan Z. Estrogen-associated severe hypertriglyceridemia with pancreatitis. *J Clin Lipidol.* 2017;11(1):297-300. PMID: 28391900

Lufkin EG, Ory SJ. Relative value of transdermal and oral estrogen therapy in various clinical situations. Mayo Clin Proc. 1994;69(2):131-135. PMID: 8309263

Rosenthal SM. Approach to the patient: transgender youth: endocrine considerations. *J Clin Endocrinol Metab.* 2014;99(12):4379-4389. PMID: 25140398

Thyroid Board Review

Elizabeth N. Pearce, MD, MSc ● Boston University

1 ANSWER: D) Thyroid lobectomy

Nondiagnostic FNAB results describe samples that contain only cyst fluid or in which there are insufficient cells for diagnosis; this occurs in 2% to 16% of FNAB attempts. Repeated FNAB is typically recommended when this occurs, and repeated aspiration is diagnostic 60% to 80% of the time when nodules are not predominantly cystic. The risk of malignancy in repeatedly nondiagnostic nodules with suspicious ultrasonographic features such as irregular margins, taller-than-wide shape, hypoechogenicity, or microcalcifications is approximately 25%, whereas the risk of malignancy is only about 4% in nodules lacking those concerning features.

If this nodule did not have a high-suspicion ultrasonographic pattern, either continued close observation (Answer A) or diagnostic lobectomy (Answer D) would be appropriate options. However, in the presence of both high-suspicion ultrasonographic features and significant nodule growth (20% in at least 2 dimensions), thyroid surgery is the more appropriate choice.

[18]F-fluorodeoxyglucose PET/CT uptake (Answer C) in thyroid nodules confers an increased risk for thyroid cancer (about 33%), but this imaging would not provide a definitive diagnosis. Molecular markers (Answer B) are unlikely to provide additional diagnostic information in the absence of an adequate cellular biopsy. Whether serum calcitonin (Answer E) should be routinely measured in the workup of thyroid nodules remains controversial, but this will not provide a definitive diagnosis in the case. In some studies, core-needle biopsy, an option that was not provided in this vignette, may improve rates of diagnosis in nodules with repeatedly nondiagnostic FNAB.

EDUCATIONAL OBJECTIVE
Manage thyroid nodules that have repeatedly nondiagnostic cytopathology.

REFERENCE(S)

Haugen BR, Alexander EK, Bible KC, et al. 2015 American Thyroid Association management guidelines for adult patients with thyroid nodules and differentiated thyroid cancer: the American Thyroid Association guidelines task force on thyroid nodules and differentiated thyroid cancer. *Thyroid.* 2016;26(1):1-133. PMID: 26462967

Moon HJ, Kwak JY, Choi YS, Kim EK.How to manage thyroid nodules with two consecutive non-diagnostic results on ultrasonography-guided fine-needle aspiration. *World J Surg.* 2012;36(3):586-592. PMID: 22228400

Park CJ, Kim EK, Moon HJ, Yoon JH, Park VY, Kwak JY. Thyroidnodules with nondiagnostic cytologic results: follow-up management using ultrasound patterns based on the 2015 American Thyroid Association Guidelines. *AJR Am J Roentgenol.* 2018;210(2):412-417. PMID: 29091005

2 ANSWER: A) Thyroid hormone therapy with a target TSH level between 0.5 and 2.0 mIU/L

In this vignette, a solitary microcarcinoma was identified at the time of thyroid lobectomy. The patient has no evidence of metastatic disease or aggressive histology. The risk of tumor persistence or recurrence in unifocal, intrathyroidal micropapillary carcinoma (tumor size ≤1 cm) is extremely low—on the order of 1% to 2%. The risk for tumor-related mortality is essentially zero. Thyroid lobectomy provides sufficient treatment. The 2015 American Thyroid Association guidelines on the management of thyroid nodules and thyroid cancer explicitly recommend against the use of radioiodine remnant ablation in this setting because it has not been shown to improve either overall or disease-free survival. Completion thyroidectomy with or without remnant ablation with radioiodine (Answers B and C) is overly aggressive for this clinical circumstance. The guidelines also specifically recommend against ablation of a remaining lobe without completion thyroidectomy in any patient with thyroid cancer (Answer D) because long-term outcomes of this approach are unknown. Levothyroxine therapy with a low-normal TSH target (Answer A) is the best option.

EDUCATIONAL OBJECTIVE
Manage unifocal papillary microcarcinoma.

REFERENCE(S)
Pacini F. Thyroid microcarcinoma. *Best Pract Res Clin Endocrinol Metab*. 2012;26(4):421-429. PMID: 22863385

Haugen BR, Alexander EK, Bible KC, et al. 2015 American Thyroid Association management guidelines for adult patients with thyroid nodules and differentiated thyroid cancer: the American Thyroid Association guidelines task force on thyroid nodules and differentiated thyroid cancer. *Thyroid*. 2016;26(1):1-133. PMID: 26462967

Tarasova VD, Tuttle RM. Current management of low risk differentiated thyroid cancer and papillary microcarcinoma. *Clin Oncol (R Coll Radiol)*. 2017;29(5):290-297. PMID: 28087101

3 **ANSWER: C) Expected changes in euthyroid patients on amiodarone**

Apart from drug-induced hyperthyroidism (5% of treated patients) or hypothyroidism (7%), amiodarone has dramatic effects on thyroid function tests in clinically euthyroid patients. A large iodine load (74 mg total iodine, 7.4 mg of free iodine per 200 mg tablet) is delivered with each dose. Amiodarone inhibits both peripheral and central (intrapituitary) conversion of T_4 to T_3 through its action on type 1 and type 2 5´-monodeiodinase, respectively. Lastly, amiodarone has T_3 antagonistic effects at the nuclear level. The common pattern shown in euthyroid patients is a high free and total T_4, a low-normal T_3, and a high-normal TSH (thus, Answer C is correct). These changes tend to persist over time, although serum TSH values may gradually normalize in some patients.

Amiodarone and its metabolites are not known to cause artifactual interference with thyroid function assays (Answer D). This patient's normal TSH and lack of symptoms exclude thyrotoxicosis (Answers A and B). Also, he is not acutely ill, so euthyroid sick syndrome (Answer E) is incorrect.

EDUCATIONAL OBJECTIVE
Distinguish expected changes in thyroid function parameters in patients taking amiodarone from amiodarone-induced thyroid dysfunction.

REFERENCE(S)
Danzi S, Klein I. Amiodarone-induced thyroid dysfunction. *J Intensive Care Med*. 2015;30(4):179-185. PMID: 24067547

Basaria S, Cooper DS. Amiodarone and the thyroid. *Am J Med*. 2005;118(7):706-714. PMID: 15989900

4 **ANSWER: C) Resistance to TSH**

This patient has the classic features of pseudohypoparathyroidism type 1a (Albright hereditary osteodystrophy). This is an autosomal dominant disorder with a loss-of-function mutation in the *GNAS* gene, which results in the inability to activate adenyl cyclase when PTH is bound to its receptor. Resistance to PTH in the renal tubule causes hyperphosphatemia and hypocalcemia and leads to secondary hyperparathyroidism. In order to manifest pseudohypoparathyroidism type 1a, there must be maternal transmission (individuals with paternal mutations have the phenotype of Albright hereditary osteodystrophy but have normal serum calcium concentrations; this condition is termed "pseudo-pseudohypoparathyroidism"). Because *GNAS* from the maternal allele is expressed in the thyroid, gonads, and pituitary, patients with pseudohypoparathyroidism type 1a are resistant to other G-protein–coupled hormones, including TSH, GnRH, LH, and FSH. This patient's hypothyroidism is most likely due to TSH resistance (Answer C). Such patients typically do not have goiter or detectable TPO antibodies, and peripheral thyroid hormone levels are normal to slightly low. Hashimoto thyroiditis (Answer B) is not the most likely cause of TSH elevation in a patient with pseudohypoparathyroidism type 1a. TSH-secreting pituitary adenoma (Answer D) does not occur in pseudohypoparathyroidism type 1a.

Heterophilic antibody interference with the TSH assay (Answer A) occurs in patients possessing antibodies that recognize the mouse monoclonal antibody used in the sandwich assay for TSH, creating a link between the capture and signal antibodies in the absence of antigen (in this case, TSH). Human antimouse monoclonal antibodies (HAMA) may occur naturally in up to 10% of the general population, and they result in a false elevation of serum TSH. However, in this patient, there is no reason to believe that the TSH elevation is spurious. Defects in thyroid hormone transport (Answer E) involving the monocarboxylate transporter 8 (MCT8) protein are quite rare. Although thyroid hormone was once believed to freely permeate into the intracellular space, it is now known to be actively transported by proteins such as MCT8. Defective MCT8 transport is an X-linked recessive disorder, seen nearly exclusively in males. The phenotype is profound intellectual impairment and congenital hypotonia.

EDUCATIONAL OBJECTIVE
Identify resistance to TSH as the cause of hypothyroidism in pseudohypoparathyroidism type 1a.

REFERENCE(S)

Balavoine AS, Ladsous M, Velayoudom FL, Vlaeminck V, Cardot-Bauters C, d'Herbomez M, Wemeau JL. Hypothyroidism in patients with pseudohypoparathyroidism type Ia: clinical evidence of resistance to TSH and TRH. *Eur J Endocrinol.* 2008 Oct;159(4):431-437. PMID: 18805917

Mantovani G, Elli FM, Corbetta S. Hypothyroidism associated with parathyroid disorders. *Best Pract Res Clin Endocrinol Metab.* 2017;31(2):161-173. PMID: 28648505

5 **ANSWER: E) Continued monitoring for compressive symptoms**

This patient's ultrasound demonstrates a low-risk pattern (an isoechoic solid thyroid nodule with regular margins) and the nodule was benign on FNAB on 2 occasions. The risk of false-negative FNAB results is believed to be less than 3%, and the risk that a nodule will have false-negative results on more than one occasion is very close to zero. The risk of malignancy does not differ in thyroid nodules with low-risk ultrasonographic characteristics that grow compared with low-risk nodules that do not grow. There is no clear rationale for continued ultrasonographic surveillance (Answer C) of nodules with repeatedly benign FNAB and low-risk ultrasonographic characteristics, and certainly no rationale for repeated ultrasound in such a short timeframe. Despite continued nodule growth, the risk of malignancy is very low in this patient and repeated FNAB (Answer B) is not warranted. Core biopsy (Answer D) may be considered in patients with nodules that are repeatedly nondiagnostic on FNAB, but there is no reason to pursue core biopsy in this patient who has had diagnostic results on FNAB. Thyroid lobectomy (Answer A) may ultimately be required if the patient develops compressive symptoms, but he is currently asymptomatic. Continued monitoring for compressive symptoms (Answer E) is reasonable, since such symptoms would prompt consideration of surgery.

EDUCATIONAL OBJECTIVE
Guide the appropriate follow-up of benign thyroid nodules.

REFERENCE(S)

Haugen BR, Alexander EK, Bible KC, et al. 2015 American Thyroid Association management guidelines for adult patients with thyroid nodules and differentiated thyroid cancer: the American Thyroid Association guidelines task force on thyroid nodules and differentiated thyroid cancer. *Thyroid.* 2016;26(1):1-133. PMID: 26462967

Rosário PW, Purisch S. Ultrasonographic characteristics as a criterion for repeat cytology in benign thyroid nodules. *Arq Bras Endocrinol Metabol.* 2010;54(1):52-55. PMID: 20414548

Kim YY, Han K, Kim EK, et al. Validation of the 2015 American Thyroid Association management guidelines for thyroid nodules with benign cytologic findings in the era of the Bethesda system. *AJR Am J Roentgenol.* 2018;210(3):629-634. PMID: 29323546

Bahn RS, Castro MR. Approach to the patient with nontoxic multinodular goiter. *J Clin Endocrinol Metab.* 2011;96(5):1202-1212. PMID: 21543434

6 ANSWER: D) Restoration of ovulatory menstrual cycles

Patient education is important at the time of hypothyroidism diagnosis. Overt hypothyroidism is frequently associated with irregular menses, which should normalize with treatment (Answer D). It is important to counsel this patient that she should avoid pregnancy until the hypothyroidism is well controlled, since overt hypothyroidism is associated with adverse obstetric and fetal outcomes, including miscarriage, stillbirth, gestational hypertension, preterm delivery, low birth weight, and decreased child intelligence.

Contrary to popular opinion, weight loss following initiation of treatment for overt hypothyroidism is modest and is primarily due to diuresis rather than loss of fat mass (Answer A). Restoration of euthyroidism should lead to a rapid decrease in total and LDL-cholesterol levels. However, serum HDL cholesterol (Answer B) is not typically affected by thyroid status. Because hyperlipidemia often resolves with treatment of hypothyroidism and there is a theoretic concern for increased rhabdomyolysis risk when statins are used in the setting of overt hypothyroidism, levothyroxine should be initiated before considering statin therapy in any overtly hypothyroid patient. Overt hypothyroidism is associated with hyperhomocysteinemia, which improves, not worsens (Answer C), with treatment.

Driving simulation studies show that severe hypothyroidism slows reaction times similar to the effects of intoxication; therefore, this patient should be advised to avoid driving until her overt hypothyroidism has resolved.

EDUCATIONAL OBJECTIVE
Educate patients in the setting of newly diagnosed overt hypothyroidism, including counseling regarding the importance of avoiding both driving and conception.

REFERENCE(S)

Chaker L, Bianco AC, Jonklaas J, Peeters RP. Hypothyroidism. *Lancet.* 2017;390(10101):1550-1562. PMID: 28336049

Karmisholt J, Andersen S, Laurberg P. Weight loss after therapy of hypothyroidism is mainly caused by excretion of excess body water associated with

myxoedema. *J Clin Endocrinol Metab.* 2011;96(1):E99-E103. PMID: 20926526

Alexander EK, Pearce EN, Brent GA, et al. 2017 guidelines of the American Thyroid Association for the diagnosis and management of thyroid disease during pregnancy and the postpartum. *Thyroid.* 2017;27(3):315-389. PMID: 28056690

7 ANSWER: B) Ethanol injection of the cyst

Simple cysts are, by definition, benign, and do not require FNAB to exclude malignancy. Fluid reaccumulation after aspiration occurs in 60% to 90% patients with cystic nodules. In controlled studies, percutaneous ethanol injection of a cyst (Answer B) is less likely to result in fluid reaccumulation than simple cyst aspiration (Answer A) and is now considered the first-line therapy. Up to 3 treatments may be required. Adverse effects are relatively minor, but may include local pain and dysphonia. Thyroid function is not affected.

Radiofrequency ablation (Answer C) is relatively new and is not routinely being used in the United States. Studies to date suggest that this is a promising nonsurgical option for reduction of the size of cold or hyperfunctioning solid or mixed solid-cystic nodules, but this is not considered a first-line treatment for a simple cyst because it is more expensive and requires more treatments to achieve the same results as percutaneous ethanol injection. Laser ablation (Answer D) can decrease the size of solid nodules by about 50%, but it does not effectively reduce cyst size. Radioactive iodine therapy (Answer E) would not be expected to affect cyst size and would most likely cause hypothyroidism. Thyroid lobectomy would be a reasonable option, but this patient prefers to avoid surgery.

EDUCATIONAL OBJECTIVE
Explain nonsurgical treatment options for benign nodules with compressive symptoms.

REFERENCE(S)

Gharib H, Hegedüs L, Pacella CM, Baek JH, Papini E. Clinical review: nonsurgical, image-guided, minimally invasive therapy for thyroid nodules. *J Clin Endocrinol Metab.* 2013;98(10):3949-3957. PMID: 23956350

Bennedbaek FN, Hegedüs L. Treatment of recurrent thyroid cysts with ethanol: a randomized double-blind controlled trial. *J Clin Endocrinol Metab*. 2003;88(12):5773-5777. PMID: 14671167

Cesareo R, Palermo A, Pasqualini V, et al. Radiofrequency ablation for the management of thyroid nodules: a critical appraisal of the literature. *Clin Endocrinol (Oxf)*. 2017;87(6):639-648. PMID: 28718950

8 ANSWER: A) Recommend radioactive iodine treatment at least 6 months before pregnancy with normalization of TSH on levothyroxine before conception

Preconception counseling is very important for women with Graves hyperthyroidism and should include a discussion of the risks and benefits of all treatment options and the patient's desired timeline to conception. All of the listed approaches could be appropriate in individual patients, depending on circumstances and the severity of hyperthyroidism. The safety and effectiveness of these approaches have not been directly compared in studies to date.

Methimazole use in pregnancy is associated with a syndrome of fetal anomalies, including dysmorphic facies, choanal or esophageal atresia, abdominal wall defects such as umbilical abnormalities, eye defects, urinary system defects, ventricular septal defects, and aplasia cutis. Recent studies have shown that these complications are more common than previously thought, affecting 2% to 4% of children exposed to methimazole in early pregnancy, especially during gestational weeks 6 through 10. Propylthiouracil was not previously considered teratogenic. However, a recent Danish study demonstrated that 2% to 3% of children exposed to propylthiouracil in utero developed defects, including face cysts, neck cysts, and urinary tract abnormalities (in boys). Although propylthiouracil-associated birth defects appear to be less severe than methimazole-associated birth defects, they are not negligible. If antithyroid drugs are continued until pregnancy is diagnosed, there is still some first-trimester exposure. Infants of women who are switched from methimazole to propylthiouracil during the first trimester (Answer C) are at risk for both types of birth defects. Therefore, Answer A, which is the only approach that would not involve any antithyroid drug exposure in pregnancy, is associated with a lower risk of fetal malformations than Answers B, C, or D. Women who undergo thyroidectomy or radioactive iodine ablation before conception still may have detectable thyroid receptor–stimulating antibodies, which could pose a risk for fetal and neonatal hyperthyroidism.

EDUCATIONAL OBJECTIVE
Counsel women about the teratogenic risks of antithyroid drugs in the first trimester.

REFERENCE(S)

Andersen SL, Olsen J, Wu CS, Laurberg P. Birth defects after early pregnancy use of antithyroid drugs: a Danish nationwide study. *J Clin Endocrinol Metab*. 2013;98(11):4373-4381. PMID: 24151287

Andersen SL, Olsen J, Laurberg P. Antithyroid drug side effects in the population and in pregnancy. *J Clin Endocrinol Metab*. 2016;101(4):1606-1614. PMID: 26815881

Alexander EK, Pearce EN, et al. 2017 guidelines of the American Thyroid Association for the diagnosis and management of thyroid disease during pregnancy and the postpartum. *Thyroid*. 2017;27(3):315-389. PMID: 28056690

9 ANSWER: D) Levothyroxine therapy with a goal TSH between 0.5 and 2.0 mIU/L

This patient's histopathology would formerly have been described as encapsulated follicular variant of papillary thyroid carcinoma, but this has recently been renamed to noninvasive follicular thyroid neoplasm with papillary-like nuclear features (NIFTP). This redefinition was an expert consensus made on the basis of a retrospective review of 109 patients with NIFTP who did not receive radioactive iodine and who were observed for 10 to 26 years; all of these patients were alive without evidence for tumor recurrence at the end of follow-up. Long-term prospective studies have not been performed. NIFTP is currently best understood as a premalignant lesion. It can only be diagnosed based on surgical pathology, when there has been close examination of the entire lesion and tumor capsule. NIFTP is believed to be associated with a very low risk for tumor recurrence. Because this is considered low-risk, completion thyroidectomy with or without radioactive iodine ablation

(Answers A and B) is not warranted. TSH suppressive levothyroxine therapy (Answer C) confers some risks of bone and cardiac toxicity and is unlikely to confer any benefit given the absent recurrence risk in these lesions. Levothyroxine therapy with a low-normal TSH target (Answer D) is the best option. The most appropriate follow-up surveillance strategy is currently unknown, although periodic ultrasonography and serum thyroglobulin assessment can be considered.

EDUCATIONAL OBJECTIVE
Identify noninvasive follicular thyroid neoplasm with papillary-like nuclear features and explain its prognostic implications.

REFERENCE(S)
Nikiforov YE, Seethala RR, Tallini G, et al. Nomenclature revision for encapsulated follicular variant of papillary thyroid carcinoma: a paradigm shift to reduce overtreatment of indolent tumors. *JAMA Oncol.* 2016;2(8):1023-1029. PMID: 27078145

Haugen BR, Sawka AM, Alexander EK, et al. American Thyroid Association guidelines on the management of thyroid nodules and differentiated thyroid cancer task force review and recommendation on the proposed renaming of encapsulated follicular variant papillary thyroid carcinoma without invasion to noninvasive follicular thyroid neoplasm with papillary-like nuclear features. *Thyroid.* 2017;27(4):481-483. PMID: 28114862

Baloch ZW, Harrell RM, Brett EM, Randolph G, Garber JR; AACE Endocrine Surgery Scientific Committee and Thyroid Scientific Committee. American Association of Clinical Endocrinologists and American College of Endocrinology disease state commentary: managing thyroid tumors diagnosed as noninvasive follicular thyroid neoplasm with papillary-like nuclear features. *Endocr Pract.* 2017;23(9):1150-1155. PMID: 28920749

10 ANSWER: D) Oral prednisone, 60 mg daily

Hashimoto encephalopathy, sometimes termed steroid-responsive encephalopathy associated with autoimmune thyroiditis (SREAT), is defined as the presence of antithyroid antibodies in patients with altered mental status who are responsive to corticosteroids. The underlying pathophysiology is unknown, but it is generally assumed that this is a form of autoimmune encephalitis in which antithyroid antibodies serve as a nonspecific marker. The alterations in mental status are not thought to be directly caused by the antithyroid antibodies, and the antibody titer is not related to disease severity. Patients may be positive for either TPO or thyroglobulin antibodies, but most affected patients have both. This is primarily a diagnosis of exclusion; it is important to rule out other causes of dementia. Most patients with this condition are euthyroid, although hypothyroidism and, less commonly, hyperthyroidism have been reported. An improvement in response to high-dosage glucocorticoids (Answer D) is one of the hallmarks of this disorder.

This patient is subclinically hypothyroid. Mild hypothyroidism is not associated with severe cognitive dysfunction. Therefore, treatment with thyroid hormone (Answers A, B, and C) would not be expected to improve her mental status. Although this patient is hypothyroid with altered mental status, she does not have myxedema coma (for which combined high-dosage levothyroxine and liothyronine [Answer A] would be appropriate) based on her mild biochemical hypothyroidism and her lack of bradycardia, hypothermia, or other clinical signs of severe hypothyroidism. SSKI (Answer E) can be used in the treatment of thyroid storm, but there is no role for high-dosage iodine therapy in the treatment of hypothyroidism. Supraphysiologic doses of iodine might induce worsen hypothyroidism in this patient with Hashimoto thyroiditis.

EDUCATIONAL OBJECTIVE
Diagnose and treat steroid-responsive encephalopathy associated with autoimmune thyroiditis (SREAT).

REFERENCE(S)

Laurent C, Capron J, Quillerou B, et al. Steroid-responsive encephalopathy associated with autoimmune thyroiditis (SREAT): Characteristics, treatment and outcome in 251 cases from the literature. *Autoimmun Rev.* 2016;15(12):1129-1133. PMID: 27639840

Samuels MH. Thyroid disease and cognition. *Endocrinol Metab Clin North Am.* 2014;43(2):529-543. PMID: 24891176

11 ANSWER: E) Octreotide

This patient underwent transsphenoidal surgery for a large TSH-secreting pituitary adenoma with invasion of the cavernous sinus. As expected, resection was incomplete and the patient, although improved, is still thyrotoxic. Octreotide therapy (Answer E) has been found to be very useful in this setting, with normalization of thyroid hormone in most patients treated (>70% of patients treated in one study) and tumor size reduction in 20% to 50% of patients. Thyroidectomy (Answer A) and methimazole (Answer B) are not indicated because of the risk of tumor growth in the absence of negative feedback of thyroid hormone. Bromocriptine (Answer C) is not as effective as octreotide therapy in this setting. Triiodothyroacetic acid (TRIAC) (Answer D) is a thyroid hormone analogue that has been used to treat some patients with thyroid hormone resistance, but which would not be an appropriate therapy for TSH-secreting adenoma.

EDUCATIONAL OBJECTIVE
Recommend treatment for secondary hyperthyroidism.

REFERENCE(S)

Beck-Peccoz P, Persani L, Mannavola D, Campi I. Pituitary tumours: TSH-secreting adenomas. *Best Pract Res Clin Endocrinol Metab.* 2009;23(5):597-606. PMID: 19945025

Socin HV, Chanson P, Delemer B, et al. The changing spectrum of TSH-secreting pituitary adenomas: diagnosis and management in 43 patients. *Eur J Endocrinol.* 2003;148(4):433-442. PMID: 12656664

Amlashi FG, Tritos NA. Thyrotropin-secreting pituitary adenomas: epidemiology, diagnosis, and management. *Endocrine.* 2016;52(3):427-440. PMID: 26792794

12 ANSWER: D) Repeat laboratory tests in 3 months

This patient has subclinical hyperthyroidism, most likely due to TSH receptor–stimulating antibodies. Her family history of autoimmune thyroid disease, her own diffuse goiter, and the mildly positive thyroid-stimulating immunoglobulin are all consistent with this etiology. Patients with mild degrees of subclinical hyperthyroidism, particularly when it is due to thyroiditis or mild Graves disease, very often experience spontaneous resolution. Thus, the best course of action for this patient would be to repeat laboratory tests in 3 months (Answer D). Predictors of reversibility include having detectable (albeit subnormal) TSH values and having etiologies other than nodular hyperthyroidism (toxic adenoma or toxic multinodular goiter), such as thyroiditis or mild Graves disease, as is illustrated by the current case. Among patients with subclinical hyperthyroidism, the rate of progression to overt hyperthyroidism is 0.5% to 7% annually. Up to half of patients may spontaneously revert to normal TSH levels over time.

It is premature to start methimazole (Answer A) in this young patient who has a high likelihood of remission, but this could be considered in an elderly patient with similar findings because of the increased risk of arrhythmia, although the dosage of 20 mg daily would be excessive for this situation. This patient does not require atenolol (Answer B) because she is asymptomatic and has a resting pulse rate less than 90 beats/min. Although treatment with radioiodine therapy (Answer C) could be considered, it would most likely result in permanent hypothyroidism, and she may not require therapy at all with further observation.

EDUCATIONAL OBJECTIVE
Describe the natural history of nonnodular causes of subclinical hyperthyroidism.

REFERENCE(S)

Mai VQ, Burch HB. A stepwise approach to the evaluation and treatment of subclinical hyperthyroidism. *Endocr Pract.* 2012;18(5):772-780. PMID: 22784850

Ross DS, Burch HB, Cooper DS, et al. 2016 American Thyroid Association guidelines for diagnosis and management of hyperthyroidism and other causes of thyrotoxicosis. *Thyroid.* 2016;26(10):1343-1421. PMID: 27521067

13   ANSWER: B) Iodine

Patients with underlying nodular autonomy are at risk for the development of hyperthyroidism in response to high levels of iodine exposure (Answer B). The tolerable upper limit for daily iodine intake is 1100 mcg, but some supplements contain amounts greatly in excess of this.

Perchlorate (Answer D) is a competitive inhibitor of thyroidal iodine uptake, and it would be expected to cause hypothyroidism rather than hyperthyroidism. Thyroid hormone (Answer C) is found illegally in some over-the-counter US supplements, but serum thyroglobulin would be expected to be low, rather than elevated, in a patient taking exogenous thyroid hormone. Selenium excess (Answer A) does not cause hyperthyroidism. The use of biotin supplements (Answer E) can cause artifactual interference with commonly used biotin-streptavidin immunoassays for TSH, thyroid hormone, and anti–thyrotropin receptor antibodies. A high-dose biotin supplement could cause assay changes similar to those seen in this patient, but the biotin would not actually be associated with symptomatic hyperthyroidism, or with elevated serum thyroglobulin. High circulating biotin levels cause falsely low measurements in immunometric sandwich assays (such as that for TSH), but falsely high measurements for competitive immunoassays (such as those for free T_4, T_3, and thyroid-stimulating immunoglobulin). Thus, patients taking biotin may have laboratory results identical to those found in Graves hyperthyroidism. Artifactual thyroid function results have been reported in patients taking at least 1500 mcg of biotin daily, and test results normalize 2 to 7 days after stopping the biotin.

EDUCATIONAL OBJECTIVE
Describe potential effects of iodine excess.

REFERENCE(S)

Leung AM, Braverman LE. Consequences of excess iodine. *Nat Rev Endocrinol.* 2014;10(3):136-142. PMID: 24342882

Kang GY, Parks JR, Fileta B, et al. Thyroxine and triiodothyronine content in commercially available thyroid health supplements. *Thyroid.* 2013;23(10):1233-1237. PMID: 23758055

Kummer S, Hermsen D, Distelmaier F. Biotin treatment mimicking Graves' disease. *N Engl J Med.* 2016;375(7):704-706. PMID: 27532849

14   ANSWER: A) Continue current levothyroxine

This patient has had an incomplete biochemical response to therapy for her thyroid cancer, with persistently elevated serum thyroglobulin levels in the absence of localizable disease. Based on the lack of uptake on her most recent posttreatment scan, her disease does not appear to be radioactive iodine-avid and repeated radioiodine therapy (Answer D) is unlikely to be helpful. She has no evidence for measurable structural disease, her disease is not currently symptomatic or progressive, and kinase inhibitor therapy is associated with significant adverse effects; therefore, sorafenib therapy (Answer C) is not warranted at this time. Studies overall demonstrate a survival benefit for TSH-suppressive levothyroxine dosing in patients with high-risk tumors. However, TSH suppression is also associated with increased morbidity and mortality, particularly in patients who are elderly or who have cardiovascular disease, cardiovascular risk factors, or osteoporosis. Of the available options, maintaining a moderate degree of TSH suppression (Answer A) is preferable to complete TSH suppression (Answer B) in this older patient with osteoporosis, whose thyroglobulin has been stable and who does not have known structural disease. It would also be appropriate to consider other bone-protective therapies in this patient, such as calcium, vitamin D, and bisphosphate treatment.

EDUCATIONAL OBJECTIVE

Identify clinical characteristics informing the choice of TSH targets in the long-term follow-up of patients with differentiated thyroid cancer.

REFERENCE(S)

Biondi B, Cooper DS. Benefits of thyrotropin suppression versus the risks of adverse effects in differentiated thyroid cancer. *Thyroid.* 2010;20(2):135-146. PMID: 20151821

Parker WA, Edafe O, Balasubramanian SP. Long-term treatment-related morbidity in differentiated thyroid cancer: a systematic review of the literature. *Pragmat Obs Res.* 2017;8:57-67. PMID: 28553154

Haugen BR, Alexander EK, Bible KC, et al. 2015 American Thyroid Association management guidelines for adult patients with thyroid nodules and differentiated thyroid cancer: the American Thyroid Association guidelines task force on thyroid nodules and differentiated thyroid cancer. *Thyroid.* 2016;26(1):1-133. PMID: 26462967

15 ANSWER: D) Orbital decompression followed by strabismus surgery

This patient has moderately severe Graves ophthalmopathy manifested by proptosis and extraocular muscle dysfunction. In terms of active inflammation as assessed using the clinical activity score, this would be considered inactive and therefore unlikely to respond to immunomodulatory therapy. The clinical activity score assigns 1 point each for spontaneous retroocular eye pain, pain with eye movement, eyelid swelling, eyelid redness, conjunctival redness, conjunctival edema (chemosis), and caruncle edema, for a maximum of 7 points.

Clinical activity scores greater than 3 or 4 suggest active inflammatory disease that will most likely respond to immunomodulatory therapy such as glucocorticoids. Because this patient does not have active inflammatory changes, the primary treatment options are surgical. He will require both orbital decompression surgery to reduce the degree of proptosis and extraocular muscle surgery to correct his dysconjugate gaze (Answer D).

Orbital radiotherapy (Answer A), which may have modest beneficial effects on extraocular eye muscle function, will not relieve his excessive proptosis and it is therefore not the best approach.

Rituximab therapy (Answer B), which leads to B-lymphocyte depletion, has recently been studied in 2 randomized prospective trials (showing net benefit in one trial but not the other), and it would not be expected to provide benefit in the absence of active inflammation. Likewise, corticosteroid therapy (Answer C) would not be expected to be beneficial in this setting. Finally, strabismus surgery alone (Answer E) would not relieve the patient's excessive proptosis, which, in addition to a cosmetic defect, is causing exposure keratitis.

EDUCATIONAL OBJECTIVE

Recommend surgical treatment of inactive Graves ophthalmopathy that is unlikely to respond to immunomodulatory therapy.

REFERENCE(S)

Bartalena L, Tanda ML. Clinical practice. Graves' ophthalmopathy. *N Engl J Med.* 2009;360(10):994-1001. PMID: 19264688

Novaes P, DinizGrisolia AB, Smith TJ. Update on thyroid-associated Ophthalmopathy with a special emphasis on the ocular surface. *Clin Diabetes Endocrinol.* 2016;2:19. PMID: 28702253

[No authors listed]. Classification of eye changes of Graves' disease. *Thyroid.* 1992;2(3):235-236. PMID: 14222347

16 ANSWER: E) Nephrotic syndrome

Nephrotic syndrome (Answer E) is the cause of this patient's progressive increase in levothyroxine dosage requirement, due largely to loss of thyroid-binding proteins (with thyroid hormone still bound) in the urine. Clues to this etiology include her lower-extremity edema, low albumin, and high lipid levels. This case and similar cases have been reported in the literature. In the setting of reversible nephrotic syndrome, levothyroxine dosage requirements return to baseline as the proteinuria resolves. Other sources of unexpected changes in levothyroxine dosage requirements include starting new medications that interfere either with absorption (iron, calcium, and binding resins) or with clearance (phenytoin, phenobarbital, and possibly sertraline) of thyroid hormone, weight gain or loss, and, of course, nonadherence to therapy.

Metformin therapy (Answer A) is associated with slight decrease in serum TSH concentrations in levothyroxine-treated patients. It does not increase the levothyroxine dosage requirement. Although medication nonadherence (Answer B) and celiac disease (Answer C) could both increase the levothyroxine dosage requirement, they would not explain the clinical stigmata of nephrotic syndrome in the vignette. The patient is not acutely ill, so euthyroid sick syndrome (Answer D) does not pertain to this patient, and even if it did, this syndrome does not result in an increased thyroid hormone dosage requirement.

EDUCATIONAL OBJECTIVE
Explain the effect of thyroid-binding protein loss in urine on the thyroid hormone dosage requirement.

REFERENCE(S)
Karethimmaiah H, Sarathi V. Nephrotic syndrome increases the need for levothyroxine replacement in patients with hypothyroidism. *J Clin Diagn Res.* 2016;10(12):OC10-OC12. PMID: 28208903

Halma C. Thyroid function in patients with proteinuria. *Neth J Med.* 2009;67(4):153. PMID: 19581660

Lupoli R, Di Minno A, Tortora A, Ambrosino P, Lupoli GA, Di Minno MN. Effects of treatment with metformin on TSH levels: a meta-analysis of literature studies. *J Clin Endocrinol Metab.* 2014;99(1):E143-E148. PMID: 24203069

17 **ANSWER: A) Sunitinib**
Sunitinib (Answer A) and other tyrosine kinase inhibitors may cause de novo primary hypothyroidism or worsen preexisting primary hypothyroidism. In patients treated with tyrosine kinase inhibitors who do not have preexisting thyroid dysfunction, overt hypothyroidism has been reported in 32% to 85%, and subclinical hypothyroidism has been reported in up to 100%. Transient hyperthyroidism has also been reported to occur in up to 24% of patients treated with tyrosine kinase inhibitors.

Bexarotene (Answer C), which is rarely used for the treatment of late-stage cutaneous T-cell lymphoma, and other retinoic acid X receptors have been associated with severe central hypothyroidism in up to 70% of patients. Effects are reversible with discontinuation of treatment. Other pituitary function is not affected. Denileukin diftitox (Answer B), a recombinant protein that contains both interleukin-2 and fragments of diptheria toxin, is approved for the treatment of cutaneous T-cell lymphoma. It has been associated with thyroiditis. If this patient had recently started denileukindiftitox, thyrotoxicosis rather than hypothyroidism would be expected. Ipilimumab (Answer D), an immune-modulating monoclonal antibody directed against CTLA-4, is used in patients with advanced melanoma. It has been associated with the development of irreversible central hypothyroidism in up to 17% of patients.

EDUCATIONAL OBJECTIVE
Explain the thyroidal effects of drugs used for cancer treatment.

REFERENCE(S)
Graeppi-Dulac J, Vlaeminck-Guillem V, Perier-Muzet M, Dalle S, Orgiazzi J. Endocrine side-effects of anti-cancer drugs: the impact of retinoids on the thyroid axis. *Eur J Endocrinol.* 2014;170(6):R253-R262. PMID: 24616413

Torino F, Barnabei A, Paragliola R, Baldelli R, Appetecchia M, Corsello SM. Thyroid dysfunction as an unintended side effect of anticancer drugs. *Thyroid.* 2013;23(11):1345-1366. PMID: 23750887

18 **ANSWER: E) Heterophilic antibody interference with the TSH assay**
This pattern is typical of heterophilic antibody interference with the TSH assay (Answer E). The interference occurs in patients possessing antibodies that recognize the mouse monoclonal antibody used in the sandwich assay for TSH, creating a link between the capture and signal antibodies in the absence of antigen (in this case, TSH). The human antimouse monoclonal antibodies (HAMA) may occur naturally in up to 10% of the general population (not just laboratory workers with mouse exposure, as was first described), and they result in a false elevation of serum TSH. Preincubation of the patient's serum with nonimmune mouse antibodies is an added step in the assay intended to eliminate the effect of HAMA. Clues to the presence

of HAMA in this case are the unchanged serum TSH despite progressively increasing free T_4 values as the levothyroxine dosage was increased. If the patient were absorbing levothyroxine poorly (Answer A), or were poorly adherent to therapy (Answer D), free T_4 values would not increase with an increasing levothyroxine dosage. If this patient had resistance to thyroid hormone (Answer B), the free T_4 level would have been elevated, rather than normal, at baseline. In a TSH-secreting pituitary adenoma (Answer C) the patient would be expected to be clinically hyperthyroid.

EDUCATIONAL OBJECTIVE
Identify heterophilic antibody interference with the thyrotropin assay.

REFERENCE(S)
SanthanaKrishnan SG, Pathalapati R, Kaplan L, Cobbs RK. Falsely raised TSH levels due to human anti-mouse antibody interfering with thyrotropin assay [published correction appears in *Postgrad Med J*. 2007;83(977):186]. *Postgrad Med J*. 2006;82(973):e27. PMID: 17099084

Ross HA, Menheere PP; Endocrinology Section of SKML (Dutch Foundation for Quality Assessment in Clinical Laboratories), Thomas CM, Mudde AH, Kouwenberg M, Wolffenbuttel BH. Interference from heterophilic antibodies in seven current TSH assays. *Ann Clin Biochem*. 2008;45(Pt 6):616. PMID: 18782812

19 ANSWER: B) Reduce the methimazole dosage

This patient has a history of thyrotoxicosis and is being treated with methimazole. Her thyroid scan from 2 years ago clearly shows a pattern of toxic multinodular goiter. Unlike Graves disease, which may enter a lasting remission after completion of a 12- to 18-month course of antithyroid drug therapy, toxic multinodular goiter will continue to require either medical therapy with low dosages of antithyroid drugs or definitive therapy with radioactive iodine or thyroidectomy. Because the patient is currently biochemically hypothyroid, her methimazole dose should be reduced (Answer B) or definitive therapy should be considered.

There is no reason to perform another scan with radioactive iodine uptake (Answer A) because it is unlikely to have changed. Discontinuing methimazole (Answers C and D) would result in resurgent thyrotoxicosis. The 2016 American Thyroid Association guidelines for the management of hyperthyroidism state that long-term therapy with low-dosage antithyroid drugs is an acceptable option for patients who prefer to avoid definitive therapy, and a recent meta-analysis concluded that long-term antithyroid drug use is safe.

EDUCATIONAL OBJECTIVE
Recommend continued therapy with a low-dosage antithyroid drug in a patient with toxic multinodular goiter and distinguish this approach from that used to treat Graves disease, which may enter remission.

REFERENCE(S)
Ross DS, Burch HB, Cooper DS, et al. 2016 American Thyroid Association guidelines for diagnosis and management of hyperthyroidism and other causes of thyrotoxicosis. *Thyroid*. 2016;26(10):1343-1421. PMID: 27521067

Azizi F, Malboosbaf R. Long-term antithyroid drug treatment: asystematic review and meta-analysis. *Thyroid*. 2017;27(10):1223-1231. PMID: 28699478

20 ANSWER: A) Thyroid hormone resistance

This patient has discordant TSH and free T_4 values, suggesting inappropriate TSH release. The α-subunit-to-TSH molar ratio less than 1.0 favors thyroid hormone resistance (Answer A) rather than a TSH-producing pituitary tumor (Answer B) (pituitary MRI is also normal and most TSH-producing tumors are macroadenomas). The prevalence of thyroid hormone resistance is about 1 in 40,000 live births. Another possible cause is heterophilic antibodies (Answer C), but serial dilutions would not be expected to yield linear results if these were present. T_4 antibodies tend to increase the measured value of free T_4 (thus, Answer D is incorrect). Surreptitious use of thyroid hormone (Answer E) might cause thyrotoxicosis but would not produce this pattern of thyroid function tests or the diffuse goiter.

EDUCATIONAL OBJECTIVE
Identify clinical features of thyroid hormone resistance.

REFERENCE(S)
Ortiga-Carvalho TM, Sidhaye AR, Wondisford FE. Thyroid hormone receptors and resistance to thyroid hormone disorders. *Nat Rev Endocrinol.* 2014;10(10):582-591. PMID: 25135573

Macchia E, Lombardi M, Raffaelli V, et al. Clinical and genetic characteristics of a large monocentric series of patients affected by thyroid hormone (Th) resistance and suggestions for differential diagnosis in patients without mutation of Th receptor β. *Clin Endocrinol (Oxf).* 2014;81(6):921-928. PMID: 25040256

21 ANSWER: A) Figure A

The correct answer to this question is best arrived at by exclusion of the nodules with benign ultrasound appearances. The nodule in Figure B is a simple cyst—a hypoechoic, thin-walled structure with "enhancement," or an increased echo pattern behind it. The nodule in Figure C has a classic spongiform appearance, which has been shown to be very low risk for malignancy. The nodule in Figure D is hyperechoic relative to the surrounding thyroid parenchyma, and it has an intact halo, making it most likely a benign lesion. That leaves the nodule shown in Figure A. This nodule is hypoechoic, has irregular borders, and has visible microcalcifications, which are strongly associated with malignancy.

EDUCATIONAL OBJECTIVE
Identify ultrasound patterns characteristic of malignant nodules.

REFERENCE(S)
Brito JP, Gionfriddo MR, Al Nofal A, et al. The accuracy of thyroid nodule ultrasound to predict thyroid cancer: systematic review and meta-analysis. *J Clin Endocrinol Metab.* 2014;99(4):1253-1263. PMID: 24276450

22 ANSWER: E) Parathyroid cyst

The classic description of parathyroid cyst fluid is clear, colorless liquid containing extremely high PTH levels (Answer E). When such fluid is obtained during biopsy of what appears to be a thyroid nodule, the fluid should be sent for PTH analysis and no further aspirations should be performed. Serum calcium levels may also be elevated if the patient has hyperparathyroidism.

Branchial cleft cysts (Answer A) are located laterally in the neck, and thyroglossal duct cysts (Answer C) are generally located at the midline adjacent to the hyoid bone. Follicular thyroid cancer (Answer B) is not generally prone to cystic change, but conversely this is a common finding in patients with papillary thyroid cancer. Aberrant salivary gland tissue with cystic degeneration (Answer D) is a very rare disorder and cases do not occur within or juxtaposed to the thyroid.

EDUCATIONAL OBJECTIVE
Recognize the typical presentation of a parathyroid cyst.

REFERENCE(S)
Wani S, Hao Z. Atypical cystic adenoma of the parathyroid gland: case report and review of the literature. *Endocr Pract.* 2005;11(6):389-393. PMID: 16638726

Xu P, Xia X, Li M, Guo M, Yang Z. Parathyroid cysts: experience of a rare phenomenon at a single institution. *BMC Surg.* 2018;18(1):9. PMID: 29409478

23 ANSWER: C) Neck ultrasonography

Medullary thyroid cancer accounts for fewer than 5% of thyroid cancer cases in the United States; approximately 80% of these cases represent sporadic, nonfamilial disease. The 2015 American Thyroid Association guidelines for the management of medullary thyroid cancer recommend that *RET* proto-oncogene testing be offered to all patients with a preoperative (or postoperative) diagnosis of medullary thyroid cancer. The guidelines state that "patients presenting with a thyroid nodule and a cytological or histological diagnosis of medullary thyroid cancer should have a physical examination, determination of serum levels of calcitonin and CEA, and genetic testing for a *RET* germline mutation. The presence of a pheochromocytoma and hyperparathyroidism should be excluded in patients with hereditary medullary thyroid cancer." This patient's plasma metanephrine levels are normal, which effectively rules out pheochromocytoma, and thus she does not need adrenal imaging (Answer B). Hyperparathyroidism has also been ruled out, and therefore a sestamibi scan (Answer D) is not warranted.

Neck ultrasonography (Answer C) to assess for the presence of local metastases is important before thyroidectomy in order to determine whether neck dissection is warranted. This patient's baseline serum calcitonin level less than 500 pg/mL suggests that distant metastases will not be present. However, if this patient's preoperative ultrasound demonstrates extensive disease in the neck, or if she had signs or symptoms suggestive of distant metastases, imaging with chest CT to detect lung or mediastinal metastases and imaging with MRI or 3-phase contrast-enhanced multidetector CT to detect liver metastases would be recommended.

Fluorodeoxyglucose-PET (Answer A) is poorly sensitive for medullary cancer and is not recommended for the detection of distant disease.

EDUCATIONAL OBJECTIVE
In a patient with medullary thyroid cancer, perform neck ultrasonography before proceeding to thyroid surgery.

REFERENCE(S)
Wells SA Jr, Asa SL, Dralle H, et al; American Thyroid Association Guidelines Task Force on Medullary Thyroid Carcinoma. Revised American Thyroid Association guidelines for the management of medullary thyroid carcinoma. *Thyroid.* 2015;25(6):567-610. PMID: 25810047

Moraitis AG, Martucci VL, Pacak K. Genetics, diagnosis, and management of medullary thyroid carcinoma and pheochromocytoma/paraganglioma. *Endocr Pract.* 2014;20(2):176-187. PMID: 24449662

24 ANSWER: A) No radioactive iodine
Current guidelines call for risk stratification postoperatively to inform decision-making about radioactive iodine and other additional therapies. This patient's tumor is considered low-risk because it is a classic papillary cancer smaller than 4 cm without aggressive histologic features (such as tall-cell or columnar variant), there was no tumor invasion of local structures, the tumor was fully resected, and there was no vascular invasion. The presence of fewer than 5 micrometastases (<0.2 cm) in cervical lymph nodes does not confer additional risk.

In patients determined to have low-risk tumors according to the American Thyroid Association criteria, radioactive iodine ablation has not been shown to reduce risk for disease recurrence or mortality and is not routinely recommended. Therefore, Answer A is correct and the other answers are incorrect because this patient's tumor does not meet criteria for intermediate or high risk. Radioactive iodine ablation has been associated with decreased risk for both tumor recurrence and for disease-specific mortality in patients with high-risk tumors (those with gross extrathyroidal extension, incomplete tumor resection, and known distant metastases or postoperative thyroglobulin levels suggesting distant metastasis). In patients with intermediate-risk tumors (microscopic extrathyroidal extension, vascular invasion, aggressive histologic features, or metastases in the neck), the evidence for benefit is less clear, but radioactive iodine should be considered and treatment should be individualized on the basis of patient and tumor characteristics.

EDUCATIONAL OBJECTIVE
Recommend the most appropriate postoperative therapy for thyroid cancer classified as low risk.

REFERENCE(S)
Haugen BR, Alexander EK, Bible KC, et al. 2015 American Thyroid Association management guidelines for adult patients with thyroid nodules and differentiated thyroid cancer: the American Thyroid Association guidelines task force on thyroid nodules and differentiated thyroid cancer. *Thyroid.* 2016;26(1):1-133. PMID: 26462967

Lamartina L, Durante C, Filetti S, Cooper DS. Low-risk differentiated thyroid cancer and radioiodine remnant ablation: a systematic review of the literature. *J Clin Endocrinol Metab*. 2015;100(5):1748-1761.PMID: 25679996

Nixon IJ, Ganly I, Patel SG, et al. The results of selective use of radioactive iodine on survival and on recurrence in the management of papillary thyroid cancer, based on Memorial Sloan-Kettering Cancer Center risk group stratification. *Thyroid*. 2013;23(6):683-694. PMID: 23742290

25 ANSWER: B) Propranolol

This patient has thyrotoxic periodic paralysis. Both thyrotoxic and familial varieties of periodic paralysis are caused by an intermittent intracellular shift of potassium, resulting in ineffective sarcolemmal activity within muscle fibrils. The severity of attacks is linked to the severity of hypokalemia. Serum potassium levels return to normal between episodes—hence the normal level in this patient at the time of testing. Attacks may be precipitated by ingestion of large carbohydrate loads or intense physical exertion followed by a period of rest during which paralysis occurs. Whereas alterations in specific genes have been implicated in the familial varieties of periodic paralysis, the nature of the genetic predisposition for the thyrotoxic variety remains unclear. The predominance in Asian males suggests an X-linked abnormality with additional ethnicity-specific genetic influences. Thyroid hormone and adrenergic stimulation are known to stimulate the Na-K-ATPase pump, which contributes to the intermittent hypokalemia.

During an episode, judicious potassium therapy assists with recovery of normal muscle function, but it is recommended that the total dose given should be less than 50 mEq in order to avoid rebound hyperkalemia. There is no evidence that a daily potassium supplement (Answer C) prevents subsequent attacks because total body potassium stores are normal in these patients. Controlling thyrotoxicosis is important; in fact, attacks stop with restoration of a euthyroid state, but this will take many weeks, so methimazole (Answer A) is incorrect. Propranolol (Answer B) inhibits adrenergic stimulation of the NA-K-ATPase pump and has been found to help rapidly prevent recurrent episodes of periodic paralysis. As noted, vigorous exercise may actually precipitate attacks, so an exercise program (Answer D) would not be a useful intervention at this time. Pyridostigmine (Answer E) is used to treat myasthenia gravis, not periodic paralysis.

EDUCATIONAL OBJECTIVE
Diagnose periodic paralysis and recommend treatment.

REFERENCE(S)
Lin SH. Thyrotoxic periodic paralysis. *Mayo Clin Proc*. 2005;80(1):99-105. PMID: 15667036

Vijayakumar A, Ashwath G, Thimmappa D. Thyrotoxic periodic paralysis: clinical challenges. *J Thyroid Res*. 2014;2014:649502. PMID: 24695373

26 ANSWER: D) Repeated FNAB with flow cytometry

The image shows multiple uniform-appearing lymphocytes. Features of anaplastic carcinoma, another potential cause of very rapid thyroid growth, are not seen. Thyroid lymphoma is rare, comprising 2% or less of all thyroid malignancies. The mean age at presentation is 65 to 75 years, and this occurs more frequently in women. The risk for thyroid lymphoma is 40 to 80 times higher in individuals with Hashimoto thyroiditis than in the general population. The most common presentation of thyroid lymphoma is a rapidly enlarging, painless goiter, often with compressive symptoms. The enlargement may be nodular or diffuse. Cytopathology showing uniform-appearing lymphocytes may be consistent with either Hashimoto thyroiditis or thyroid lymphoma. FNAB with flow cytometry (Answer D) is typically needed to confirm a diagnosis of lymphoma. Treatment of thyroid lymphoma usually consists of chemotherapy with or without radiation. The role of thyroidectomy (Answer B) is controversial, but it has not been demonstrated to improve survival. Radioactive iodine scan (Answer A) may demonstrate a cold nodule, but it would not be helpful in making the diagnosis of thyroid lymphoma. Gene classifier testing (Answer C) can be useful to predict the risk of differentiated thyroid cancer when an FNAB result is indeterminate, but is not of utility in distinguishing between Hashimoto thyroiditis and thyroid lymphoma.

27 ANSWER: B) Lenvatinib

This patient has rapidly progressive metastatic differentiated thyroid cancer that is becoming increasingly symptomatic. She is not a good candidate for additional radioactive iodine treatment because the absence of uptake on her post-treatment scans indicates that her disease is ^{131}I refractory. Cytotoxic chemotherapy (Answer A) is generally of limited utility in differentiated thyroid cancer. Given that her disease is refractory to radioactive iodine, diffuse, progressive, and symptomatic (which would be expected to produce morbidity or mortality within 6 months), she is a candidate for kinase inhibitor therapy. This treatment has been shown in several trials to improve progression-free survival. Although several other kinase inhibitors are currently being studied in differentiated thyroid cancer (see table), only 2, lenvatinib (Answer B) and sorafenib, are currently FDA approved for the treatment of differentiated thyroid cancer in patients with extensive local disease or distant metastases. Palbociclib (Answer D) is a kinase inhibitor used for metastatic breast cancer; it has not been studied in thyroid cancers. Ipilimumab (Answer C) is a monoclonal antibody that blocks the cytotoxic T-cell receptor 4 (CTLA-4) on activated T cells. It is used for the treatment of metastatic melanoma, but it has not been studied in differentiated thyroid cancer. Offering no treatment (Answer E) is inappropriate given the potential for improved progression-free survival with kinase inhibitor therapy.

Table. Tyrosine Kinase Inhibitors Currently Approved for Use in Advanced Thyroid Cancer.

Tyrosine Kinase Inhibitor	Type of Thyroid Cancer	Effectiveness: Progression-Free Survival Compared With Placebo*
Vandetanib	Medullary	30.5 vs 19.3 months
Cabozantinib	Medullary	11.2 vs 4 months
Sorafenib	Differentiated	10.8 vs 5.8 months
Lenvatinib	Differentiated	18.3 vs 3.6 months

*Note: enrolled populations were different; efficacy cannot be compared directly across studies. Many other multikinase inhibitors are currently being investigated for use in advanced thyroid cancer.

28 ANSWER: B) Refer for immediate total thyroidectomy with neck dissection

Current guidelines for the management of thyroid disease in pregnancy suggest that in general it is safe to wait until after delivery to perform thyroid surgery for thyroid cancer discovered early in pregnancy. The exception, however, is in patients demonstrating a more aggressive course, including growth by 50% of nodule volume (or 20% in 2 dimensions) or aggressive baseline features, such as local invasion. This patient had a doubling of her tumor size and the new appearance of metastatic disease to lymph nodes; therefore, thyroidectomy should not be deferred (thus, Answer B is correct and Answers C and D are incorrect). If thyroid surgery is required during pregnancy, the second trimester is thought to be safest because anesthetic agents may have a teratogenic effect during organogenesis in the first trimester, and surgery in the third trimester has the potential to induce premature labor. Initiating levothyroxine suppressive therapy (Answer A) might be helpful, but it would not be an acceptable substitute for thyroidectomy.

EDUCATIONAL OBJECTIVE
Recommend options for thyroid cancer treatment in pregnant women.

REFERENCE(S)

Alexander EK, Pearce EN, Brent GA, et al. 2017 Guidelines of the American Thyroid Association for the diagnosis and management of thyroid disease during pregnancy and the postpartum. *Thyroid.* 2017;27(3):315-389. PMID: 28056690

Gibelli B, Zamperini P, Proh M, Giugliano G. Management and follow-up of thyroid cancer in pregnant women. *Acta Otorhinolaryngol Ital.* 2011;31(6):358-365. PMID: 22323846

29 **ANSWER: D) Atenolol**
This patient has developed what appears to be painless thyroiditis while taking interferon alfa. β-Adrenergic blockade (Answer D) is indicated to control his rapid pulse, but the other measures listed are unnecessary. Patients with hepatitis C have a higher prevalence of positive TPO antibodies, even before treatment with interferon alfa, than do patients with other forms of viral hepatitis (11.2% vs 3.6%, respectively). The most common thyroid manifestation of interferon alfa therapy is hypothyroidism, which occurs in approximately 5% of all treated patients but in 36% of patients with positive TPO antibodies before treatment. Women are twice as likely as men to develop this disorder (8.7% vs 3.4% in one study). A smaller number of patients develop thyrotoxicosis during interferon alfa therapy; this is more often painless thyroiditis rather than Graves disease, although both have been described. The percentage of patients with positive TPO antibodies increases after treatment with interferon alfa (from 3.7% to 9.7% in one study). Most patients (60%) with interferon alfa–associated thyroid dysfunction improve after drug discontinuation.

Methimazole therapy (Answer A) would not be effective for thyroiditis. Prednisone therapy (Answer B) is sometimes used to treat painful subacute thyroiditis, but it is not indicated for painless drug-induced thyroiditis. Intravenous immunoglobulin (Answer C) is not indicated for the treatment of thyroiditis.

EDUCATIONAL OBJECTIVE
Diagnose and manage drug-induced thyroiditis.

REFERENCE(S)

Nair Kesavachandran C, Haamann F, Nienhaus A. Frequency of thyroid dysfunctions during interferon alpha treatment of single and combination therapy in hepatitis C virus-infected patients: a systematic review based analysis. *PLoS One.* 2013;8(2):e55364. PMID: 23383326

Carella C, Mazziotti G, Amato G, Braverman LE, Roti E. Clinical review 169: interferon-alpha related thyroid disease: pathophysiological, epidemiological, and clinical aspects. *J Clin Endocrinol Metab.* 2004;89(8):3656-3661. PMID: 15292282

30 **ANSWER: C) Atypia of undetermined significance**
The Bethesda System for Reporting Thyroid Cytopathology, which was introduced in 2007 and updated in 2017, distributes thyroid FNAB results into 1of 6 categories: I = nondiagnostic or unsatisfactory (Answer A); II = benign (Answer B); III = atypia of undetermined significance (AUS) or follicular lesion of undetermined significance (FLUS) (Answer C); IV = follicular neoplasm or suspicious for a follicular neoplasm; V = suspicious for malignancy (Answer D); and VI = malignant (Answer E). The atypia category includes several different subtype descriptions, one of which applies in this patient's case, consisting of focal features suggestive of papillary thyroid carcinoma, including nuclear grooves, prominent nucleoli, elongated nuclei or cytoplasm, and/or intranuclear cytoplasmic inclusions in an otherwise predominantly benign-appearing sample (thus, Answer C is correct). The malignancy rate for such lesions is expected to be 6% to 18%, assuming that noninvasive follicular thyroid neoplasm with papillary-like nuclear features (NIFTP) is not classified as a malignancy. If NIFTP is instead considered to be a cancer, then the risk for malignancy in this group is 10% to 30%.

Nodules suspicious for malignancy (Answer D) are characterized by the presence of some suspicious features, but not enough to lead to a definitive diagnosis. The risk of malignancy in these nodules is 50% to 75% (45%-60% if NIFTP is not considered to be malignant). Nodules interpreted as malignant (Answer E) have classic papillary cancer features such as true papillae, psammoma bodies, and intranuclear cytoplasmic inclusions and, in contrast to nodules with atypia of undetermined significance, cells throughout the specimen, not just focally, exhibit nuclear grooves, prominent nucleoli, and elongated nuclei. The risk for malignancy in these lesions is 97% to 99%.

EDUCATIONAL OBJECTIVE
Classify results from thyroid fine-needle aspiration biopsy according to the Bethesda System for Reporting Thyroid Cytopathology.

REFERENCE(S)

Cibas ES, Ali SZ. The 2017 Bethesda System for Reporting Thyroid Cytopathology. *Thyroid.* 2017;27(11):1341-1346. PMID: 29091573

www.ingramcontent.com/pod-product-compliance
Lightning Source LLC
Chambersburg PA
CBHW061411210326
41598CB00035B/6175